Computers in
Stereotactic Neurosurgery

Contemporary Issues in Neurological Surgery

GENERAL SERIES EDITORS

Harold J. Hoffman MD, FRCSC
Professor of Surgery, University of Toronto;
Neurosurgeon-in-Chief, Hospital for Sick Children,
Toronto, Ontario, Canada

Julian T. Hoff MD
Professor of Surgery;
Chief, Section of Neurosurgery,
University of Michigan,
Ann Arbor, Michigan

Contemporary Issues in Neurological Surgery

Computers in Stereotactic Neurosurgery

EDITED BY

Patrick J. Kelly MD
Professor of Neurosurgery,
Department of Neurosurgery,
Mayo Clinic,
Rochester, Minnesota

AND

Bruce A. Kall MS
Senior Analyst,
Section of Patient Care Systems,
Mayo Clinic,
Rochester, Minnesota

BOSTON

BLACKWELL SCIENTIFIC PUBLICATIONS

OXFORD LONDON EDINBURGH

MELBOURNE PARIS BERLIN VIENNA

© 1992 by
Blackwell Scientific Publications, Inc.
Editorial offices:
3 Cambridge Center, Cambridge
   Massachusetts 02142, USA
Osney Mead, Oxford OX2 0EL, England
25 John Street, London WC1N 2BL
   England
23 Ainslie Place, Edinburgh EH3 6AJ
   Scotland
54 University Street, Carlton
   Victoria 3053, Australia

Other editorial offices:
Arnette SA
2, rue Casimir-Delavigne
75006 Paris
France

Blackwell Wissenschaft
Meinekestrasse 4
D-1000 Berlin 15
Germany

Blackwell MZV
Feldgasse 13
A-1238 Wien
Austria

First published 1992

Set by Setrite Typesetters, Hong Kong
Printed and bound in the
United States of America by
Hamilton, Castleton, New York

92 93 94 95   5 4 3 2 1

DISTRIBUTORS

USA
   Blackwell Scientific Publications, Inc.
   3 Cambridge Center
   Cambridge, Massachusetts 02142
   (*Orders*: Tel: 800 759−6102)

Canada
   Times Mirror Professional Publishing, Ltd
   5240 Finch Avenue East
   Scarborough, Ontario, M1S 5A2
   (*Orders*: Tel: 416 298−1588)

Australia
   Blackwell Scientific Publications
   (Australia) Pty Ltd
   54 University Street
   Carlton, Victoria 3053
   (*Orders*: Tel: 03 347 0300)

Outside North America and Australia
   Marston Book Services Ltd
   PO Box 87, Oxford OX2 0DT
   (*Orders*: Tel: 0865 791155
              Fax: 0865 791927
              Telex: 837515)

Library of Congress
Cataloging-in-Publication Data

Computers in stereotactic neurosurgery
   edited by Patrick J. Kelly and Bruce A. Kall.
         p.   cm. — (Contemporary issues in
   neurological surgery)
      Includes bibliographical references and index.
      ISBN 0−86542−145−5
      1. Stereoencephalotomy — Data processing.
   2. Image processing.   3. Robotics.
   I. Kelly, Patrick J., 1941−   . II. Kall, Bruce A.
   III. Series.
      [DNLM: 1. Computer Systems.
      2. Diagnosis, Surgical — methods.
      3. Image Interpretation, Computer-Assisted.
      4. Image Processing, Computer-Assisted.
      5. Neurosurgery — instrumentation.
      6. Neurosurgery — methods.
      7. Stereotaxic Techniques. WL 368 C738]
   RD594.C654 1992   617.4'8059 — dc20

Contents

List of Contributors

Farhad Afshar BSc, MD, FRCS, Consultant in Charge, Department of Neurosurgery, St. Bartholomew's Hospital, London, England

Beatrice Alagna, Division of Neurosurgery, National Institute of Neurology, Milan, Italy

Bernhard Bauer-Kirpes PhD, Fischer Company, Freiburg, Germany

Alim L. Benabid MD, PhD, Professor of Biophysics, Head of Neurosurgery, Grenoble University Hospital, France

Bruce Bronson, The Lovelace Medical Center, Albuquerque, New Mexico

Laura Brynildson BCE, Computer Engineering Consultant to the Department of Neurosurgery, The Lovelace Medical Center, Albuquerque, New Mexico

Davide S. Casolino, Division of Neurosurgery, National Institute of Neurology, Milan, Italy

Ugo Cerchiari, Department of Physics, National Institute of Tumors, Milan, Italy

Philippe Cinquin MD, PhD, Professor of Biomathematics, UFR of Medicine, Grenoble University Hospital, France

John A. Clark MSc, MD, McConnell Brain Imaging Unit, Montreal Neurological Institute, Montreal, Quebec, Canada

D. Louis Collins MEng, McConnell Brain Imaging Unit, Montreal Neurological Institute, Montreal, Quebec, Canada

M. John Cookson MSc, MPhil, MBCS, AFIMA, Senior Lecturer, Computer Science, The London Hospital Medical College, London, England

François Danel PhD, Engineer, Grenoble, France

Dudley H. Davis MD, Assistant Professor of Neurological Surgery, Mayo Medical School; Department of Neurosurgery, Mayo Clinic, Rochester, Minnesota

Jacques Demongeot MD, PhD, Professor and Head of Biomathematics, UFR of Medicine, Grenoble University Hospital, France

Jonathan O. Dostrovsky PhD, Professor, Department of Physiology, University of Toronto, Toronto, Ontario, Canada

Manuel Dujovny MD, Department of Neurosurgery, Henry Ford Neurosurgical Institute, Detroit, Michigan

E. Dykes PhD, Senior Lecturer, Department of Electrical and Electronic Engineering, Hatfield Polytechnic, Hatfield, England

Erin Fagan MEng, Thayer School of Engineering, Dartmouth College, Hanover, New Hampshire

Eric M. Friets MEng, Thayer School of Engineering, Dartmouth College, Hanover, New Hampshire

Cesare G. Giorgi MD, Division of Neurosurgery, National Institute of Neurology, Milan, Italy

Stephan J. Goerss BS, Department of Neurologic Surgery, Mayo Clinic, Rochester, Minnesota

Joseph H. Goodman MD, Department of Surgery, Division of Neurological Surgery, The Ohio State University Hospital, Columbus, Ohio

Jan M. Gybels MD, PhD, Professor of Neurology and Neurosurgery; Chief of Clinic of the Department of Neurosurgery; Director of the Laboratory of Experimental Neurology; University of Leuven, Belgium

Tyrone L. Hardy MD, FACS, FICS, Chief Stereotactic Surgeon, Department of Neurosurgery, The Lovelace Medical Center; Clinical Assistant Professor of Neurosurgery, The University of New Mexico, Albuquerque, New Mexico

M. Peter Heilbrun MD, Professor and Head, Division of Neurological Surgery, University of Utah School of Medicine, Salt Lake City, Utah

Christopher J. Henri MSc, McConnell Brain Imaging Center, Department of Neurosurgery, Montreal Neurological Institute, Montreal, Quebec, Canada

Dominique Hoffmann MD, Assistant, Department of Neurosurgery, UFR of Medicine, Grenoble University Hospital, Grenoble, France

John G. Holman MA, DPhil, Lecturer, The London Hospital Medical College, London, England

Bruce A. Kall MS, Senior Analyst, Mayo Clinic, Section of Patient Care Systems, Rochester, Minnesota

Patrick J. Kelly MD, Professor of Neurosurgery, Department of Neurosurgery, Mayo Clinic, Rochester, Minnesota

Yik S. Kwoh PhD, Department of Neurosurgery, University of California, Orange, California

Stéphane Lavallée PhD, Research Fellow, UFR of Medicine, Grenoble University Hospital, France

Jean F. Le Bas MD, PhD, Professor of Biophysics, Head of Magnetic Resonance Imaging, Grenoble University Hospital, France

Louis Lemieux PhD, Department of Medical Physics, Royal Postgraduate Medical School, London, England

Hans-Gerd Lipinski PhD, Institut für Medical Informatics, University of Lübeck, Germany

Guy Marchal MD, Professor of Radiology, Department of Radiology; Research Director, Interdisciplinary Research Unit Radiological Imaging, University of Leuven, Belgium

André Olivier MD, PhD, Department of Neurosurgery, Montreal Neurological Institute, Montreal, Quebec, Canada

John D. Pavlidis MEng, Thayer School of Engineering, Dartmouth College, Hanover, New Hampshire

Terry M. Peters PhD, FCCPM, McConnell Brain Imaging Unit, Montreal Neurological Institute, Montreal, Quebec, Canada

G. Bruce Pike MEng, Department of Radiology, Stanford University, California

Gary L. Rea MD, PhD, Department of Surgery, Division of Neurological Surgery, The Ohio State University Hospital, Columbus, Ohio

Richard A. Robb PhD, Professor of Biophysics, Director, Mayo Biomedical Imaging Resource, Mayo Foundation, Rochester, Minnesota

David W. Roberts MD, Associate Professor of Surgery (Neurosurgery), Dartmouth Medical School, Dartmouth-Hitchcock Medical Center, Hanover, New Hampshire

John W. Strohbehn PhD, Sherman Fairchild Professor of Engineering Sciences, Thayer School of Engineering, Dartmouth College, Hanover, New Hampshire

Albrecht Struppler MD, PhD, Professor emeritus of Neurology and Clinical Neurophysiology, Klinikum R.d. Isar, Technical University of Munich, Munich, Germany

Paul Suetens MSc, PhD, Professor, Department of Electrical Engineering (ESAT); Research Director, Interdisciplinary Research Unit Radiological Imaging, University of Leuven, Belgium

Ronald R. Tasker MD, FRCS(C), Professor, Department of Surgery, University of Toronto; Division of Neurosurgery, Toronto Western Hospital, Toronto, Ontario

Dirk Vandermeulen MSc, PhD, Researcher, Interdisciplinary Research Unit Radiological Imaging, Department of Neurology and Neurosurgery, University of Leuven, Belgium

Heinz G. Wieser MD, Professor of Neurology, Neurology Clinic, University Hospital of Zurich, Switzerland

Guy Wilms MD, PhD, Professor of Radiology, Adjunct Clinical Head of the Department of Radiology, University of Leuven, Belgium

Daniel Yakar MD, Department of Radiation Oncology, Henry Ford Neurosurgical Institute, Detroit, Michigan

Masafumi Yoshida MD, DMSci, Lecturer, Department of Neurosurgery, Kurume University School of Medicine, Kurume; Chief, Department of Neurosurgery, Saiseikai Hita Hospital, Hita, Japan

Ronald F. Young MD, Professor and Chief, Division of Neurological Surgery, University of California Irvine Medical Center, Orange, California

Lucia Zamorano MD, PhD, Associate Professor, Department of Neurological Surgery, Chief, Divisions of Neuro-oncology, Stereotaxis, Skull Base and Radiosurgery, Wayne State University, Detroit, Michigan

Preface

Radiography-based stereotactic surgery as practiced for the treatment of movement disorders was relatively simple. Target points extrapolated from stereotactic atlases onto positive contrast ventriculograms were converted to stereotactic coordinates, corrected for magnification, and stereotactic frame coordinates were then derived. This required simple mathematics: addition, subtraction, multiplication, and division. Most stereotactic frames were also simple. Simple Cartesian systems, arc-quadrant systems, or arc-phantom systems were the most popular. However, some stereotactic frames did require simple trigonometry. That, too, was uncomplicated.

The advent of computer-based imaging technology expanded the scope and applications of stereotactic procedures, but also complicated them. The surgeon now has multiple databases to consider: computed tomography, magnetic resonance imaging, stereotactic angiography, physiologic data, and stereotactic atlas data, as well as intraoperative radiographs. In addition, target points from one imaging study should be cross-correlated to other imaging studies. For example, target points within tumors undergoing stereotactic biopsy or resection should be cross-correlated to other imaging modalities, such as angiography, so that safe trajectories can be determined.

Certainly there are manual methods for doing all of this. These are accurate but not time efficient. Surgeons may be tempted to not use all of the available data on a given patient. However, the incorporation of a computer system into the operating room environment allows rapid target point calculations and imaging-based cross-correlations, which can make surgery safer and more time efficient. In addition, computer-based stereotactic procedures can provide surgical options to patients who harbor lesions which may be considered inoperable by other means.

Over the past 20 years we have seen a virtual explosion in computer technology which has supplied us with a variety and ever increasing supply of powerful and capacious computer systems. The cost/performance ratio of these machines has progressively decreased with each advancing year. Nonetheless, the development of specific stereotactic software remains a major expense, and is frequently an unknown factor in determining the developmental cost of any computer-based project in general and computer-based stereotaxis in particular. However, software may be developed more efficiently if a specific goal is known and the steps to that endpoint are well defined. For this reason, exposure to solutions developed by our colleagues may help each of us in the further development of our own computer-based stereotactic surgical systems.

The purpose of this book is to provide an overview of state-of-the-art computer-based stereotactic surgery with regard to computer systems and application of these systems to stereotactic image processing, database manipulation, surgical planning, and intraoperative utilization. It is our belief that computers and specific software will ultimately make stereotaxis so convenient, time efficient, and cost effective that it will be irresistible in all aspects of clinical neurosurgery.

P.J.K., B.A.K.

Disclaimer. The indications and dosages of all drugs in this book have been recommended in the medical literature and conform to the practices of the general medical community. The medications described do not necessarily have specific approval by the Food and Drug Administration for use in the diseases and dosages for which they are recommended. The package insert for each drug should be consulted for use and dosage as approved by the FDA. Because standards for usage change, it is advisable to keep abreast of revised recommendations, particularly those concerning new drugs.

Computer-based
Image Processing

A

Overview of Computers and Imaging

The Impact of Computer and Imaging Technology on Stereotactic Neurosurgery

Bruce A. Kall

Introduction

Computers and medical imaging technology have significantly increased the efficacy and types of neurosurgical procedures that may be performed. Stereotaxis was originally developed in the early twentieth century as a mechanical means of precisely placing probes and electrodes to explore or destroy specific areas of the brain. Localization was performed by measuring the relationship of the target to intracranial landmarks using teleradiography and manual graphical measurement techniques.

It is now possible to precisely localize any target or volume within the brain, using new stereotactic localization techniques and recent high-resolution, computer-based scanning techniques, such as computed tomography (CT), magnetic resonance imaging (MRI), and digital subtraction angiography (DSA). This technique is also amenable for use with positron emission tomography (PET). These imaging devices create digital data that can be rapidly and meaningfully manipulated by computers in a stereotactic coordinate system.

Stereotactic software has been created as a tool for the surgeon to integrate and reformat the data from multiple modalities, simplify stereotactic coordinate and trajectory calculations, and model in three dimensions the individual patient undergoing surgery. Therapeutic computer-assisted interventions are now possible, not only to localize a small, deep-seated lesion in three dimensions for biopsy, but to precisely resect it, utilizing computer-imaging guidance. A variety of other neurosurgical procedures have been facilitated by development of these imaging techniques, stereotactic localization, and computers.

This chapter will review the current state of computer and imaging technology as it relates to the rapidly evolving field of stereotactic neurosurgery. The important features of a computer-interactive stereotactic system will also be discussed.

Historical perspective

STEREOTAXY

R. H. Clarke defined the notion of defining intracranial structures in a three-dimensional (3-D) coordinate system in 1906, and devised a special stereotactic instrument for this purpose [1]. His colleague, Sir Victor Horsley, dismissed Clarke's recommendation to apply this technology to human neurosurgery; hence this technique was only applied to neurophysiologic studies on small animals [2]. The first stereotactic atlas of the human brain was developed in 1918 by a neurophysiologist from the Montreal Neurologic Institute, who also devised a stereotactic frame for use with these maps [3]. Unfortunately, no neurosurgeons adopted these inventions.

Spiegel and Wycis reported the first human stereotactic procedures in 1947 [4]; they combined a technique called positive contrast ventriculography and the stereotactic technique proposed by Clarke to perform a dorsomedial thalamotomy. This was quickly followed by the development of human stereotactic systems, most notably by Talairach in France, and Leksell in Sweden. Many other centers around the world began performing human stereotaxy, with each surgeon developing stereotactic instruments to meet their particular needs.

Stereotactic procedures were mostly focused on the treatment of movement disorders. Localization was performed using positive contrast ventriculography and anatomic relationships. Imprecise localization and inaccurate lesioning techniques often resulted in poorly-located, often unnecessarily large lesions, and unacceptable complications.

With the development of L-dopa in 1968, stereotactic procedures were rarely performed at most institutions. Nevertheless, Talairach and Leksell continued to perform a significant number of their procedures under stereotactic control. Leksell was also developing the principles of radiosurgery, which is only now finding widespread acceptance.

In 1946, J. P. Eckert and J. W. Mauchly developed the first electronic calculator, the ENIAC (Electronic Numerical Integrator and Calculator) at the Moore School of Engineering, University of Pennsylvania. Ironically, this was only one year before the first human stereotactic procedure. The UNIVAC I (Universal Automatic Computer) was the first commercially available computer in 1951. Approximately 20 years later, computer technology was applied with standard X-ray imaging to produce computed axial tomography or CT scanning. Digital medical imaging had been born and was widely accepted. It was this particular development that dramatically altered the course of stereotactic surgery.

Principles of computers

Computing devices are generally composed of hardware and software.

Hardware is the physical component of a computer system that rapidly and repetitiously manipulates voluminous amounts of information. The hardware components that generally make up a computer are: (1) the central processing unit or CPU; (2) memory; (3) input and output (I/O) devices; and (4) high-speed data paths, or "buses."

Central processing unit

The CPU is, for lack of a better word, the "brain" of the system. It is composed of a series of switches and circuits, which allow it to perform arithmetic (e.g. add, subtract) and logic functions (e.g. if correct, then go on) with both numeric and symbolic information. Computers may have more than one internal CPU, which act in parallel to solve a problem. Computers may also have subsidiary processors, which perform specific functions, such as manipulating matrices of numbers (i.e. an array processor). Subsidiary processors usually perform in hardware what could be done in software, but much faster.

Computer calculations are performed using the binary number system (base 2). A *bit* represents the two possible states of a switch, either on (1) or off (0). Eight contiguous bits make up a *byte*, and can represent 2^8, or 256, different numeric values. Each of the alphanumeric characters used in computers has a representation in one byte of space. One of 256 gray levels in a digital image can also be represented in one byte. There are other, less popular groupings of contiguous bits: (1) a *nybble*, which is four contiguous bits (encoding up to 16 different variations); and (2) a *word*, which usually contains 16 bits (and 65 536 variations). Computers utilized in stereotactic neurosurgery today generally manipulate bits in groups of 32, known as double words, and can represent an integer number from $-2\,147\,483\,648$ to $+2\,147\,483\,647$, or a real number from as small as $1.401298e-45$ to as large as $3.402823e+38$.

The CPU performs arithmetic and logical instructions that are encoded in various-sized groupings of bits, which are usually executed in one or more clock cycles or ticks. The clock in a CPU ticks so many times a second to maintain its tempo, currently measured in megahertz (MHz — million cycles per second). The speed of a CPU is usually specified by the number of instructions per second it performs, since it may not always execute one instruction per cycle (one million instructions per second = 1 MIP). Neither of these measurements may be an accurate indicator by which to compare two computers. Megahertz may not be useful because of the number of cycles needed to execute an instruction. MIPS may also not be an accurate gauge, as a computation that takes 10 instructions on one computer architecture may take 15–20 on another.

The main architecture of computers, until recently, has been known as complex instruction set computing (CISC). In this type of architecture, a computer instruction is more flexible (has variable lengths and many options), but may take 10 or more clock cycles to execute. Intel 80486 and Motorola 68040 are examples of CPU processors that implement this architecture. A recent computer architectural development, reduced instruction set computers (RISC), has one specific goal: to streamline the job of the CPU, whereby all instructions have a fixed length (e.g. 32 bits) and are trimmed down to the most essential frequently executed functions. This results in a tempo whereby the CPU has less idle time and ideally should execute one or more instructions every clock cycle. The end result (still being debated) should be increased computational speeds. Sun SPARC, Intel i860 and Motorola 8800 are examples of RISC-based processors.

Memory

Memory is generally categorized into read-only (ROM) and random access (RAM). ROM is usually contained on one silicon chip (see WORM and CD-ROM below) and may be pre-programmed as sets of instructions grouped, for instance, to automatically start (or boot) a computer when it is turned on. ROM does not lose its content when the computer power is turned off. There are variations of ROMs, for instance EPROM, which may be modified under certain conditions, but retain their contents when power is removed.

RAM can be thought of as a large piece of scratch paper. (RAM has also been called "core"

memory.) Its contents are continually modified by the system, and can be grouped in almost any combination of bits, bytes, words, etc. Memory is usually categorized in thousands of bytes (Kbytes), millions of bytes (Mbytes), and more recently in gigabytes (Gbytes) which are groupings of billions of bytes. Each bit of memory can usually be accessed in less than 80 ns (80 billionths of a second) in most computers used in stereotactic neurosurgery today. The cost and size of RAM memory has decreased so dramatically in the last few years that the amount of RAM memory in a computer is generally not a constraining factor.

Floppy and hard disks can also be thought of as memory. These are soft or hard platters, coated with magnetic materials. A read/write head and interfacing electronics are used to convert magnetic properties into bits of information as the platters spin. Information on these types of devices is usually accessed in milliseconds, which is much slower than RAM. Not only do these types of devices have a delay caused by the relatively slow rotation of the medium, but the read/write heads delay the transfer operations, because they have to move to (or seek) different tracks in the disks (like the grooves in an audio record).

Optical disks, operating on much the same principle as a laser audio compact disk, are also available for many computers, but accesses its stored information much slower than even hard disks. Most optical disks are categorized as write-once-read-many (WORM) or compact disk read-only memory (CD-ROM). Both devices are usually used for long-term storage of data and programs, and may be read into and out of hard disks or directly into RAM as the need arises. CD-ROM disks are usually written by a manufacturer to distribute their software. WORM disks are usually written by the user for storage of user data. Rewritable optical drives are now just becoming reliable, but one interchangeable format has not been adopted. These will probably be augmented by digital audio tape (DAT) technology which is now available for recording computerized information in digital form.

Information is *swapped* into and out of RAM from time to time. For instance, a program may need to write something onto a printer, which in terms of computer speed is very slow. The

CPU could be performing many calculations while the paper advances just one line. The CPU would swap this program out of memory and run another program or task during this interval. This allows a computer to do many tasks, apparently at once. Swapping from RAM to disk is also used to make the RAM memory appear larger that its actual capacity, which is known as *virtual memory*. Sometimes there is also an intermediate fast memory, known as *cache memory*, which holds small portions of information coming in and out of RAM or the CPU that has a high probability of been needed again very soon. This can be used, for example, to speed up access to data from the disk.

Input and output devices

These devices allow data to be transferred into and out of computers. Keyboards, touch screens, light pens, trackballs, mice, and frame grabbers (video digitizers) are input devices; while cathode ray tubes (CRTs), graphic screens, printers, and plotters are output devices. Networks are also an I/O mechanism. Floppy, hard, and optical disks, as well as cartridge and reel-to-reel nine-track magnetic tapes, are also input and output devices, in that they are utilized for long-term storage and transfer of computerized data.

Buses

Buses are the "highways" by which data is transferred into, out of, and within various parts of a computer. A bus is used to transfer data between the CPU and RAM, between the CPU and I/O devices, and between memory and I/O devices. Buses have a width, as measured by the number of bits that can pass through the bus simultaneously. Furthermore, buses move data at a certain speed. Together, the width and speed of the bus is one of the constraining factors when using inexpensive computers for image processing where huge amounts of information need to be manipulated rapidly.

SOFTWARE

Software is a mechanism for translating a hu-man idea into the language of zeros and ones of the computer. An algorithm, or program, is a set of steps that sequence the computer through a series of operations, manipulating the hardware to perform a desired operation. There are several layers of software in most computers: (1) machine language; (2) assembly language; (3) high-level languages; (4) operating systems; and (5) applications and utility programs.

Machine language

The combinations of zeros and ones that mimic the switching mechanism of the electronics of a computer is known as the machine language. The first computers built were programmed specifically using this language. Huge amounts of manpower were consumed programming what today would be considered trivial tasks.

Assembly language

Assembly languages were developed to facilitate machine language programming by representing a series of steps with symbols (or mnemonics). Programs written in these languages are translated into machine language by an assembler. This is the closest method to programming computers above the machine language. Assembly language programming is utilized less frequently today, but remains the language of choice for some programmers to squeeze out the best performance from a computer when necessary. Assembly language programs are not usually portable from one machine to the next.

High-level languages

High-level languages (C, C++, FORTRAN, PASCAL) are a mechanism for taking a human idea in a pseudo-natural language and converting it into instructions for the computer. Language translators, or compilers, are developed to automatically convert the high-level language program into machine language. Compilers follow a set of translation algorithms to generate machine code as optimal as the compiler's algorithm. High-level language programs are usually portable from one machine to another. Most languages, though, have *extensions* introduced by the manufacturer or the computer or compiler/developer that may not be supported on another computer. Furthermore, even some of the standard features of languages may have deviations, and are not always 100% portable, but they remain the closest to maintaining portability at present.

Operating systems

An operating system is a combination of a command language and a variety of utility programs that are utilized to control the basic functions and manage the resources of a computer. Operating system *commands* are available, for instance, to perform basic file manipulations (create or delete files), format and edit text, compile programs, and so on. The *command language* is usually interpreted on the fly, and allows the user to tailor the actions of the commands and the operating system's environment to meet their specific needs. Operating systems are controlled by typing commands into a keyboard, storing a series of commands in a (command) file to execute when needed, and by window-mouse graphical user interfaces (GUIs).

Application and utility programs

Application programs are usually written in high-level languages to perform a certain process. Stereotactic software is an application program. *Utility programs* can be a series of operating system commands and/or combination of high-level language programs to perform certain tasks. A program to copy information from a floppy disk onto a hard disk would usually be a utility program.

Which type of software is to be used for a specific purpose is highly dependent on the task to be performed. Most stereotactic software is programmed in high-level languages, but may also utilize small programs that are a series of operating system commands. Care should be taken to develop application programs under a language that is portable from machine to machine, since stereotactic software is very complex and takes years to develop and test. This software will need to be transferred from obsolete equipment to faster and newer hardware as it becomes available.

Evolution of computers

The performance of a computer that filled a large auditorium several years ago is now available in a unit that sits on a desk. Nevertheless, this does not mean that the technology will stand pat. Users, and the computational tasks that they execute on computers, are becoming more sophisticated, utilize more memory, and require an increasingly higher amount of computing power. Large, room-sized mainframe computers are still being built today to perform the most sophisticated tasks that tomorrow will be performed on much smaller hardware.

Increased performance in computers can be traced to evolving technology. The ENIAC and first generation computers utilized vacuum tubes. (The term computer "bug" was actually coined during this period, because bugs would get into these computers and cause failures.) Second generation computers used integrated transistors, and third generation systems were constructed with integrated circuits (ICs). Evolving technology is still increasing the density of circuits. Large-scale integration (LSI) was replaced by very-large-scale integration (VSLI) and so on. A large computer filling a small office 10 years ago is now capable of being miniaturized onto a single chip!

Software development and user interaction and development tools have not kept pace with the near-exponential rate of growth in hardware. First generation computers only allowed one programmer to access the machine at a time. Several users could submit decks of punch cards containing their algorithm and data in the second generation, and they would be executed one at a time in a "batch." It was not uncommon to wait several hours or longer for results. Interactive sessions or "time sharing" was introduced late in the second generation. Many terminals would be connected to a large computer and it would swap between users very quickly, giving each a small number of clock cycles or "time slices" several times a second. This gave many users an illusion of interactivity.

Many algorithms (programs) require true real-time processing, such as patient monitoring. Real-time systems monitor incoming data from some type of sensor, detect undesirable deviations, and then immediately provide feedback by, for instance, adjusting an infusion pump. These single-user real-time systems were also developed late in the second generation.

Newer third and fourth generation computers introduced *parallel* and *distributed* processing. Parallel processing entails splitting an algorithm into several, usually distinct, steps which can each be performed on a separate CPU, and the results merged to make the whole. Computers with hundreds of parallel CPUs are now being developed in research laboratories: perhaps millions will be combined in the future. Distributed processing is analogous to parallel processing, in that several parts may be performed simultaneously. Distributed processing, though, relocates or distributes computations at other computers over interconnected networks. The current limiting feature of both parallel and distributed processing is in developing "smart" compilers that can separate an algorithm in parts, freeing the programmer from this task.

Classification of computers today

There are several classifications of computers amenable to stereotactic neurosurgery. The boundaries between these classes are becoming less distinct. These are: (1) mainframes; (2) minicomputers; (3) microcomputers; (4) microprocessors; and (5) workstations. The enormous cost of mainframes, or super-computers, prohibits their use in this field.

MINICOMPUTERS

Minicomputers, whose boundaries are slowly disappearing with the advent of powerful microcomputers, are general purpose computers. They are available with a wide variety of configurations and are very expandable. Minicomputers support many simultaneous users and today are usually employed as departmental computers to perform many varied tasks. The Digital Equipment Corporation VAX would be the most popular example of a minicomputer.

MICROCOMPUTER

A *microprocessor* is a single chip CPU. They may be designed to perform a specific function (e.g. connected with appropriate sensors to control an infusion pump), or be the building block for microcomputers, workstations, and X-terminals (see below). Microprocessors are categorized and rated by the number of bits their architecture manipulates, and clock speed (e.g. 32 bits, 25 MHz).

A *microcomputer* contains a microprocessor, memory, and I/O capabilities. Home and personal computers are all microcomputers (e.g. Apple Macintosh SE, IBM PC-AT, PS1). Generally, home computers are a single user device consisting of a box containing the electronics (microcomputer, floppy and/or hard disks), a monitor, a keyboard, a mouse, and a small printer. Early home computers utilized 8-bit architecture CPUs. Systems today generally use a 16-bit CPU (e.g. Intel 80286).

Personal computers are not necessarily home computers. Other generations of micro-computers (Apple Macintosh IIs, IBM PS2s) provide substantial performance and may be configured (but are not usually used) to support more than one user. These are often used in office environments and provide interconnectivity between other personal computers and departmental minicomputers in order to share resources and data. These personal computers also use 16-bit CPUs and buses, but are slowly being replaced by 32-bit CPUs and buses (e.g. Intel 80386, 80486, and 80586).

Both home and personal computers require strong compatibility between the software and hardware. Vendors usually only add technical advancements when they do not result in a compatibility conflict with their own line of systems. For example, most microprocessor improvements integrated into one manufacturer's line usually provide upward but not downward compatibility. Compatibility between home and personal computer vendors is not likely to exist because of competitive constraints. This means a program written for one will not run on another without modifications and vice versa. Furthermore, much software for home and personal computers is developed by third-party companies. These programs are not always guaranteed to run on an upward compatible machine from a particular vendor.

WORKSTATIONS

A workstation is usually a single user, high performance, stand-alone microcomputer, which employs a 32-bit CPU and one or more buses. Workstations are as easy to use as personal computers. They are standardly packaged with multitasking (multiple operations appear to be performed simultaneously by fast swapping), virtual-memory operating systems (e.g. UNIX), and have an integrated high resolution graphics device that utilizes a window-mouse graphical user interface (GUI), as well as built in networking and connectivity tools. Workstations are often interconnected in large networks. Many workstations now employ RISC technology and are available at speeds of 10–76 MIPS. The speed of workstations continues to be the fastest growing niche in the computer field.

Workstations are currently employed mostly for scientific purposes and are the most amenable to stereotactic neurosurgery. Workstation vendors stress standards among their lines of systems. Sun Microsystems is a good example of a vendor making its standards openly available. Nevertheless, standards between competitors do not currently exist, although they are being discussed.

A personal computer (PC) may be designed, *ad hoc*, with higher performance coprocessors, high resolution graphics, multitasking operating systems, networking electronics, and software, as well as other features, to be similar to a workstation. Nonetheless, this "build it up yourself" approach usually results in integration nightmares, and may eventually cost more than a workstation itself. Workstations are generally capable of much more performance, storage, and graphics, with all items available from one vendor. The distinction between home/personal computers and workstations may disappear, or be merged in the future, although price and performance will probably maintain the separation.

Workstation environments

The X Windowing System was developed at the Massachusetts Institute of Technology as a portable software environment for workstations, implemented using distributed network computing. The X system offers the hope of portability of software to systems from different vendors which previously had proprietary interfaces. X is being ported to a variety of work-

stations and some PCs. Two popular graphical user interfaces using X Windowing Systems for workstations are currently known as Open Look and Motif.

In addition to workstations, low-cost devices known as X-terminals run the X system and are now on the market. X-terminals implement the X environment on a high-resolution "smart terminal" and are, in a way, technologically one step backwards and one step forwards. X-terminals are a part of a network whereby multiple windows, each containing a running program, are controlled by a remote computer. X-terminals are much less expensive than PCs and workstations, because they do not contain devices like disk drives. Furthermore, they can be centrally administered, resulting in more security of data, and require less manpower to manage the entire group of systems, as compared to each user having a stand-alone PC or workstation.

Nevertheless, the jury is still out on X-terminals. Most office environments have moved away from a strongly-centralized environment, where one computer services all of the users from many terminals. Presently, many users have PCs on their desks, and only share a departmental computer for storage and interconnectivity purposes.

Digital medical imaging

No field has led to greater advancement in stereotactic neurosurgery than digital medical imaging. Digital medical images are made up of thousands of picture elements (or pixels — a dot on the screen), each containing some property of some portion of the scanned item. (A pixel having a 3-D depth is known as a voxel or volume element.) Each pixel of a 512×512 pixel resolution CT image is a function of the X-ray attenuation of tissue at a specified location.

Medical images are viewed on high resolution screens. A single image is stored in a RAM memory called a "frame buffer." The image on the screen is refreshed onto the phosphor of the screen 30, 60, or more times per second by a digital-to-analog converter (DAC). This convertor translates a digital number into an analog value to fire an electron beam across the screen's phosphor.

Most screens can display up to 256 shades of

gray, even though the human eye can only distinguish about 16 at one time. Therefore, the DAC would be an 8-bit converter. Nevertheless, the images have more inherent information in them. The way in which a system handles this reduction of data onto the screen is a very important mechanism of the system.

Display devices have a spatial resolution, which is measured by the number of pixels on the screen (e.g. 512×512 pixels, 1024×1024 pixels, etc.) and an intensity resolution, which is defined as the number of bits in the frame buffer capable of storing the original image. Some of these bits may be reserved for graphics overlays, as in annotation, menus, cursors, etc. High-intensity-resolution grayscale displays usually commit one 16-bit word for each pixel on the screen, and encode a wide range of intensity values (usually 12 bits for data (4096 values) and 4 bits for graphics).

Lower resolution displays utilize one byte (8 bits) for each pixel, but can only encode 256 intensity values. These systems utilize an 8-bit frame buffer and the amount of information in the original image must be reduced before it is placed in the buffer. This results in a loss of dynamic range in the image.

Both high- and low-intensity-resolution devices enable the user to modify the contrast and brightness (window and level) by a mechanism known as a look-up table (LUT). This rapid translation mechanism converts the image in the frame buffer into values amenable to display on the screen. In other words, the LUT is the means for the user to manipulate what is white, what is black, and what is in between on the screen.

For example, consider a CT image which contains 12 bits of intensity information in its original form. The phosphor gun requires a voltage from 0.0 V for black to 1.0 V for white. This would require a 12-bit to 8-bit LUT and an 8-bit DAC that would then convert values from 0, in the 8-bit range, into a 0.0 V voltage, and a value of 255 into a voltage of 1.0 V. Every value in the original 12-bit image (4096 values) requires a direct mapping into the 8-bit range (256 values) before the DAC converts it into a voltage. There is one window and level LUT responsible for modifying all the values on the entire screen.

The window and level together define the range by which the scales from 0 to 255 and hence the voltages of 0.0 to 1.0 V are defined. All pixel values below the bottom of the window are mapped to black (or 0.0 V), and all values above the top of the window are mapped to 255 (or 1.0 V). Everything in between is mapped, usually on a linear ramp, to values between 0 and 255, and hence from 0.0 V to 1.0 V.

Windowing is performed by defining how many of the original range of 4096 values are encompassed into the linear ramp. Varying contrast is provided by narrowing or widening the range and thereby the mapping of the original values into 0 and 255. *Leveling* (or centering) is performed by moving the current window width within the original intensity range to focus in on values of particular interest. Different window and level settings are required for soft tissue and bone, since they may be at opposite ends in the original intensity range. Furthermore, different window and level settings are required for CT, MRI, and DSA images, and even for MRI images collected at the same level but with quite different pulse sequences.

Most CT and DSA images are usually 512×512 pixeis, with 12 bits of property information in an intensity range of 0 to 4095. CT intensities are in Hounsfield units, and DSA intensities are dependent of the X-ray technique used. MRI images contain anywhere from 8 to 11 bits of information per pixel in a 256×256 matrix, and vary in range from one pulse sequence to the next.

Architectural considerations

There are several key variables that must be considered when selecting a computer system for handling diagnostic images, besides the speed of the CPU itself. The system must have at least the spatial resolution of the original image. This is not a concern with workstations. However, most PCs only come with a 480×640 pixel display, and necessitate adding a special purpose board in the system to display higher resolution images. The only other alternative would be to display only portions of the image at a time.

Most importantly, the system should be able to manipulate the entire original intensity range of the images it displays. A device that can only handle 8-bit images would not be able to display 12-bit CT images. One would have to reduce the original intensity values *before* the image was ever displayed on the screen, and window and leveling was performed. Also, remapping may remove the possibility, for example, of obtaining the original Hounsfield units along a biopsy specimen for study and correlation. Furthermore, today's technology only delivers one LUT for an entire screen, no matter how many windows are separately displayed.

Therefore, if CT, MRI, and DSA images were displayed simultaneously on the same screen they would be affected by the window and level at the same rate, even though they may have drastically different intensity ranges. This would perhaps obscure key features of an image from one modality, while one could view the features on another modality. This would again necessitate some remapping of the original intensity values before they were ever windowed or leveled.

A multiscreen display, with each screen having its own LUT is the current technological choice for multimodality display without loss or a priori modification of original intensity information. Single screen, multiwindow devices (each with their own LUT) should be available soon.

USES OF STEREOTACTIC DIGITAL IMAGING

Digital diagnostic images provide valuable 3-D information. Procedures have been proposed for calculation of stereotactic coordinates directly from CT images using anatomical and/or scanner table references [5]. Some have taped a radiopaque marker onto a patient's skull for reference during the scan and during surgery. Most stereotactic systems, however, employ an immobilization device (headframe) and a reference system that leaves various markings on the diagnostic images, which are then related through manual or computerized means.

The basic premise behind all stereotactic reference systems is that they provide a mechanism for calculation of coordinates from a known point or plane. This point or plane has a reference in the coordinate system of the stereotactic device used in surgery. A direct measurement

or transformation algorithm then needs to be followed to determine the stereotactic coordinates from the diagnostic image. Digital medical images collected under stereotactic conditions may be utilized for stereotaxis in a number of manners: (1) film-based; (2) scanner-dependent; and (3) scanner-independent.

Film-based

Film-based stereotactic systems generally involve having the user draw lines on the film images. (Film images, though, may introduce non-linearities and differences in aspect ratios that must be corrected for, or taken into account of, in the final calculations. Furthermore, distortion corrections have to be applied to X-ray projection images as well.) The lines can be between grids, or a set of dots superimposed on the film by the localization device. Generally, the intersection between two intersecting lines provides the stereotactic coordinate, or is a reference point from which the target coordinates are measured. Measurements are usually performed using a ruler and manual geometric correction factors. Film-based systems are adequate for the derivation of a single coordinate, but are not amenable for volumetric calculations. Furthermore, corrections for a slice's angulation and geometric distortions are not usually possible with these types of system.

Scanner-based

The method of stereotactic calculations for scanner-based systems is generally the same, or similar to film-based systems, except that they utilize the scanner's software for drawing the lines or measuring the distances. Some systems take a series of scanner-software-generated x, y coordinates and table positions for known points, and then have the user enter these in a handheld calculator, or small PC. This is not only time consuming, but presents possibilities for user transcription errors, and inaccuracies of table movements and dropoff. Often this task is given to a technician to perform after the surgeon identifies the target, possibly leading to errors not directly recognizable by the surgeon.

One advantage of scanner-based over film-based systems is that the scanner's software should (although it may not) correct for geometric distortions in the image (as in MRI), before they produce their x, y coordinates. Furthermore, scanner-based systems do not allow the possibility of film-generated distortions.

There are various limitations to scanner-based systems. If a new target needs to be calculated intraoperatively this will require a trip back to the radiology department, where the scanner is located. Furthermore, one has to go to one scanner for one calculation and another scanner for another, since the various modalities may not be available at the same site. Most importantly, scanner-based systems are not amenable for volumetric stereotaxis, or occasions where more sophisticated corrections and calculations are necessary (e.g. multimodality correlations and usage of subtraction angiograms collected with an image intensifier).

Scanner-independent

Scanner-independent systems utilize a stand-alone computer system, which is located at or near the operating room. They may be home-grown or commercially available. Imaging data are transferred into these systems by magnetic tape, video digitization, or networks. These systems vary widely in the speed, capacity, and the degree of sophistication of their software.

Image transfers

Some scanner-based systems are wheeled right into the diagnostic suite and collect the video signal off the scanner monitor. (Alternatively this type of system can be remotely located and connect to the video signal by a long cable.) These utilize an 8-bit frame grabber, and entail setting the window and level of the image before the image is acquired (with a consequent loss of original intensity information.) Furthermore, patient identification information may be displayed on the screen, but is only available to the computer for classification by user entry. This could possibly result in human error.

Magnetic tape transfers will include the entire imaging set (in full spatial and intensity resolution), as well as important demographic and other associated data describing the image's geo-

metry, acquisition mode, etc. Software must be developed to translate these data from the manufacturer's proprietary format into the format necessary for the scanner-independent display device. This may be cumbersome, but it will guarantee that all of the information available at the scanner will be available at the remote computer and can be validated to ensure that the correct patient data are utilized for the correct surgical patient.

Networks are now beginning to be used for image transfer. These can be either proprietary or an implementation of the American College of Radiology—National Electrical Manufacturers Association (ACR—NEMA) medical imaging standard. Either method would transfer the entire dataset with identification information. These techniques would still require translation from a manufacturer's proprietary or the ACR—NEMA format, to a format for the display device. ACR—NEMA standards hold out the possibility of only needing one translation program for all modalities.

There are currently two other problems with networking techniques:

1 Most diagnostic scanners utilize computing technology that is many years old and may be obsolete. They very rarely have built-in networking capabilities. They may, however, be retrofitted with network capabilities, if there is room in their chassis for an additional circuit board. Nevertheless, manufacturers are hesitant about, if not against, having foreign parts placed in their computer. This is especially relevant if the institution has a maintenance contract with the vendor for support and doesn't want to void their contract. Manufacturers are only now beginning to offer new scanners with present-day networking computer technology, or are retrofitting their old ones with networking capabilities.

2 The most important constraint in networking an operative computer with diagnostic radiology is patient data security. Radiologists are very hesitant about, if not strongly against, having data recorded on their systems transferred onto a network that may not be under their control, or introducing losses in data integrity. Additionally, networking of information out of the scanner usually requires some CPU activity and may affect the scanning of patients.

Sophistication

Scanner-independent systems provide all the capabilities of film-based and scanner-dependent systems in the operating room, and much more. They should eliminate, or at least limit, the possibilities for human error. How well they handle it when it occurs is important. They are absolutely necessary for volumetric stereotaxis and true multimodality target and volume correlations, since this requires precise quantitative analysis.

Scanner-independent, stereotactic computer systems vary in sophistication and capacity. Capacity is related to whether the system is based on PC or workstation architecture. Sophistication involves how well the software is thought-out, and how long it takes to plan a surgical case, as well as how robust, user-friendly and proven it is. Scanner-independent software should correct for geometric irregularities and angular deviations in the images it manipulates. What features it has, what procedures it provides for, how mature it is, how it is supported, whether new features will be added, and the existence of a proven track record are only some of the issues to consider.

Discussion

There can be no question that the advent of computers has dramatically broadened, if not revolutionized, the field of stereotactic surgery. Computers have made possible the entire field of digital imaging, and in particular the modalities of CT, MRI, DSA, and PET. Coinciding with the introduction of these modalities has been the development of instrumentation to collect these data under stereotactic conditions. Techniques, and associated stereotactic software, for relating points and volumes from these data into the stereotactic coordinate system of stereotactic frames has made possible more precise and comprehensive surgical procedures, thereby increasing their efficacy. Precise 3-D imaging data can be rapidly manipulated, reformatted, and correlated by computers. Volumetric stereotaxis, in particular, would not be feasible without computers.

Computers and the software that controls them are only as useful, safe, and comprehensive as they are programmed to be. Artificial intelligence (AI) techniques have been applied in the field of medical diagnosis from as early as 1976 [6]. AI techniques could be applied in the field of stereotaxy. Furthermore, process control, in the form of, for example, computer control of a stereotactically-directed CO_2 laser is not difficult. However, there are medico-legal questions that must be addressed as to "who" or "what" is performing the surgery; the surgeon or the computer.

There are many other complex issues relating to computer-assisted surgery. Software is inherently complex and may have bugs. Furthermore, computer computations must be precise, extensively validated, and intuitive for the surgeon to verify. Surgeons should not place "blind trust" in either a purchased or self-developed hardware–software package, without proof that the particular system performs to its specification today and will do so at any time in the future. Hardware errors also occur; these could possibly lead to inaccurate calculations. More sophisticated computers usually offer diagnostics and error-correction mechanisms to avoid these types of inaccuracies. Nevertheless, it is better for a computer to fail or "crash" than calculate inaccurately. Redundant calculations and fault-tolerant computers can help in regard to these matters. Scannable phantoms, and tele-radiographic and other verification mechanisms must also be provided or developed, which allow the user to prove the hardware and software are performing correctly at any time. These validation mechanisms should be used as an ongoing part of computer-assisted surgical practice.

Stereotactic hardware and software systems must be amenable to evolving technology. They should be developed in such a way that they are able to adapt to evolving hardware technology, parallel and distributed processing, or whatever new technology appears on the horizon. Furthermore, systems must have support, be expandable, provide improvements and enhancements, and have a proven track record. One cannot just buy or develop a system and expect it to always function correctly and meet future needs. There are significant issues related to software maintenance: portability to new hardware, sustainability of code by someone other than the person who wrote it, and whether the developer of the software will even be around in the future. Vendors *must* provide support for their products.

Stereotactic hardware and software systems are usually like buying a car; you often get what you pay for. The costs of developing it oneself are not usually inexpensive. Hardware is easy to purchase (assuming one can determine the correct combination and fit), but software development is (and should be) a methodical (and often long) and expensive process. There are significant hardware integration issues related to piecing together a system from multiple vendors: (1) who do you call for support when one aspect fails?; and (2) not all pieces may be compatible. Manufacturer specifications are not always reliable, are subject to change, and there are often incompatibilities in hardware revisions even among the same products.

This "you get what you pay for" statement does not imply that throwing expensive technology at a problem always solves it, and if it does it may not always be optimal. A balance must be found between the needs of the user in specific solutions and the costs of the available technology. This is relevant to developing a system oneself, purchasing one or doing without the technology at all. The latter, in today's age, is becoming less and less an option, if not medico-legally unwise.

Purchasing or developing a system for stereotactic neurosurgery deserves significant consideration. Assuming the technology is warranted, at least the following three issues should be considered: *quality*, *cost*, and *speed*. In most cases, one can only obtain two of these items. If the technology is of high quality, and either runs fast or is developed quickly, it usually

will not be cheap, because a lot of expensive technology and/or personnel will be required to develop it. If the technology is cheap and is developed fast, the quality will not usually be high or the system will not be very robust. Finally, if the quality is high and it is developed inexpensively it will not be developed quickly or the system will run slowly.

Inexpensive development is usually limited in personnel, but software usually also takes longer to develop if the correct development tools are unavailable, or it must be developed in assembly language to attain higher performance. Users and developers of computer-assisted or computer-aided stereotactic systems should strive to meet all three criteria: the systems should be affordable for the user's caseload and requirements, run fast, and be available quickly, and most of all be of highest quality.

References

1 Horsley, V. & Clarke, R.H. The structure and function of the cerebellum examined by a new method. *Brain* **31**: 45–124 (1980).

2 Ingram, W.R., Ransom, S.W., Hannet, F.I., *et al.* Results of stimulation of the tegmentum with Horsley–Clarke stereotaxic apparatus. *Arch. Psychiatr.* **28**: 513–41 (1932).

3 Pecard, C., Olivier, A. & Bertrand, G. The first stereotaxic apparatus: the contribution of Aubrey Musser to the field of stereotaxis *J. Neurosurg.* **59**: 673–6 (1983).

4 Spiegel, E.A., Wycis, H.T., Marks, O.R., *et al.* Stereotaxic apparatus for operations on the human brain. *Science* **106**: 349–50 (1947).

5 Gildenberg, P., Kaufman, H.H. & Murthy, K.S.M. Calculation of stereotactic coordinates from the computed tomography scan. *Neurosurgery* **10**: 580–6 (1982).

6 Shortcliff, E.H. *Computer-based medical consultations: MYCIN.* New York: Elsevier North-Holland (1976).

chapter 2

Interactive and Quantitative Analysis of Biomedical Images

Richard A. Robb

Introduction

Human vision provides an extraordinarily powerful and effective means for acquiring information. Much of what we know about ourselves and our environment has been derived from images — images produced by various instruments, ranging from microscopes to telescopes which extend the range of human vision into realms beyond that which is naturally accessible. However, the full scientific, educational, and/or biomedical value of these images, although profoundly significant, remains largely unexploited. This is due primarily to the lack of objective, quantitative methods to fully analyze the intrinsic information contained in the images. We have largely relied on subjective interpretations, and only recently have begun to recognize and unearth the rich treasures of image recordings.

The traditional disciplines of biologic and medical science are significantly grounded in the observation of living structures and in the measurement of various properties of these structures (e.g. their functions). These observations and measurements are often recorded as images. Ever since the invention of the microscope and discovery of X-rays, physicians, surgeons, and life scientists have been using images to diagnose and treat disease and to better understand basic physiology and biology. The value of biomedical images depends upon the context in which they are obtained, and the scientific or medical interests and goals which motivate their production and use.

The imaging modalities used in biology and medicine are based on a variety of energy sources, including light, electrons, lasers, X-rays, radionuclides, ultrasound, and nuclear magnetic resonance. The objects imaged span orders of magnitude in scale, ranging from molecules and cells to organ systems and the full body. The advantages and limitations of each modality are primarily governed by the basic physical and biologic principles which influence the way each energy form interacts with tissues, and by the specific engineering implementation for a particular medical or biologic application. The variety of disease processes and abnormalities affecting all regions of the human body are so numerous and different that each imaging modality possesses attributes that make it uniquely helpful in providing the desired understanding and/or discrimination of the disease or abnormality, and therefore no single method has prevailed to the complete exclusion of others. In general, the methodologies are complementary, together providing a powerful armamentarium of clinical diagnostic, therapeutic, and biomedical research capabilities, which has potential advance significantly the practice of medicine and the frontiers of biologic understanding.

The process of forming an image involves the

mapping of an object, and/or some property of an object, into or onto what is called "image space". This space is used to visualize the object and its properties, and may be used to quantitatively characterize its structure and/or its function. "Imaging science" may be defined as the study of these mappings and development of ways to understand them better, to improve them and to use them productively. There are four postulates fundamentally important in imaging science, which derive from this definition: (1) image mappings, varied as they are, provide a *direct* measurement of form and/or function; (2) an image, especially a digital or computer image, is truly synergistic — that is, the "gestalt" or whole of an image is greater than the sum of its parts; (3) the contextual "glue" that holds discrete images together contains important information — therein is contained subtle details fundamental to understanding the mapping of the real object and its properties into image space; and (4) there are many ways, mostly arbitrary, to manipulate and use images — a rational basis for their selection is important to the biomedical scientist and clinician alike.

The challenge of imaging science is to provide advanced capabilities for acquisition, processing, visualization, and quantitative analysis of biomedical images in order to significantly increase the faithful extraction of both scientific and clinical information which they contain. This is a formidable task, one which consistently suggests that existing approaches and constructs are not adequate to address it effectively. The need for resolution of this problem will become increasingly important and pressing as advances in imaging and computer technology enable more complex objects and processes to be imaged and simulated. The system described in this chapter represents a software paradigm sufficiently robust and flexible to meet this need.

Background

The revolutionary capabilities provided by new three-dimensional (3-D) and four-dimensional (4-D) imaging modalities (computed tomography (CT), magnetic resonance imaging (MRI), positron emission tomography (PET), single photon emission computed tomography (SPECT), ultrasound, confocal microscopy, etc.) now provide data for direct visualization and study of structure and function of internal organs and organelles. However, the ability to extract objective and quantitatively accurate information from 3-D biomedical images has not kept pace with the ability to produce the images themselves.

Modern advances in the microelectronics industry have provided remarkable hardware capabilities to help close this gap [1]. We now can put the supercomputers of the recent past on our desktops for a fraction of their previous cost. Powerful graphics and image display hardware, recently the exclusive purview of high-end computer-aided design/computer-aided manufacture (CAD/CAM) or image-processing workstations, are now available on personal desktop computers. What is needed additionally is comprehensive, integrated software for *interactive and quantitative* display and analysis of multimodality, multidimensional biomedical images.

Techniques for processing and displaying 3-D information include integrated projections of the volume onto the display screen, sometimes with prior dissolution of structures from the volume [2], stereo displays generated from projection images [3,4], shaded surface display [5–7], and volume rendering [8–12]. One of the most popular techniques for presenting 3-D structures is to use depth shading of object surfaces. An important precursor to shaded surface display is the extraction of a 3-D surface descripton from a raw 3-D volume image. This segmentation step is often required not only for display but for measurement as well. However, the segmentation step is an area which is in need of improved algorithms [7,13–16], particularly for the extraction of soft tissue structures, and for images such as those produced by MRI and ultrasound. Shaded surface display algorithms for medical applications have been based on conventional polygonal models [17], a cuberille model for the surface [18], a contour model for the surface [19], and an octtree model of the 3-D object [18]. Another 3-D display technique, often called ray casting or volume rendering, has been implemented in several applications [5,8–12,20–21]. This technique features the advantage of using the entire 3-D data set ("volume image") in the process. The challenge heretofore has been to exploit this powerful technique in an interactive implementation. This chapter describes and illustrates a solution to this problem.

The Biotechnology Computer Resource and the Biodynamics Research Unit (BRU) at the Mayo Clinic has been involved in the development of biomedical image display and analysis algorithms for 3-D and 4-D images since the early 1970s. The successful development of the Dynamic Spatial Reconstructor [22,23] has provided a ready source of 3-D and 4-D imagery from a variety of biomedical investigative and clinical studies. During this time, several unique and useful analysis techniques were developed. These include projection displays [3], stereo displays [2,3], interactive oblique sectioning algorithms [24], shaded surface display algorithms [19], and space-filling virtual 3-D display using a vibrating mirror system [25,26]. Many of these capabilities have been developed on different computer systems as the need for them arose. The programs were developed, to a large extent, independent of one another. These established tools and several new important capabilities have now been generalized and made applicable to a wide variety of multidimensional biomedical images (e.g. CT, MRI, PET, ultrasound, microscopy, etc.) and have been integrated into a single comprehensive software package which runs on dedicated, powerful image analysis workstations and networks [1,12,27].

Software design considerations

Architecture and implementation

The implementation of a software package to effectively integrate multidimensional, multimodality image display and analysis capabilities requires the design of an efficient shell to synergistically relate such programs. The primary design goal has been to provide the user with an integrated, interactive means of accessing all of the display and analysis tools required to completely evaluate multidimensional image data sets, and to realistically simulate manipulation on these (e.g. surgery). The key features of such a package include an intuitive user interface, access to all of the programs necessary to complete any particular application task (with intermediate steps stored in memory rather than other storage media), and efficient implementation of each of the program tasks to provide truly interactive display and analysis. Furthermore, from a software development perspective, certain standards are required for the representation of image data and program formats to facilitate and accommodate development by multiple programmers. To allow for expandability, the architecture of any such package should be designed in a modular fashion.

The ANALYZE software system is a manifestation of this design criterion. Each ANALYZE program presents the user with a common base of functions and a common user interface and display format. These functions are the basic building blocks of all the ANALYZE programs, and are contained in libraries that can be linked to each of the individual programs when they are compiled. This organization provides a common implementation style for the ANALYZE modules, and facilitates parallel program development.

Program organization and user interface

The ANALYZE software package is written entirely in the "C" programming language and runs on many standard UNIX workstation systems. There are over 60 programs in the package, made up of over 250 000 lines of source code. The subprogram structure is modular and parallel, with each display and analysis function incorporated as a separate program. This architecture permits systematic enhancements and modifications, which has fostered development of a readily extensible and portable package.

The infrastructure of the ANALYZE architecture is based on a hierarchical arrangement of display, manipulation, and measurement tools, through which the user invokes single processes from the main ANALYZE menu. Each process or program has access to one or more image data sets loaded by the user. Major emphasis has been placed on optimizing the tradeoffs between speed (interactivity) and accuracy (image fidelity) in all ANALYZE procedures.

Pop-down menus for selection of individual processes is provided. The interface tools include numeric field entries (using sliders, if desired), scroll bars for selection of items from a list, and confirmation messages. Other user interface tools include the use of "hot keys" for invoking selected options, such as interactive windows for the display, review, and editing of text files. ANALYZE uses color extensively and intelligently to facilitate clarity and ease of use.

System features

Image data management

The ANALYZE system consists of modules which share image memory segments and which communicate with each other to pass related image information. The integration of these subprocesses allows for multiple analyses, whereby the output of one process may be in the input to another. Image data is input and output in the system using the programs in Move. Several image data formats archivally stored on $\frac{1}{2}$ inch tape can be loaded onto an ANALYZE image database file, using the *tape in* program. Similarly, image database files can be written out to $\frac{1}{2}$ inch tape, using the *tape out* program. The *load volume* program allows the interactive selection of database files, review of selected image data by displaying the images on the screen prior to loading, and control of the word size and dimensions of the image data when loading into memory. The *save volume* program stores image data in memory to a new or existing image database file on disk, with control over the spatial region of the data in memory that is saved.

The ANALYZE image database supports the following image data types: 1-bit binary (packed 8 bits/byte); 8-bit unsigned integer; 16-bit signed integer; 32-bit signed integer; 32-bit single precision floating point; 64-bit double precision floating point; and 64-bit complex (32 bit real and 32 bit imaginary). These image data types are further supported by representations in the shared image memory, i.e. ANALYZE programs know and can work with images composed of any of these data types. The ANALYZE image database currently supports up to four dimensions, e.g. three spatial dimensions plus time, or three spatial dimensions plus modality, etc. When loading or storing image data, the bounds of all dimensions can be con-trolled along with specified increments within each dimension. A "bounding box" can be used to automatically reduce the data array to the smallest subregion containing non-zero data. A robust *file manager* program provides image database file management utilities, including backup and restore, delete, copy, rename, compress, and uncompress.

Ancillary utilities

A rich set of useful ancillary utilities is available in ANALYZE. Some of these are loaded under the *other* option on the root menu. A *configure* program allows the user to design the ANALYZE working environment to specific preferences, including font size and type, colors for text highlights and background, single/double click for mouse selections, specification of networked resources to be used, and the numeric format of any computed data for compatibility with popular statistical analysis packages. The *screen edit* program provides extensive capabilities for screen preparation, including generation of text and graphics, image scaling and coloring, cut-and-paste, and file merging, all of which can be formatted and displayed in a variety of ways. Textual, numeric, graphic and image information can be printed on a variety of supported printers using the *hardcopy* program. The *macros* tools can be used to generate repetitive routines, customized processing, tutorials, and demonstrations. This tool provides capabilities for interactive input from the operator upon playback of the *macros* (e.g. pauses, entry of file names, numbers, etc.). Programs and utilities that exist outside of the ANALYZE shell can be run by using the *special* options. Upon selection of this tool, another menu is generated, giving the user selections for these external programs. This menu is generated from a text file that can be easily edited to add new programs.

A helpful Tooltable can be invoked from any screen in ANALYZE to provide even more tools. A *magnifying glass* can be invoked for magnification of any region of the screen (see Fig. 2.1). The mouse buttons control the size of the area being magnified and the magnification factor. The magnifying mode can be toggled to display histograms or numeric pixel values in the region selected. The *interactive color* tool can be used to

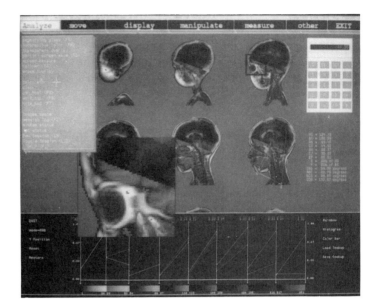

FIGURE 2.1 A montage of Tooltable utilities including *magnifying glass, interactive color, caliper,* and *calculator.* From Robb & Hanson [31] © 1990 IEEE.

interactively and flexibly specify the mapping of colors to images (see Fig. 2.1). The *transparent overlay* tool allows the user to select a region of the screen and transparently move it around to another area on the screen. The *screen measure* tool makes distance measurements in pixels along an interactively specified straight line or curvilinear trace. A line profile for the line or trace can also be interactively displayed. Another screen measuring tool, called *caliper*, can be used to measure linear segment distances and angles between specified lines (see Fig. 2.1).

The *C-shell* tool can be used to enter operating system (UNIX) commands, such as deleting files, moving files, checking process status, etc. Several different *status* tools are available to display run-time information. The *new session* and *toggle session* options can be used to start multiple sessions of the ANALYZE package and allow the user to rapidly switch between these sessions. This allows multiple tools to be run on the same or different image data set(s) loaded into memory. A complete, on-screen *text editor* has been developed for entry and review of text notes typed into a specific notepad file. Extensive *help* is available throughout ANALYZE. A comprehensive Users' Manual has been developed for the ANALYZE package, and the pages of this manual have been converted into ANALYZE image files and placed on-line. The electronic

manual is context-sensitive — that is, the pages describing the program currently running are automatically displayed, and the pages for that section can be turned using the mouse buttons. Keyboard options exist to allow the user to change to any portion of the ANALYZE manual, including the Introduction and Appendices.

Image display

The Display routines in ANALYZE provide capabilities for a variety of graphic presentations of multiformatted 2-D sections and of computed 3-D objects extracted from the volume image data sets. Included in each display module are tools for interactive manipulation of the presentation style and format.

The *normal sections* program permits 2-D images to be arbitrarily sized, flexibly formatted, and rapidly displayed on the screen. Multiple sections through a 3-D volume image can be displayed by selection of a starting position and automatic increment. Figure 2.2 shows a different way to display orthogonal sections, provided by the *ortho sections* program — a cubic volume with interactive scaling (both geometric and intensity), rotation about any axis, and dissection at any depth in the transverse, coronal, and/or sagittal planes. In Fig. 2.2, 3-D chest data has been rotated, orthogonally sectioned, and intensity-windowed so as to better

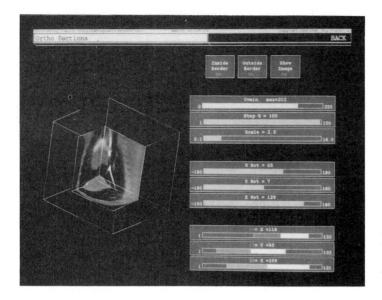

FIGURE 2.2 Interactive orthogonal sectioning and 3-D visualization using the *ortho sections* program. From Robb & Hanson [31] © 1990 IEEE.

visualize the contrast-filled heart and pulmonary arteries. The *oblique sections* program provides an interactive method for arbitrary viewpoint selection by providing the user with pictorial feedback cues to indicate the current orientation of the volume image data. Newly oriented 3-D images can be stored in the data base for subsequent analysis. The *curved sections* module permits a curved line to be drawn on one of the standard orthogonal planes (transverse, coronal, or sagittal), and sections perpendicular to this line, interactively computed and displayed adjacent one to another to yield an image of any curvilinear section through the volume. Modes that can be used to generate the output image include *free-hand trace*, *rubber band*, and *rays*.

Frequently the output of segmentation programs (described subsequently) are contours defined by 3-D coordinates on the surface of the segmented structures. ANALYZE supports a data structure of this type, called a "surface description file," wherein the 3-D coordinates are stored along with a normal to the surface at each point. The *connect* and *extract edges* programs automatically format such 3-D coordinate files into *contour* files. The *contours* program provides interactive display capability for these data files. The *surface* program takes as input any number of surface description files for multiple objects in an image data set and produces a shaded surface display of this data. The surface descrip-

tion algorithm [19] uses flat patches, of a user-defined size, which can be oriented in many directions to generate faces for each point in the surface description file. Sequences of shaded surface displays can be generated and stored in an image database file for later display in the *movie* program in order to visualize sequences of parameter changes, i.e. rotation. The *surface* program has been used extensively for visualization of objects to convey shape and relative dimensions, and for verifying that a given object has been properly identified.

One of the most versatile and powerful image display and manipulation tools in ANALYZE is the *volume render* program. Volume rendering techniques [8–12] are able to display surfaces with shading, and other parts of the volume simultaneously. An important advantage is to display data directly from the grayscale volume. The selection of the data which will appear on the screen is done during the projection of the voxels (sometimes called ray casting). A function of different attributes of the voxels, such as their density or gradient values and/or spatial coordinates, can be invoked during the projection process to produce "on the fly" segmented surfaces, cutting planes anywhere in the volume, and/or selected degrees of transparency/opacity within the volume. Volume set operations (union, intersection, difference of volume) can also be invoked during the projection process. Angle of view and illumination direc-

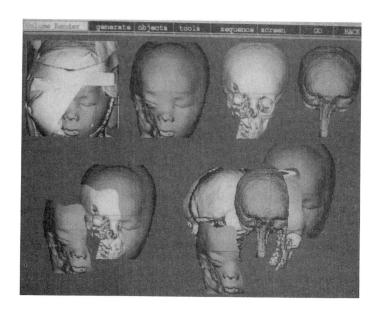

FIGURE 2.3 Montage of images demonstrating the capability to segment and color objects in *volume render* and individually manipulate them (see text). From Robb & Hanson [31] © 1990 IEEE.

tion can be interactively adjusted. The implementation of volume rendering in ANALYZE has several unique features and advantages in comparison to shaded surface display and other volume rendering methods. The algorithm is optimized to be fast without compromising fidelity [12]. The goal of the ray-tracing implementation is to interactively render an anatomical volume with different degrees of segmentation, and with image quality sufficient to convey the information in the data set, no more or no less.

The *volume render* program includes tools for individual object discrimination and manipulation. Figure 2.3 illustrates this capability. The images in the top row have been rendered from the raw X-ray CT data, using an object map to render, from left to right, the full image, remove the bandage and head holder, remove the skin, and finally remove the bone to reveal the brain. The bottom left image in Fig. 2.3. illustrates the capability to translate a section of the skin away from the rest of the image, exposing the underlying skull. The bottom right image illustrates a combination of translation and rotation of multiple objects to visualize interior structures. These images depict the capability of the *volume render* module to interactively explore 3-D images, much as a surgeon or pathologist would explore an actual organ or body part. Each image in Fig. 2.3 required less than 2 seconds to compute from a volume image of dimensions $160 \times 160 \times 160$ pixels.

There are utilities in the *volume render* module for interactively positioning mutually orthogonal or arbitrary oblique planes, which represent the raw X-ray CT data and which intersect familiar surfaces in the 3-D volume. Figure 2.4 shows clipping planes in the front and back of the current viewing angle, interactively adjusted to cut through the 3-D surface image (top center and right). Masked regions defined on the surface image by interactive tracing (bottom row), and any selected rendering parameters, can be applied exclusively to this region to visualize "inlaid" structures surrounded by the current image.

Both the *surface* program and the *volume render* programs can automatically generate sequences of images stored in an image file where consecutive images differ by selected combinations of rendering parameters applied in specified increments, such as thresholding, dissecting, rotating, etc. The *movie* program provides the capability to rapidly display these sequences of images in a cine-movie loop. This program is also useful for redisplay of images acquired through time in order to visualize changes in the images.

Image manipulation

Image processing functions for enhancement of images or as a precursor to application of segmentation tools are important components of

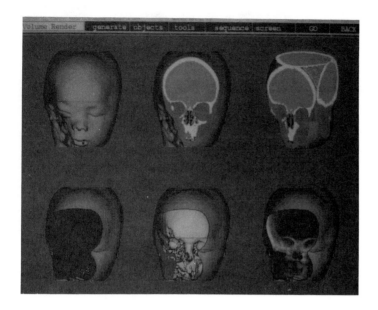

FIGURE 2.4 Arbitrary clipping planes and windows can be interactively placed in volume-rendered images to visualize internal values (see text). From Robb & Hanson [31] © 1990 IEEE.

an image display and analysis package. The programs in the Manipulate group of modules in ANALYZE allow the user to apply several types of image processing and segmentation algorithms to the image data.

The *transform* program allows the user to enter any desired formula, where the operands are variables assigned to image files or constants, and the operators are the standard arithmetic or logical operators (a limited set of transcendental functions are also included), to form a linear combination of image sets, i.e. to do "image algebra." Several common image transforms can also be applied in the *transform* program. These include trilinear interpolation, image rotation and translation, intensity windowing and scaling, and image volume subregioning and flipping.

A variety of 3-D convolution and frequency space filters can be applied to the image data using the *filter* program. Several edge enhancement filters (e.g. Sobel) and histogram equalization can be performed on 2-D or 3-D image data sets. Clipped adaptive histogram equalization can also be applied to the image data for contrast enhancement. The package provides both forward and inverse Fourier transforms on image data, and can represent frequency space as a complex image (i.e. magnitude and phase, real and imaginary) in the shared image memory. Filters can be applied non-destructively

(without altering the image memory) and inversely applied to display the spatial domain. An interactive, versatile *digital filter design* tool is also available for customized processing of images.

The *slice edit* program provides both efficient manual segmentation tools as well as capabilities for semi-automated object definition and feature extraction. The top row of images in Fig. 2.5 illustrate two of the techniques available, including "painting" on the image data with a selected cursor shape and size and tracing area(s) to be deleted. A depth can be set in both of these modes to cause the edit to penetrate into the volume image. Interactive thresholding can also be used as a precursor to editing. A semi-automatic mode for finding structure boundaries is also available. The user defines a seed point from which region-growing is to originate, and then moves a slider to alter the threshold range within which pixels will be included in the growth region. The center row of images in Fig. 2.5 depicts this technique applied to multiple MRI sections of the head leaving only the segmented structure of interest, as shown in the bottom row.

Image mensuration

The programs in Measure are all interactive, and provide quantitative sampling capabilities,

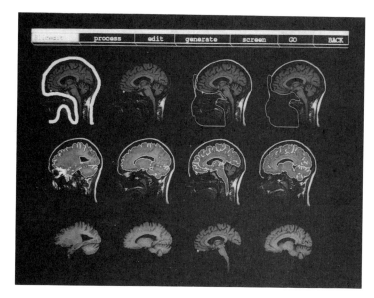

FIGURE 2.5 Examples of image editing and segmentation using *slice edit*. Both manual (top row) and automatic (center row) methods are available (see text). From Robb [32].

making no assumptions about the significance of these measurements, which must be determined by the application. Each program can produce output that is stored in an ANALYZE data file structure called a "stats" file. Stats files can be generated in several different formats which match the formats accepted as input to some of the common numerical analysis packages, such as SAS, RS/1, S, and DIF files for PC programs.

The *project trace* program provides a method of unambiguously tracing 3-D tree structures, such as dye-filled coronary arteries or pulmonary arteries. Interactive traces on any one projection are simultaneously displayed on all projections to generate the trace. Such traces can be used to compute segment lengths, branching angles, and oblique images.

Single dimension profiles can be interactively sampled from image data and plotted using the *profile* program. The line profiles can be applied to multiple images. In automatic sampling mode, multiple lines through multiple images can be sampled and stored in a stats file. The *volume estimate* program measures and estimates the volume of an arbitrarily shaped three-dimensional object using a probabilistic model [28]. A user-specified number of voxels are randomly marked in the volume image, and a cursor of varying size is then used to interactively select the marked voxels overlying the

structure for which the volume is to be calculated. The ratio of the selected voxels in each section to the total number of marked voxels is used to estimate the volume of the desired object. A significant advantage in speed of volume estimation is realized by comparison to manual tracing of the structure of interest, with similar accuracy (greater than 95% [28]).

The *biopsy* program can be used to interactively define and sample regions of interest (ROIs) on the image data. Regions can be defined using analytic shapes (e.g. rectangles and ellipses), by tracing a free-form area on the image, or by semi-automated boundary definition using region-growing. Information provided by the area sampling includes the maximum and minimum values, mean and standard deviation of the values, the calibrated area within the region, and the integrated brightness—area product, as shown in the stats panel in the upper right of Fig. 2.6. Areas can be automatically sampled through a series of sections to provide a volumetric sampling function if the third dimension is spatial, or a time sampling function if the third dimension is time. Individual ROIs can be summed together to provide an arbitrary shaped volumetric sample through the multidimensional image data.

Another measurement provided by the *biopsy* program is the fractal signature for ROIs. The fractal dimension [29] is calculated for the speci-

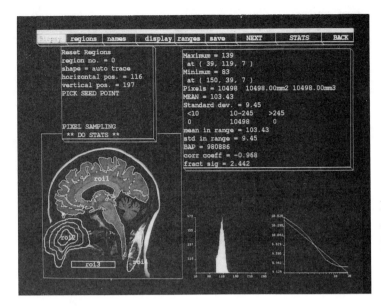

FIGURE 2.6 A screen from the *biopsy* program showing different types of regions of interest and quantitative sampling of regions, including fractal signatures/graphs. From Robb & Hanson [31] © 1990 IEEE.

fied regions by placing an envelope both above and below the grayscale surface, and then calculating the volume that is contained between them. This value is a scalar multiple of the enclosing surface area, which is logarithmically proportional to the fractal dimension. The distance between the "blankets" of the envelope and the surface can be varied to generate values at different scales. When these calculations are completed over a desired range of scales, a log–log plot of surface area versus scale is generated, and a least squares estimate of the linear regression line for this plot is calculated, as shown in the lower right of Fig. 2.6. The linear correlation coefficient of this fit is given in the stats output, and the slope of the fit is reported as the fractal signature for the region. These data can be used as input to the *plot* program for data plotting and numerical analysis. The *plot* program is very flexible and provides the user with many options for data manipulation and graphing.

Multimodality applications

The ANALYZE software is being used in a wide variety of applications in a number of institutions. These applications include both basic science and clinical investigations, ranging from exploring the world of the living cell to simulating surgery (i.e. planning an actual operation with a computer). ANALYZE has been used extensively for analysis of many organ systems and their function — heart, lungs, kidneys, brain, etc. There are several potential applications of ANALYZE that are non-medical — for example, in oil exploration, meteorology, and industrial inspection. The following sections indicate only some of the ongoing biomedical uses of ANALYZE.

3-D microscopy

New technologies in digital microscopy can generate tomographic images of serial sections of specimens. Therefore, the study of microscopic structures such as cells and tissue sections can now be significantly facilitated with 3-D visualization tools. The ANALYZE volume rendering program has been applied to several microscopic structures obtained from different microscopy modalities, including digital scanning fluorescence microscopy, standard light transmission microscopy, and confocal microscopy.

X-ray computed tomography

Since the advent of X-ray CT in the early 1970s, a great deal of research into display and analysis techniques for CT data has been undertaken. As scanning resolutions in all dimensions became

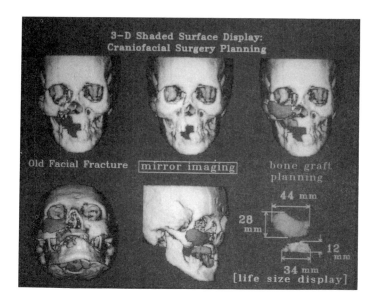

FIGURE 2.7 Examples of object manipulation in *volume render* for prosthesis design (see text). From Robb & Hanson [31] © 1990 IEEE.

higher, the possibility of accurately rendering 3-D structure from X-ray CT became real.

Figure 2.7 shows the application of the ANALYZE volume rendering program to X-ray CT data acquired for craniofacial surgery planning and simulation. The images show data from a preoperative scan of a patient with a facial feature. Linear and curvilinear distance measurements and volume calculations can be performed directly on these 3-D images. Through the use of the editing, measurement, and display tools available in the volume rendering program, a surgical procedure for this patient was planned and simulated using ANALYZE, including completion of a prosthesis. ANALYZE has been used to plan many such craniofacial surgery cases, both within Mayo Foundation and at other institutions.

Magnetic resonance imaging

Magnetic resonance imaging (MRI) has proved useful for detailed visualization of soft tissue structures often unrevealed by X-ray CT imaging. For instance, MRI can be used to image white versus gray matter in the brain, or to image soft tissue structures in joints, including the muscles and ligaments.

New scanning modes in MRI have allowed for the acquisition of isotropic 3-D image data sets at high spatial resolution. Figure 2.8 shows volume-rendered images from a 3-D acquired

MRI scan of a head for visualization of brain structures. At the left of Fig. 2.8, the editing tools in ANALYZE have been used to segment the brain from the other tissues, and rendered to visualize the brain in position with the facial soft tissue as reference. The objects can be rotated together, or can be separately manipulated, as shown by the image depicting the brain lifted out of the soft tissue and rotated opposite of the facial structures. The striking detail in the convolutions of the brain has been the impetus for use of this kind of data acquisition and rendering in the planning of neurosurgery cases at Mayo Foundation, including mapping of epileptic foci in the gyri for therapeutic resection. Another new scanning mode being developed in MRI imaging can be used to image vasculature structures through which blood is flowing. This "MR angio" acquisition method was used to produce the data used for the 3-D rendered images of brain vasculature at the right of Fig. 2.8. The vessels in the brain have been rendered from multiple angles of view to generate a rotational movie for visualizing the 3-D anatomic relationships of these vessels.

Nuclear medicine imaging

Physiologic and metabolic imaging of the body has been accomplished using radioactively-labeled chemicals that are preferentially

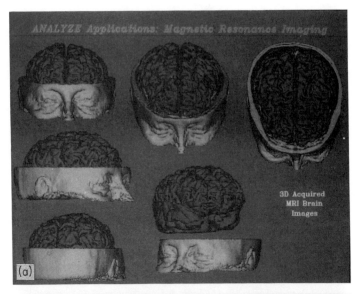

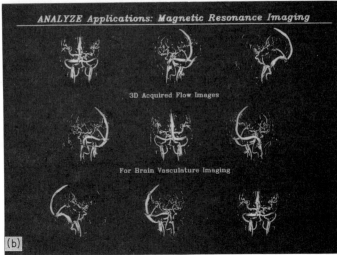

FIGURE 2.8 (a) Volume-rendered images from 3-D MRI head scan showing segmentation, rotation, and object manipulation. From Robb & Hanson [31] © 1990 IEEE. (b) 3-D images of brain vasculature rendered by ANALYZE from 3-D acquired MRI angiographic images (see also text). From Robb [32].

absorbed by certain tissues. The radioactive emissions are measured with detectors specific to the radiation type and tomographic images produced. Such imaging devices form pictures of physiologic and metabolic function of organs and organ systems of the body but do not generally form highly detailed images of the structures of these organs. ANALYZE has been used in nuclear medicine imaging to visualize these areas of activity and, in conjunction with the other imaging modalities, can be used to compare the functional images with detailed anatomic images obtained from other scan modalities.

Figure 2.9 shows colored images acquired using positron emission tomography (PET) scanning to study cerebral oxygen utilization in stroke victims. The images are multiple serial sections of a brain, where the images are generated using radiolabeled oxygen, with colors corresponding to levels of activity in the brain. The PET images have been merged with MRI images to illustrate both structure and function.

Dynamic spatial reconstructor

The Dynamic Spatial Reconstructor (DSR) is a unique X-ray scanning device, developed in the

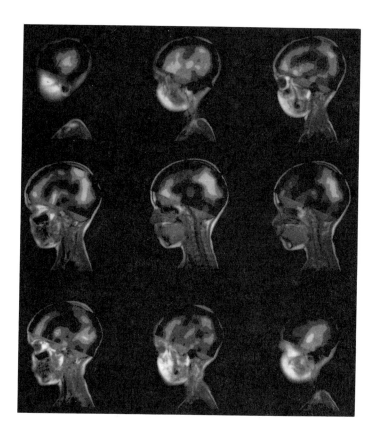

FIGURE 2.9 Positron emission tomography (PET) images of cerebral oxygen uptake (see text). From Robb [32].

Biodynamics Research Unit at Mayo to generate time sequences of synchronous 3-D volume images in studies of structural/functional relationships in moving organs. The DSR is capable of generating an isotropic 3-D volume image 60 times per second, truly a 4-D imaging system.

Figure 2.10 is a montage of images demonstrating the 4-D scanning capabilities of the DSR. Each image is a 3-D shaded surface display of the major chambers of the heart, red being the left ventricular chamber and blue the right ventricular chamber (essentially the surface of the blood pool in the chambers). Since multiple

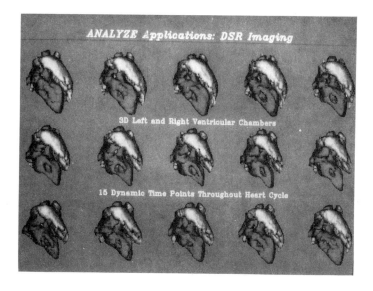

FIGURE 2.10 Time sequence of 3-D shaded surface displays of heart chambers throughout one complete heart cycle (see text). From Robb & Hanson [31] © 1990 IEEE.

volume images can be acquired through time, these shaded surface displays can be generated for multiple time points throughout the cardiac cycle. Here 15 time points through a single heart beat are depicted, starting at end diastole, going through end systole (approximately image 11), and back to near end diastole. The "hole" in the left ventricular chamber is caused by invagination of the papillary muscle from the surrounding myocardium. These images are part of a movie sequence that shows the change in 3-D structure of the heart through time from several different viewing angles. Such a movie is more than just a picture of the heart, it is a picture of the heart beat, a study of structure and function simultaneously.

Workstation implementations

ANALYZE has been successfully ported to a number of workstation platforms. Generally these implementations are straightforward if the platform has a standard UNIX operating system and C compiler. It is only required to modify the ANALYZE graphics libraries to read and write screen pixels. (Some minor nuances in compiled code may need to be reconciled in different vendor products.) Typically ANALYZE, which is composed of over 250 000 lines of C source code, can be ported to a new workstation platform within 2–3 weeks. If special system constraints exist, as presented by some special graphics options (e.g. a windows manager), the port may take longer. Table 2.1 provides a listing of some of the workstation platforms to which ANALYZE has been successfully ported, along with comparative performance measures for several of the modules in ANALYZE. These ANALYZE-specific benchmarks test rates of (1) disk transfer; (2) screen display; (3) integer computation; and (4) floating point computation, in various ANALYZE processes. Table 2.1 also indicates an "overall performance" factor obtained by applying certain weights to different performance functions and normalizing to unity (the higher the number, the better the performance rating). Changing the values of weights would change the overall outcome, but the values selected for Table 2.1 are those considered to be appropriate in prioritizing func-

TABLE 2.1 Performance of some ANALYZE program functions on different systems

System	Disk Xfer[1] (Mbytes s^{-1})	Pixel display[2] (Mpixels s^{-1})	Integer[3] (images s^{-1})	Float Pt[4] (images s^{-1})	Overall average[5]
DECStation 3100	0.27	0.83	0.18	2.08	0.19
HP 360	0.27	0.24	0.20	0.63	0.14
IBM RS 6000/530	3.36	1.40	1.01	5.86	0.68
MIPS RS2030	0.43	3.76	0.62	2.94	0.54
SGI 4D-25 Pers. Iris	0.84	1.17	0.69	2.66	0.42
SGI 4D-70/GT	0.42	0.56	0.46	1.73	0.25
SGI 4D-120/GTX	Not tested	0.90	0.55	2.20	0.31
Solbourne 4/602	1.03	1.54	0.33	0.99	0.28
Sun 3−160	0.39	1.48	0.11	0.05	0.16
Sun 3−280	1.66	2.13	0.22	0.08	0.31
Sun 3−470	2.98	3.33	0.36	0.17	0.51
Sun 386i−250	0.14	2.41	0.17	0.38	0.22
Sun SPARCStation1+	0.82	4.73	0.69	1.69	0.67
Sun 4−260	0.97	1.36	0.46	1.02	0.32
Sun 4−330	2.87	4.57	0.73	2.05	0.75
Sun 4−490	2.90	6.67	1.00	3.08	0.99

1 *Load* program timing in Mbytes s^{-1} to transfer 4 Mbyte volume image.
2 *Movie* program timing in Mbytes s^{-1} to display 5-cycle sequence of 160×160 pixel size images.
3 *Volume render* program timing in images s^{-1} for $160 \times 160 \times 160$ pixel size images.
4 *Adaptive histogram equalization* program timing in images s^{-1} for 256×256 pixel images.
5 Averaged performance with weighting on disk transfer = 20%, pixel display = 40%, integer computation = 30%, and floating point = 10%.

tions used in typical ANALYZE applications (e.g. speed of display is critical for interactive usage).

New developments

The ANALYZE software package has been developed and continues to be refined and extended to provide comprehensive, detailed quantitative investigations and evaluation of 3-D and 4-D biomedical images. Under development are two customized applications, one to facilitate use of ANALYZE specifically for simulation of surgical procedures employed in many aspects of craniofacial and orthopedic surgery planning, and the other for interactive manipulation and display of "beam's eye" views (the views along the path of the treatment beam) of 3-D treatment plans in radiation therapy. Both extended and new user interfaces (based on X windows) with comprehensive databased management capabilities, including a structured query language, are in development. Arguably, the two most important problems inhibiting major progress in biomedical imaging are automated segmentation of features of interest, and accurate fusion of information from multiple modality images. New algorithms for these "differentiation and integration" problems in imaging science are being developed and evaluated. All of these capabilities will combine, in an evolutionary way, to provide increased sensitivity and specificity in quantitative analyses of cells, tissues, organs, and complete biologic systems.

Summary

Major segments of the biologic sciences and the practice of medicine are based on the study and knowledge of the relationships of anatomic structure to biologic function. Traditionally, this knowledge has been gained either indirectly or by inference and, in the final analysis, by direct surgical vivisection or by post mortem examinations. Direct visualization and study of anatomic structure and function of internal organ systems in man have, up to the present, been the preserve of the surgeon and pathologist. The revolutionary capabilities provided by new 3-D and 4-D imaging modalities [30] for obtaining similar information non-invasively, non-destructively, and painlessly can now provide these data to the physician, surgeon, and researcher, for direct reproducible examinations of individual patients or experimental subjects without disturbing the physiology of the organ system under study, or altering its normal integration into the physiology of the body as a whole. The ANALYZE software system facilitates comprehensive exploitation of these capabilities.

References

1 Robb, R.A. A workstation for interactive display and analysis of multi-dimensional biomedical images. In: Lemke, H.U., Rhodes, M.L., Jaffee, C.C. & Felix, R. (eds), *Computer Assisted Radiology. Proceedings of the International Symposium Computer-assisted Radiology 87*, pp. 642−56 (1987).

2 Harris, L.D., Robb, R.A., Yuen, T.S. & Ritman, E.L. Non-invasive numerical dissection and display of anatomic structure using computerized X-ray tomography. *Proceedings of the Society of Photo-optical Instrumentation Engineering* **152**: 10−18 (1978).

3 Harris, L.D., Robb, R.A., Johnson, S.A. & Khalafalla, A.S. Stereo display of computed tomographic data. In: Emlet, H.A. Jr. (ed.), *Challenges and Prospects for Advanced Medical Systems*. Symposia Specialists, Inc., Miami. (1978).

4 Hodges, L.F. & McAllister, D.F. Stereo and alternating-pair techniques for display of computer-generated images. *Institute of Electrical and Electronics Engineers Computer Graphics and Applications* **5**: 38−45 (1985).

5 Hohne, K.H., Riemer, M., Tiede, U. & Bomans, M. Volume rendering of 3-D tomographic imagery. *Proceedings of the Xth Information Processing in Medical Imaging International Conference, Utrecht, The Netherlands*, pp. 403−12 (1987).

6 Herman, G.T. Computer produced stereoscopic display in radiology. *Proceedings National Computer Graphics Association '86*, **3**: 71−79 (1986).

7 Heffernan, P.B. & Robb, R.A. Display and analysis of 4-D medical images. *Proceedings of the International Symposium Computer-assisted Radiology '85*, pp. 583−92 (1985).

8 Drebin, R., Carpenter, L. & Harrahan, P. Volume rendering. *SIGGRAPH '88* pp. 65−74 (1988).

9 Levoy, M. Display of surfaces from volume data. *Computer Graphics and Applications* **8**(3): 29−37 (1988).

10 Robb, R.A. & Barillot, C. Interactive 3-D image display and analysis. In: *Proceedings of the Society of Photo-optical Instrumentation Engineering, Hybrid Image and Signal Processing* **939**: 173−202 (1988).

11 Hohne, K.H. & Bernstein R. Shading 3-D images from CT using grey-level gradients. *Institute of Electrical and Electronics Engineers Trans. Med. Imag.* **MI-15**: 45−7 (1986).

12 Robb, R.A. & Barillot, C. Interactive display and analysis of 3-D medical images. *Institute of Electrical and Electronics Engineers Trans. Med. Imag.* **MI-8**: 217−26 (1989).

13 Pizer, S.M., Oliver, W.R. & Bloomberg, S.H. *Hierarchial Shape Description via the Multi-resolution Symmetric Axis Transform.* Technical Report, Department of Computer Science, University of North Carolina (1986).

14 Pizer, S.M., Gauch, J.M. & Lifshitz, L.M. *Interactive 2-D and 3-D Object Definition in Medical Images Based on Multiresolution Image Descriptions.* University of North Carolina, Technical Report 88−005 (1988).

15 Peleg, S., Naor, J., Hartley, R. & Avnir, D. Multiple resolution texture analysis and classification. *Institute of Electrical and Electronics Engineers Pattern Analysis and Machine Intelligence* **6**(4): 518−32 (1984).

16 Grossberg, S. & Mingolla, E. Neural dynamics of perceptual groupings: textures, boundaries, and emergent segmentation. *Percept. Psychophys.* **38**: 141−71 (1985).

17 Fellingham, L.L., Vogel, J.H., Lau, C., & Dev, P. Interactive graphics and 3-D modeling for surgical planning and prosthesis and implant design. *Proceedings of the National Computer Graphics Association '86,* **3**: 132−42 (1986).

18 Herman, G.T. & Liu, H.K. Display of three-dimensional information in computed tomography. *J. Comput. Assist. Tomogr.* **1**: 155−60 (1977).

19 Heffernan, P.B. & Robb, R.A. A new method for shaded surfaced display of biological and medical images. *Institute of Electrical and Electronics Engineers Trans. Med. Imag.* **4**: 26−38 (1985).

20 Talton, D.A., Goldwasser, S.M., Reynolds, R.A. & Walsh, E.S. Volume rendering algorithms for the presentation of 3-D medical data. *Proceedings of the National Computer Graphics Association '87* **III**: 119−28 (1987).

21 Farrell, E.J., Watson, T.J., Zappulla, R.A. & Spigelman, M. Imaging tools for interpreting two and three dimensional medical data. *Proceedings of the National Computer Graphics Association '87* **III**: 60−68 (1987).

22 Ritman, E.L., Kinsey, J.H., Robb, R.A., Gilbert, B.K., Harris, L.D. & Wood, E.H. Three-dimensional imaging of heart, lungs, and circulation. *Science* **210**: 273−80 (1980).

23 Robb, R.A. High-speed three-dimensional X-ray computed tomography: the Dynamic Spatial Reconstructor. *Proceedings of the Institute of Electrical and Electronics Engineers* **71**: 308−19 (1983).

24 Harris, L.D. Identification of the optimal orientation of oblique sections through multiple parallel CT images. *J. Comput. Assist. Tomogr.* **5**: 881−7 (1981).

25 Harris, L.D., Camp, J.J., Ritman, E.L. & Robb, R.A. Three-dimensional display and analysis of tomographic volume images utilizing a varifocal mirror. *Institute of Electrical and Electronics Engineers Trans. Med. Imag.* **5**: 67−72 (1986).

26 Camp, J.J., Stacy, M.C. & Robb, R.A. A system for interactive volume analysis (SIVA) of 4-D biomedical images. *J. Med. Sys.* **2**: 287−310 (1987).

27 Robb, R.A., Hanson, D.P., Karwoski, R.A., Larson, A.G., Workman, E.L. & Stacy, M.C. ANALYZE: a comprehensive, operator-interactive software package for multidimensional medical image display and analysis. *Comput. Med. Imag. Graph.* **13**: 433−54 (1989).

28 Bentley, M.D. & Karwoski, R.A. Estimation of tissue volume from serial tomographic sections: a statistical random marking method. *Invest. Radiol.* **23**(10): 742−7 (1988).

29 Mandelbrot, B.B. *Fractals: Form, Chance, and Dimension.* San Francisco, CA: Freeman (1977).

30 Robb, R.A. *Three-Dimensional Biomedical Imaging.* Boca Raton, FL: CRC Press, Inc. (1985).

31 Robb, R.A. & Hanson, D.P. ANALYZE: A software system for biomedical image analysis. *Proceedings of the First Conference on Visualization in Biomedical Computing, May 22−25 1990, Atlanta Georgia,* pp. 507−18 (1990).

32 Robb, R.A. A software system for interactive and quantitative analysis of biomedical images. In: Höhne, K.H., Fuchs, H. & Pizer, S.M. (eds) *3-D Imaging in Medicine. NATO ASI series Vol. F* **60**: 333−61.

section

B

Stereotactic Image Manipulation

3

Display and Graphic Manipulation of Neurodiagnostic Images

Joseph H. Goodman

Introduction

Neurosurgical decision-making depends on neurodiagnostic images created to depict both normal and abnormal conditions of the central nervous system. Images frequently used in neurosurgery include plain X-rays, computed axial tomography, magnetic resonance imaging, digital subtraction angiography, and positive contrast, plain film angiography. Images that are useful but not as commonly available include positron emission tomography, single photon emission computed tomography, and electroencephalographically-generated brain maps.

Surgeons relate neurodiagnostic images to their own visual image of the patient, and this information, evaluated through training and familiarity, is adequate for most purposes. Precise dimensioning of image data becomes critical for stereotactic procedures involving functional stereotaxis, as well as instrumentation of subcortical mass lesions and implantation of brachytherapy sources. Performing this type of surgery depends on geometric information contained in imaged data. As the area of interest is not visible, coordinates established in three-dimensional (3-D) space become the basis for planning such procedures. The coordinates become an integral component of a mechanical pointing device for directing surgical instruments into the cranial compartment. Localizing deep structures requires a method of transferring geometric data to stereotactic equipment with confidence that the coordinates being used accurately reflect the individual patient's anatomy.

Stereotactic coordinate system conversion

To use imaged data for stereotactic surgery, one must convert information contained in the image into a workable coordinate system, which is determined by the type of stereotactic apparatus being used. Several coordinate systems have been applied to stereotactic procedures, and all are capable of establishing accurate spatial geometry [1]. The use of 3-D coordinates is convenient in conjunction with orthogonal stereotactic radiographs. This particular approach involves identifying the x, y, and z position of any point within the image and correlating that point with its position in stereotactic space. The reason for choosing such a coordinate system rests with the principle that *given any three values x_1, y_1, and z_1 of the variables x, y, and z, a corresponding point in space P_1 is uniquely determined with respect to a 3-D system of rectangular coordinates.*

Establishing spatial geometry with 3-D rectangular coordinates allows multiple data sets to be integrated in a uniform fashion. These principles apply to geometric shapes such as those found with neurodiagnostic images and are the basis for using computer-generated graphics as a method of correlating the various types of images available. Image-to-graphic conversion is a convenient method of comparison of pictorial data from multiple sources. Creating points, lines, and contours to identify areas of interest makes possible the depiction of whatever information one chooses in a format that can be transformed into a compatible coordinate set. The diversity of images currently available, and the variety of ways in which they are generated, make it unlikely that commonly-used images will be displayed in the same format in the foreseeable future. Computer-generated graphics offer an interim solution to a few of the problems facing those interested in using multimodality image display for stereotactic surgical procedures.

Fundamentals of geometric handling in 3-D space

Linear transformations of graphic information in 3-D space are carried out using several basic operations: translation, rotation, scaling, and perspective view or projection [2]. Translation, rotation, and scaling are the basis for establishing concordance among drawing files created from multiple image sources. A sequence of transformations designed to match each drawing's identical position, orientation, and size in space can then, through output devices, provide a composite drawing for working purposes. The problem then is to select mutually-identifiable coordinate sets of the separate images to be subjected to routines needed to achieve the desired result. Certain anatomic landmarks such as the pituitary gland, frontal sinuses, bony protuberances of the skull, pineal gland, orbital contents, and the facial bones, are frequently identifiable in various images, and selected landmarks can be used to carry out the transformation sequences.

Sources of error

The possibility of error exists in any attempt to carry out quantitative measurements. Errors can be broadly classified as: (1) blunders; (2) constant errors; (3) systematic errors; and (4) random errors [3].

Blunders are caused by carelessness and are unpredictable. They can be of any magnitude and occur in any direction.

Constant errors occur as a result of discrepancies in calibration of measuring tools, and are usually small enough to be considered insignificant with the instruments used in stereotactic surgery. Constant errors within a computer system can be detected by direct measurement of output data from a calibrated phantom image; they require correction at the source, which is usually faulty programming or hardware malfunction.

Systematic errors occur according to some pattern and are usually known, although there may be unknown sources of this type of error. For example, the film magnification in X-rays taken at a distance less than infinity is a systematic error; film magnification artifact can be corrected by calculating image enlargement factors from known source, subject, and film distances. Another error of this type, commonly seen in magnetic resonance image film formatting, is a variance in the $x-y$ aspect ratio; this is correctable mathematically. In magnetic resonance imaging, systematic errors resulting from non-linearity of the magnetic field and eddy currents require analysis based on phantom imaging to calculate distance corrections and minimize such errors [4].

Random errors result from the inability of individuals to make exact measurements, are generally small, and relate to the care with which the measurements are done. Additional sources of error such as pixel resolution, scan slice thickness, movement during the scanning process, gantry tilt, and image interpretation can be categorized and must be considered in deciding how confident one is of being able to actually place a probe at a desired target site. The potential for error is proportional to a system's complexity and the number of steps taken in translating information to establish a target point.

Recognizing that multiple sources of error are inherent in attempting to establish precise measurements from neurodiagnostic images, one must set limits for the level of precision that may be expected. A rigorous analytic approach to this problem can be taken, using statistical evaluation of direct measurements and mathematic determination of variance and probabilities of error from each potential source of error [3]. Theoretically, those potential sources of error can be minimized so that small targets can be approached with a high degree of confidence. A practical method of establishing confidence limits with a particular system used for 3-D measurements from imaged data is to carry out a series of practice procedures using calibrated phantom targets. This not only increases one's familiarity with the components of any given system, but also realistically appraises that system's accuracy as it is used in an operative setting.

Microcomputer image display

Microcomputers can display medical images with adequate resolution and contrast so that, for practical purposes, the pictures produced are indistinguishable from those seen on dedicated scanner consoles. This capability is well established, as demonstrated by PC-based displays currently being coupled to stereotactic head frames. Image display can be accomplished by the addition of peripherals specifically designed for image processing. Both computed tomography (CT) and magnetic resonance (MR) data can be downloaded for processing with a microcomputer. Another method of image manipulation involves the use of a frame grabber to capture images with a video camera. Both methods have advantages and shortcomings, and both have some utility for image-to-graphic conversion.

Transferring scan data directly to a microcomputer by magnetic tape has the advantage of avoiding degradation of the image and the slight distortions that are inherent in the film formatting process and in optical systems used for video capture. Perhaps the greatest disadvantage in attempting to work with images in their original format is the difficulty of deciphering industrial data formats and making them compatible with the microcomputer environment. There is an understandable reluctance on the part of scan vendors to release programming source codes and, although it is possible to overcome this, there are proprietary rights which must be respected. When depending solely on original data for image analysis, one must anticipate changes in data formats and be prepared to make modifications as needed to keep a personal system working.

Once displayed, a suitable image must be converted to graphic form. One method is to use a mapping algorithm based on grayscale differences on the display [5]. Selecting the appropriate level on the contrast scale allows the creation of a polyline corresponding to the shape to be incorporated into a drawing file. Points and lines can likewise be identified in the image for transfer to the drawing file. An example of such a contour map is shown in Fig. 3.1. Transferring several contour maps that represent outlines of significant structures allows the creation of a graphic reconstruction of the image, with identifiable points and contours that can be manipulated, using

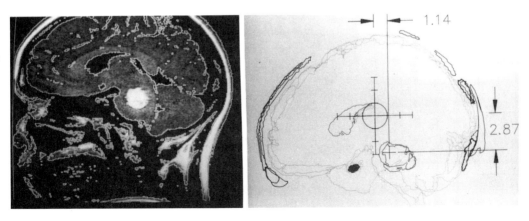

FIGURE 3.1 Image-to-graphic conversion of data points in a medical image can be accomplished by automatic or manual creation of polylines based on the pixel grayscale. Measurements to carry out headframe adjustments can then be obtained from information contained in the graphic overlay.

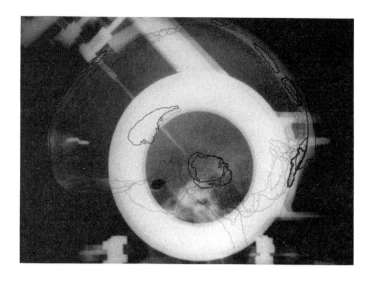

FIGURE 3.2 A target point
established from a graphic
overlay onto an operative
stereotactic radiograph is shown
from a patient undergoing
aspiration of a liquefied pontine
hematoma.

transformations included as subroutines in computer-aided design (CAD) software.

The most obvious application of this type of drawing involves correlation of the graphic image, which can be made to include a target for stereotactic probe placement, with orthogonal stereotactic radiographs. A composite contour map of the lesion, along with contours of the cranial vault as extracted from sagittal MR images of a patient with a pontine hematoma, is shown in Fig. 3.2. For illustrative purposes, the reference position of the fixed phantom of a Todd–Wells headframe (Todd–Wells Inc., South Gate, CA) is shown. Anterior–posterior and superior–inferior headframe adjustments needed to align the target with the phantom can be made to establish x and z target coordinates to correlate with a lateral stereotactic radiograph (Fig. 3.2). The y coordinate is established using graphic reconstructions of either coronal or axial scan slices, with appropriate transformations so that the drawings coincide with the operative X-ray in the anterior–posterior projection.

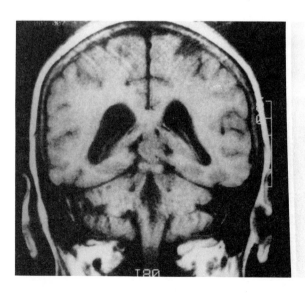
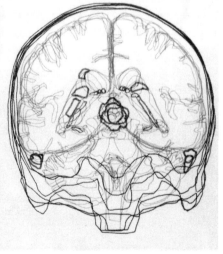

FIGURE 3.3 Graphic contours created from hard copy scan slices provide adequate information to establish geometric relationships of cranial structures. This coronal view of a pineal neoplasm was manually loaded into a drawing file using a transparent digitizing pad.

Automatically generated contours depend on gray levels of picture elements. In certain situations where contiguous structures overlap on the grayscale, cleanly outlining an area for transfer to a drawing file can be difficult. In such circumstances, the user can transfer an interpretation of the image to the file by manually digitizing the input. Manually digitizing an on-screen display or hard copy data with a digitizing pad increases the potential for random error in creation of a drawing file; nevertheless, it is an effective method of creating useful drawing files. A scaled drawing of a pineal tumor, digitized from coronal MR images, is shown in Fig. 3.3. This can be compared with automatically generated drawings of a parietal lesion taken from axial MR slices, as shown in Fig. 3.4. Both methods result in acceptable definition of important structures, and both are suitable for measuring in order to determine useful coordinates.

A 3-D drawing file, created from selected axial slices of the lesion shown in Fig. 3.4, illustrates how rotational transformations may be used to manipulate graphic outlines in 3-D space. Changing the point of view reorients the drawing file to coincide with any defined axis (Fig. 3.5). By superimposing drawing files from different image sets, it is possible to compare geometrically aligned, 3-D drawings; for example, in Fig. 3.6, coronal and axial MR scan slices are compared. This type of drawing can then serve as an overlay for use with stereotactic radiographs to establish target coordinates.

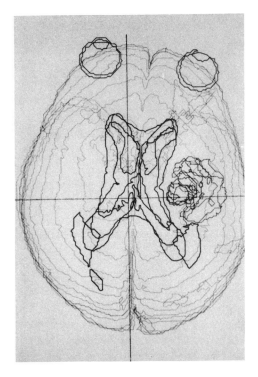

FIGURE 3.4 An automatically generated drawing file of this parietal tumor can be used for 3-D graphic manipulations. Each entity can be seen to represent a certain structure, and the contours are assigned elevations relative to the slice distance from the 0 points of x, y, and z axes.

The use of scaling and rotation allows comparison of image data from various sources. For example, one might incorporate angiographic data into a lateral stereotactic radiograph by using contours extracted from sagittal MR

FIGURE 3.5 Rotational transformation to depict a superior frontal point of view is shown to demonstrate how drawings can be spatially oriented in any desired direction relative to the drawing's central point. Extrusion and hidden line removal subroutines aid in conceptualizing 3-D relationships.

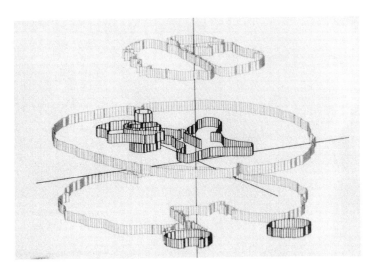

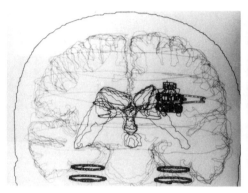
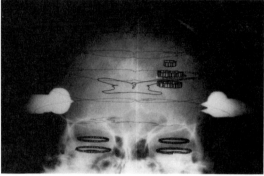

FIGURE 3.6 Composite files, such as this graphic representation of coronal and sagittal MR scan slices, can be displayed through establishing concordance of linear and rotational relationships of drawings created to identical scale. Overlays made from coronal views provide lateral dimensions for determining offset measurements needed for target point selection.

images outlining the skull, scalp, frontal sinus, orbital contents, and the pituitary gland, to create a drawing file. Measurements obtained from the angiographic plain film then allow scaling of the drawing file, so that it can be plotted on clear acetate for an overlay on the X-ray film. The combined drawing file and plain film, with a proposed target site, then can be used to digitize significant vascular structures to the drawing file (Fig. 3.7). The drawing file that now contains anatomic data from the MR scan, a possible target site, and angiographic information can be rescaled for correlation with an operative stereotactic radiograph, as described previously. This example demonstrates how

components of a microcomputer-based imaging and graphics system can be used to create and compile image and graphic information from multiple sources to establish target coordinates in stereotactic space.

Discussion

Information found in neurodiagnostic imaging modalities has been correlated for use with stereotactic surgical frames through a variety of techniques intended for practical applications [6,7]. The problems associated with achieving acceptably accurate data transformations are not unique to neurosurgical procedures.

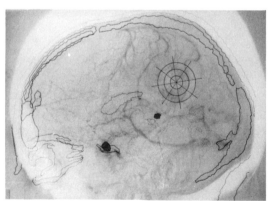
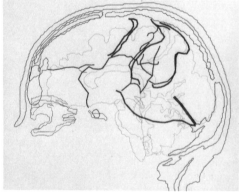

FIGURE 3.7 Arteriographic information can be incorporated into drawing files through the digitizing process. A sagittal cranial contour, generated from an MR image with a proposed target site, is shown scaled to fit a standard lateral subtraction venous phase angiogram. Significant vascular structures can then be added to the drawing for correlation with a stereotactic radiograph as shown in Fig. 3.1.

Methods of transferring tumor-localizing information from CT scans and MR images are routinely used by radiation oncologists for simulation and verification films when planning radiation therapy [8]. A radiotherapy planning technique, using radiopaque markers attached to the patient as reference points identifiable on both CT scans and simulation films, enables treatment-planning computers to calculate isodose fields to match tumor geometry. Graphic outlines of tumor margins on CT scans are manually entered into a system designed to produce transparent overlays showing the position of the markers as well as the tumor boundaries; these overlays are used to correlate information from scans and simulation films, and can be graphically manipulated for any combination of gantry angle and source-to-film distance. Scaling the overlays and correlating the reference points reproduces the tumor outline on the simulation and verification films with a high level of precision, even with the use of oblique views [9]. Projective geometry, as described here, is a powerful tool for interpretation of spatial relationships using radiographs. The precise localization of intracranial targets achieved with this methodology has clinical utility for stereotactic surgery.

Use of angiographic information in the planning of operations is intended to decrease morbidity by lessening the chances of inadvertent damage to major arterial and venous structures. Using stereotactically placed radiopaque markers to identify vascular structures during stereoscopic angiography aids in operative planning [10] and has applications for radiosurgical treatment planning [11]. Mathematic systems using projective geometry and externally placed markers to define spatial relationships avoid the constraints that X-rays be orthogonal to, or precisely aligned with, the localizing markers. Also, source-to-image and source-to-target distances need not be known. This methodology allows the incorporation of standard biplane angiography into stereotactic systems.

Microcomputer manipulation of image and graphic data can be used to combine neurodiagnostic images from multiple sources. In stereotactic surgery, this type of multimodality image management is used to identify target coordinates, establish trajectories, and place radioactive sources for brachytherapy. The diversity of images currently in use and the dynamic nature of medical imaging justify such a system. Computer-aided design software can produce graphics with acceptable accuracy to serve as a tool for precise spatial localization of intracranial structures. The capability of interactive graphic display systems to identify and transfer 3-D coordinates inherent in medical images makes them valuable tools for establishing concordance among the various types of data used for surgical decision-making. The task is complicated to some extent by the number of steps required to incorporate the necessary data collected for a given procedure, and by the potential for error that is unavoidable in any quantitative measurement scheme.

To rely on computer-generated graphics for surgical purposes requires an understanding of the limitations of any system of this type, and confidence that the data used is accurate within the limits of the system. Perhaps the best estimate of accuracy can be achieved by designing and testing an operative plan with phantom targets of known dimensions. Minimizing errors through statistical testing of known sources of error is also of value. The decision to use this approach is best made based on one's familiarity with computers, and on the feasibility of committing the necessary time and resources to establish and maintain such a system.

References

1 Friedman, W.A. & Coffey, R.J. Stereotactic surgical instrumentation. In: Heilbrun, M.P. (ed.) *Stereotactic Neurosurgery, Volume 2: Concepts in Neurosurgery*. Baltimore: Williams & Wilkins (1988).

2 Encarnação, J. & Schlechtendahl, E.G. Engineering methods of CAD. In: Encarnacão, J. & Hayes, P. (eds) *Computer-aided Design: Fundamentals and System Architectures*, pp. 219−91. Berlin: Springer-Verlag (1983).

3 Wong, K.W. Basic mathematics of photogrammetry. In: Slama, C.C., Theurer, C. & Henriksen, S.W. (eds) *Manual of Photogrammetry*, 4th edn. Falls Church, VA: American Society of Photogrammetry (1980).

4 Schad, L., Lott, L., Schmitt, F., Sturm, V. & Lorenz, W.J. Correction of spatial distortion in MR imaging: a prerequisite for accurate stereo-

taxy. *J. Comput. Assist. Tomogr.* **11**(3): 499−505 (1987).

5 Brown, R.A. A computerized tomography−computer graphics approach to stereotaxic localization. *J. Neurosurg.* **50**: 715−20 (1979).

6 Gildenberg, P.L., Kaufman, H.H. & Krishna Murphy, K.S. Calculation of stereotactic coordinates from the computed tomographic scan. *Neurosurgery* **10**(5): 580−86 (1982).

7 Sapozink, M.D., Moeller, J.M., McDonald, P.N. & Heilbrun, M.P. Improved precision of interstitial brain tumor irradiation using the BRW CT stereotactic guidance system. *Int. J. Radiat. Oncol. Biol. Phys.* **13**: 1753−60 (1987).

8 Flickinger, J.C. & Deutsch, M. Manual reconstruction of tumor volumes from CT scans for radiotherapy planning. *Radiother. Oncol.* **14**: 151−8 (1989).

9 Haynor, D.R., Borning, A.W., Griffin, B.A., Jacky, J.P. Kalet, I.J. & Shuman, W.P. Radiotherapy planning: direct tumor localization on simulation and port films using CT. *Radiology* **158**: 537−40 (1986).

10 Kelly, P.J., Alker, G.J. Jr, Kall, B.A. & Goerss, S. Method of computed tomography-based stereotactic biopsy with arteriographic control. *Neurosurgery* **14**(2): 172−7 (1984).

11 Siddon, R.L. & Barth, N.H. Stereotaxic localization of intracranial targets. *Int. J. Radiat. Oncol. Biol. Phys.* **13**: 1241−6 (1987).

4

The Evolution and Integration of Microcomputers Used with the Brown–Roberts–Wells (BRW) Image-guided Stereotactic System

M. Peter Heilbrun

Introduction

The development of the computed tomography (CT) scanner depended upon computer techniques that could expand the X-ray density scale and define gradients not normally detected by the human eye. Similarly, the Brown–Roberts–Wells (BRW) image-guided stereotactic system could not have been developed without computers that could rapidly translate a two-dimensional (2-D) position on a scan image into a three-dimensional (3-D) position in space.

The conception, development, manufacturing, and evolution of the BRW system has depended upon and mirrored the evolution of affordable microcomputers in the 1970s and 1980s. This chapter will describe the various computer interfaces to the BRW stereotactic device that evolved from 1978 to 1990 — from basic practical and functional alphanumeric devices to more sophisticated and affordable graphics environments, including a multipurpose personal computer (PC)-based operating room workstation.

Background — development of the BRW stereotactic system

In 1978, Russell A. Brown, a medical student at the University of Utah, began working under the supervision of Theodore S. Roberts, Chairman of the Division of Neurosurgery, to design a stereotactic system that would transform 2-D CT scan image points to 3-D positions in space. As an employee at Evans and Sutherland Computer Company, Brown was able to use powerful, state-of-the-art computers for his initial design experiments.

Utilizing his background in computer science and mathematics to take a fresh look at the problem, Brown applied computer-aided design and computer-aided manufacturing (CAD CAM) technology to design a reference ring with a picket fence fiducial system that could be fixed to a patient's head [1,2,3]. This method of localizing intracranial structures solved the problems of vertical coordinate inaccuracy that had been encountered when stereotactic reference systems were attached to the CT scanner table or gantry. Next, building on a project to simulate the arm motions of the space shuttle, which he had participated in as an undergraduate, Brown developed a double arc system for guiding a trajectory in stereotactic space (Figs 4.1, 4.2, and 4.3).

During the development period, Roberts called on Mr Trent Wells' engineering expertise to create a stereotactic surgical instrument from the prototype. Wells directly translated the picket-fence design into a basic headframe, which could be fixed to the skull with pins to serve both as a reference for stereotactic space and as a platform to hold localization and

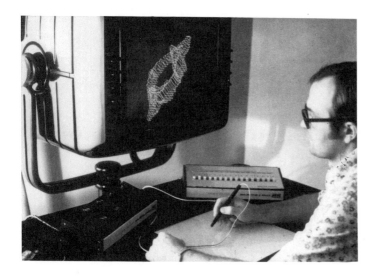

FIGURE 4.1 Vintage 1970s' Evans and Sutherland (E & S) computer graphics terminal used for design of BRW stereotactic system.

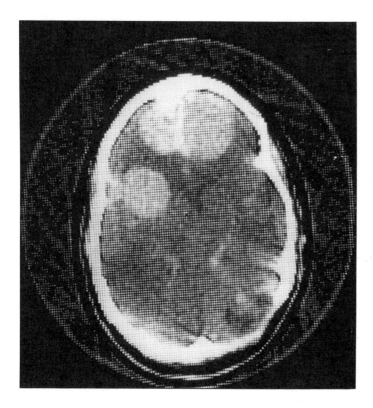

FIGURE 4.2 E & S graphics display of several superimposed CT images of a patient with multiple meningiomas.

guidance devices. Moreover, Wells improved on Brown's cumbersome double arcs by placing a single 200° vertical arc which rotated a full 360° on a horizontal arc. Wells' single vertical arc was attached to the horizontal arc by a fulcrum which permitted a 360° rotation around the horizontal arc, as well as a 40° pivot on its fulcrum. This combination of rotation and pivot created an infinite number of vertical planes within stereotactic space. Wells then attached a slide that could hold any stereotactic probe to the vertical arc. The slide also had two movements, a 200° rotation and an 110° pivot. By moving the slide along the vertical arc and pivoting it on a fulcrum at its position of attachment on the vertical arc, one could define the

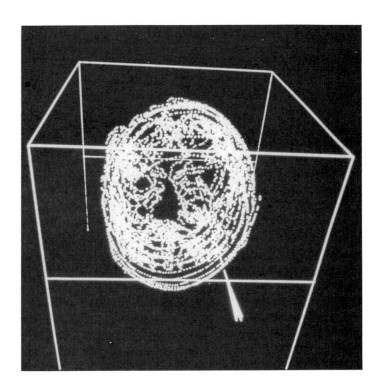

FIGURE 4.3 E & S graphics display outlines from CT images in Fig. 4.2, surrounded by a Cartesian coordinates box and a simulated probe track. Simulation capable of rotation, translation, and perspective. This displays the actual data set used by Brown to develop the BRW system.

plane of the vertical arc, which theoretically contained two points in stereotactic space, a position on the scalp or skull representing an entry point, and a position within the brain representing a stereotactic target. From a reference position of the slide, a distance from the arc to a target could be calculated [4]. In 1979, Wells delivered a working prototype to Roberts at the University of Utah. The system was first used for stereotactic biopsy in December 1979.

Computerized calculations

The calculations for the first cases were performed on the computer console of the University of Utah Varian CT scanner. The computations involved two sets of algorithms. The first algorithm set, eventually labeled the "target menu," transformed the 2-D CT scan coordinate to a 3-D coordinate within stereotactic space. The second algorithm set, labeled the "approach menu," calculated the four angular rotation and pivot settings of the guidance arc, and a distance to the target. Although the precise formulae have evolved, all variations of BRW computations have been based on algorithms

for the target and approach menu. In April 1980, Hewlett–Packard introduced the relatively inexpensive hand-held HP 41CV calculator which could support sophisticated programs. At that time, the transforming computations were transferred from the CT scanner computer [5]. However, the original mathematic program, based on matrix algebra, required too much time on the smaller calculator, so a new, faster mathematic solution based on vectors was developed [4].

Also, in 1980, a phantom simulator, which allowed the surgeon to move a pointer to any calculated position within stereotactic space, was developed to verify that the target and approach results were calculated correctly. By setting the calculated guidance angles and distances on an arc, the surgeon could simulate the operative procedure. The phantom simulator provided an important check that the target and frame values were calculated correctly by the computer and became an integral component of the system.

The HP 41CV calculator provided the means of computation until 1984, when increased computer power was available on a small laptop microcomputer, a specially configured Epson HX (Fig. 4.4). All subsequent BRW systems have used laptop microcomputer systems for computation. Recently the more powerful SCSI laptop microcomputer has replaced the Epsons.

In 1982, Heilbrun and Roberts began to look for a means of integrating computer graphics into the BRW stereotactic environment. Their plan was to expand the system, so that scan images could be displayed directly on a computer screen from standard scanner data storage formats. Such an integration would permit the fiducial marks and targets to be identified by moving a cursor around the computer screen, without using the HP 41CV or the laptop computer, which required manual entry of scan coordinates into the calculator.

A computer imaging laboratory was established within the Division of Neurosurgery, and permission was obtained to read Siemens' floppy disc CT scan data into the University of Utah computer. Since then the laboratory has expanded, with the goal of developing affordable systems that can be used in the operating room environment, and that contain a selection of functions that enhance the surgeon's capabilities in the operating room [6,7]. In 1989, Stereotactic Image Systems, Inc. was licensed through the Technology Transfer Office of the University of Utah to produce PC-based stereotactic computer systems.

During this time, Kelly was working independently to develop the concept of volumetric stereotactic surgery. He noted that modern stereotactic surgery was involved in identification of tumor volumes rather than point targets, and suggested that stereotactic surgeons should be conceptualizing not points, but volumes in space. Secondly, he developed the concept that images should be reformatted so that, in addition to standard orthogonal views, there should be a computer-generated surgeon's view, often termed the "probe view" or, by radiotherapists, the "beam's eye view" [8,9, 10,11].

The remainder of this chapter describes the computer graphics developed to date for the BRW system, and addresses some of the graphic compatibilities that will be available in the future as computers become faster and cheaper.

University of Utah computer basic graphics workstation for stereotactic surgical planning

Image-guided stereotactic surgery requires the transformation of 2-D data points from radiographic data, such as CT scans, magnetic resonance imaging (MRI) scans, angiograms, and skull radiographs. With the BRW stereotactic system, the computations are routinely performed on a laptop microcomputer and displayed as a numerical printout. All references to the image mode, whether it be CT, MRI, or angiography, are made numerically.

Obviously, the display of the numerical data can be better conceptualized by the operating surgeon if the data is displayed in a graphic mode. The PC-based computer graphics workstation developed at the University of Utah has multiple data input, manipulation, and output functions based on the standard BRW "target" and "approach" menus. Image data is entered into the computer in a digital form through a

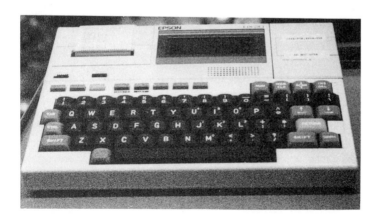

FIGURE 4.4 Laptop microcomputer with built-in printer used by the BRW system from 1985 to 1989 for computation of target and trajectory data.

standard nine inch magnetic tape storage device (Fig. 4.5). All of the images in a study can be displayed on the computer. These images can be reviewed serially to identify potential target points, and fiduciary rod positions required for the transformation of 2-D data points to 3-D stereotactic positions can be marked rapidly. Once the fiduciary rods are marked on any image, they are automatically identified and labeled on all subsequently displayed images of the study, and the conversion to stereotactic coordinates is automatically performed for all positions on all slices. When a target and entry point are chosen and marked by the surgeon, a probe track is defined graphically, so that its position can be seen on any image it intersects.

The ability to view the probe path as it passes through multiple areas of the brain is an important enhancement. This capacity allows the surgeon to change targets and positions of probe entry points on the scalp or the surface of the brain, and to recalculate probe trajectories. The new probe paths can be reviewed and accepted or rejected, depending on the surgeon's visual analysis of the position of the probe path to critical brain structures. Thus, probe paths can be readjusted in real-time until the most appropriate trajectory is visualized and accepted. The reduced morbidity from precision stereotactic approaches to biopsy intracranial lesions is well recognized. Graphic display of the data and pass-through points, coupled with the capacity of immediate recalculation of probe direction and distance, and graphic review of these data, has the potential of further increasing the safety of stereotactic surgery (Fig. 4.6).

Traditionally, radiographic image data has been viewed from accepted standard orthogonal planes, such as anterior−posterior and lateral orthogonal views. To better visualize bony structures at the base of the skull, such as foramina or petrous bone structures, other views were designed. With the advent of CT scanning, axial views which are relatively orthogonal to a vertical plane though the head and body became the accepted view. To obtain CT images comparable to accepted anterior−posterior (A/P) and lateral orthogonal views required 2-D reformatting. Such reformatted views are generally of poorer resolution than axial CT images. The capacity to view intracranial structures in multiple high-resolution orthogonal views, including axial, A/P (coronal), and lateral (sagittal), became readily available with the

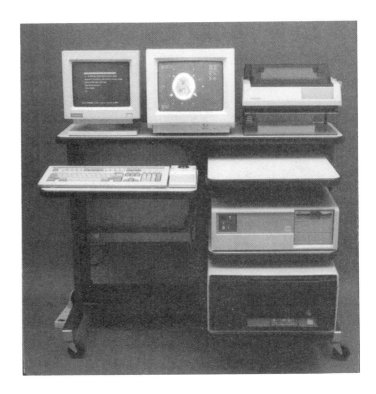

FIGURE 4.5 PC-based operating room workstation developed at the University of Utah for the graphics display of CT, MRI, and angiographic images used in stereotactic surgery.

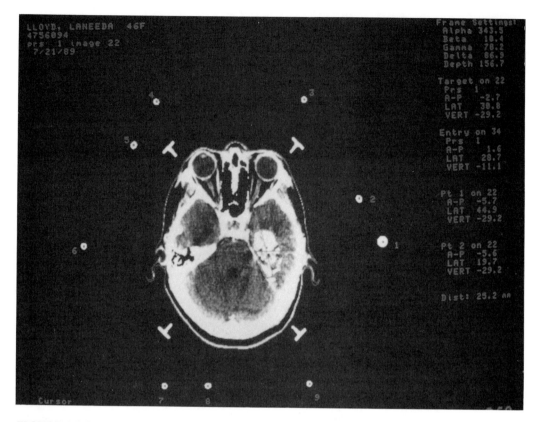

FIGURE 4.6 Computer screen of CT scan with right temporal lobe lesion, demonstrating multiple functions of the graphics computer, including display of: (1) position of cursor in scan coordinates and stereotactic coordinates; (2) alphanumeric listing of target and entry values, frame settings and distances, and lesion parameters such as anterior—posterior distances; (3) autocontouring of the scalp; and (4) manual outlining of the lesion with the cursor.

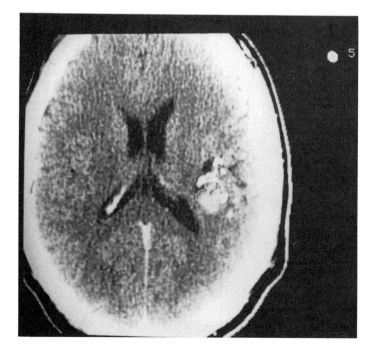

FIGURE 4.7 Enlarged view of CT scan image showing multiple manually traced outlines.

introduction of MRI scanning. Accordingly, stereotactic localization techniques for MR images in all planes are integrated into the workstation [12].

A surgeon utilizes images of brain structures from many different perspectives, and intuitively translates those images into his planned operative approach to lesions within the brain. Designing operative approaches with precision stereotactic techniques creates the possibility of using computer graphic reformatting techniques to create a surgeon's view of brain structures, along, as well as orthogonal to, the probe track. Software written by the University of Utah group has advanced Kelly's concept of visualizing brain structures along the surgeon's view. This probe track view has been adapted for computer packages for the neurosurgeon to

use for stereotactic open craniotomy, and for interstitial brachytherapy [13,14].

The outlining capacity of computer graphics allows the surgeon to identify specific structures in the brain (Fig. 4.7). Outlines of structures from multiple images from the same type of study, as well as outlines from multiple slices in different types of studies, such as CT, MRI, and angiograms, can be registered and displayed in a wireframe graphic format. This cross-registering (superimposing) of data from multiple image formats is possible because all 2-D data points derived from BRW localization techniques are transformed into a single 3-D stereotactic space, referenced to the BRW head ring fixed to the patients skull. Thus, the graphics can be a mix of actual images with outlines superimposed (Fig. 4.8). These wireframe out-

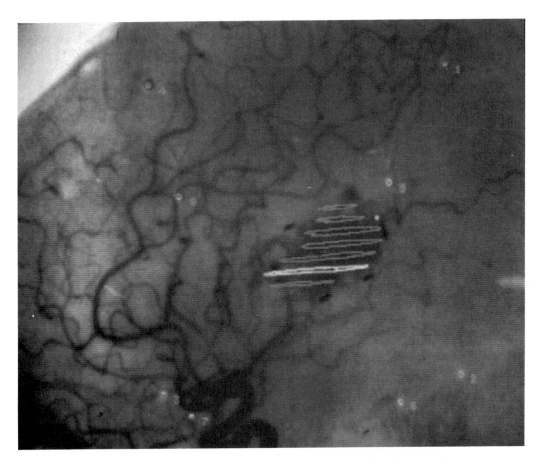

FIGURE 4.8 Stereotactic angiogram with superimposed outlines of CT borders of an arteriovenous malformation (AVM) superimposed. This cross-correlation of CT and angiographic lesions in stereotactic space is important for radiosurgical treatment planning.

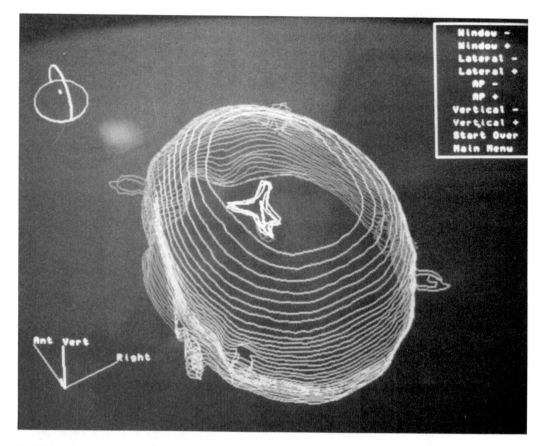

Window -
Window +
Lateral -
Lateral +
AP -
AP +
Vertical -
Vertical +
Start Over
Main Menu

Ant Vert
Right

FIGURE 4.9 Traced outlines displayed on computer monitor, and rotated and translated into a position simulating one of multiple views, from which the operating neurosurgeon can gain a graphic perspective of the position of an intracranial lesion to external landmarks, such as the scalp, and internal landmarks, such as the ventricles.

lines can be viewed in computer 3-D space, and may be rotated and translated to vary perspectives (Figs 4.9 and 4.10).

The usefulness of all of these methods in the operating suite, with computer graphics developed on relatively affordable PC-type computer systems, has been tested. The following are examples of the type of computer graphic enhancement that the surgeon finds useful in daily operative stereotactic surgery on the brain:

1 An axial CT image containing an intracranial target with:

(a) automatic marking of rod fiduciary points from which the stereotactic target position is calculated;

(b) labeling of the coordinates of the entry point on the surface of the scalp, skull, or brain;

(c) labeling of the frame settings and the

probe depth to the target from the chosen entry point;

(d) automatic outlining of the scalp or skull surface;

(e) manual outlining of intracranial structures; and

(f) measurements of distances and areas (see Fig. 4.6).

2 View of A/P and lateral angiogram, combined and registered in stereotactic space with the CT-defined outlines of a tumor registered on both angiogram views (see Fig. 4.8).

3 Wireframe view of outlined structures showing scalp outlines, tumor outlines, ventricular outlines, and the probe track (see Fig. 4.9).

4 Wireframe display in which the surgeon has eliminated the scalp outlines while retaining the outlines of the ventricles, tumor, and probe

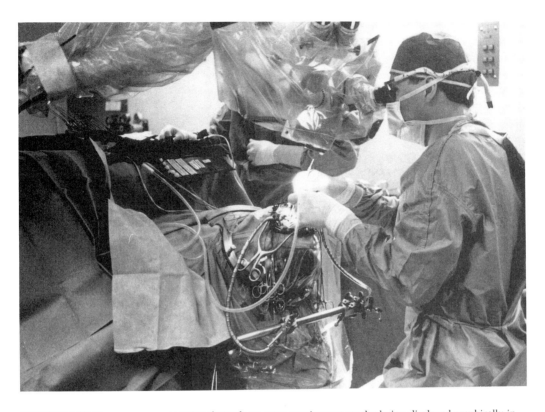

FIGURE 4.10 Neurosurgeon operating through an open craniotomy on the lesion displayed graphically in Fig. 4.9. The BRW system is in place, coupled with standard microsurgical techniques.

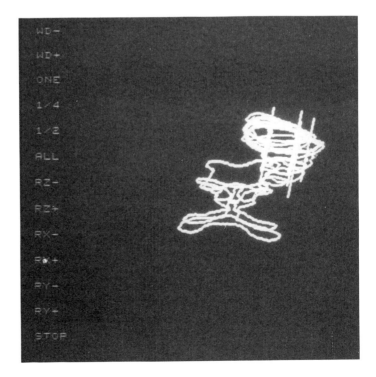

FIGURE 4.11 Graphic display of a tumor wrapped around the frontal horn, with stereotactically placed parallel catheters displaying the ^{125}I seed positions.

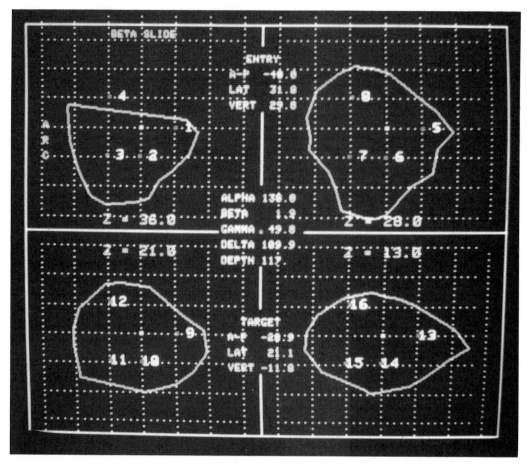

FIGURE 4.12 Two-dimensional reformatting of tumor borders at selected distances orthogonal to a stereotactic trajectory overlaid with a 10-mm spaced grid. This graphic tool is used for simulation and display of brachytherapy dosimetry. This view shows placement of seeds for radiation.

tracks, i.e. those referencing structures which will be used once the skull is opened (Fig. 4.11).

5 Orthogonal view of reconfigured tumor border perpendicular to a probe track. This displays multiple views on a single screen at chosen distances along the probe track (Fig. 4.12).

6 Image showing isodose distribution of stereotactically implanted ^{125}I seeds for interstitial brachytherapy of a malignant brain tumor (Fig. 4.13).

University of Utah advanced computer graphics workstation for stereotactic surgical planning

Future affordable graphic computer workstations will further integrate image processing and computer graphics. This capacity will provide more sophisticated analysis of images by fixing stereotactic reference of intracranial structures to external landmarks. These functions will be performed with advanced computer graphic techniques, such as combined surface and volume rendering. With surface rendering, a standard CT or MRI data set can be rapidly reformatted to a solid image of the surface of the scalp and the face, or of the surface of the skull, or the cerebral cortex. The technique of volume rendering can be used to reformat 2-D images to serially scroll through multiple planes from various perspectives, including the stereotactic probe tract. Combining surface and volume rendering allows reference of an intracranial structure, such as a tumor, to

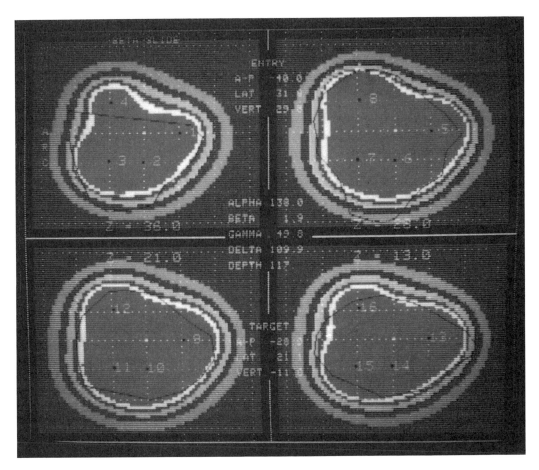

FIGURE 4.13 Dosimetry overlaid on tumor borders to simulate adequacy of seed positioning. System has ability to adjust position of seeds until best isodose contours are obtained.

external landmarks, such as the nose. With 3-D digitizing techniques, image positions can be translated into a stereotactic coordinate system without requiring preoperative fixation of a stereotactic reference device [6].

Such sophisticated computer graphics, which involve automatic surface and volume rendering of the brain in real-time, are accomplished on a Sun 3/160 graphics workstation with a TAAC graphics accelerator board. When fully developed, this system will allow instant reformatting of direct brain images along the surgeon's view path, without requiring manual outlining. Figure 4.14 demonstrates computer reformatting of a standard MRI study of the brain. Its surface rendering of the head provides detailed scalp and facial features. Figure 4.15 demonstrates computer reformatting of a standard MRI study, showing volume rendering

of reformatted 2-D images simultaneously in coronal, sagittal, and axial planes defined by the operator. This capability allows a surgeon to scroll up and down a probe track, visualizing actual brain structures continuously along the track. In addition, an operator can reference other structures in standard orthogonal views.

Conclusions

Modern stereotactic surgery is benefiting from the development of increasingly affordable advanced computer systems. All neurosurgeons should be aware that precision stereotactic localization is becoming a neurosurgical standard. In the future, most intracranial surgery will be enhanced by adjunct computer graphics for both operative simulation and actual operative procedures.

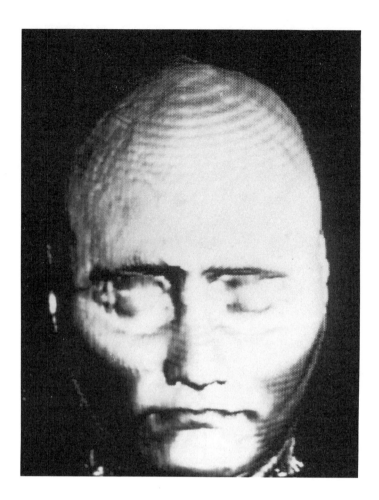

FIGURE 4.14 Surface rendering of an MRI data-set, extracting external features of the head.

References

1 Brown, R. A computed tomography–computer graphics approach to stereotaxic localization. *J. Neurosurg.* **50**: 715–20 (1979).

2 Brown, R. A stereotactic head frame for use with CT body scanners. *Invest. Radiol.* **14**: 300–4 (1979).

3 Brown, R., Roberts, T. & Osborn, A. Stereotaxic frame and computer software for CT-directed neurosurgical localization. *Invest. Radiol.* **15**: 308–12 (1980).

4 Wells, T. Jr, Cosman, E. & Ball, R. The Brown–Roberts–Wells (BRW) arc: its concept as a spatial navigation system. *Appl. Neurophysiol.* **50**: 127–32 (1987).

5 Heilbrun, M., Roberts, T., Wells, T., Ball, R. & Cosman, E. *Technical Manual: Brown–Roberts–Wells (BRW) CT Stereotaxic Guidance System.* Burlington, MA. Radionics Inc. (1982).

6 Heilbrun, M. The utilization and impact of computers on neurosurgical practice. In: Apuzzo, M.J. (ed.) *Future of Neurosurgery,* Hanley & Belfus (in press).

7 Heilbrun, M., Brown, R. & McDonald, P. Real time three-dimensional graphic reconstructions using Brown–Roberts–Wells frame coordinates in a microcomputer environment. *Appl. Neurophysiol.* **48**: 7–10 (1985).

8 Kelly, P. Stereotactic technology in tumor surgery. *Clin. Neurosurg.* **35**: 215–53 (1987).

9 Kelly, P. Volumetric stereotactic resection of intraaxial brain mass lesions. *Mayo Clin. Proc.* **63**: 1186–98 (1988).

10 Kelly, P., Kall, B. & Goerss, S. Transposition of volumetric information derived from computed tomography scanning into stereotactic space. *Surg. Neurol.* **21**: 465–71 (1984).

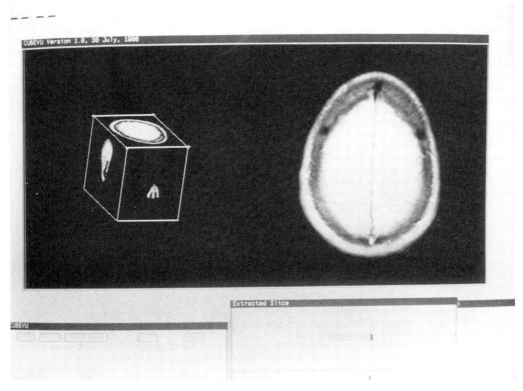

FIGURE 4.15 Advanced volume rendering of an MRI data-set with capability of viewing images from multiple perspectives within a stereotactic (Cartesian) space.

11 Kelly, P., Kall, B., Goerss, S. & Earnest, F.I. Computer-assisted stereotaxic laser resection of intra-axial brain neoplasms. *J. Neurosurg.* **64**: 427–39 (1986).

12 Heilbrun, M., Sunderland, P., McDonald, P., Wells, T. Jr, Cosman, E. & Ganz, E. Brown–Roberts–Wells stereotactic frame modifications to accomplish magnetic resonance imaging guidance in three planes. *Appl. Neurophysiol.* **50**: 143–52 (1987).

13 Sapozink, M., Moeller, J., McDonald, P. & Heilbrun, M. Improved precision of interstitial brain tumor irradiation using the BRW CT stereotaxic guidance system. *Int. J. Radiat. Oncol. Biol. Phys.* **13**: 1753–60 (1987).

14 Willis, B., Heilbrun, M., Sapozink, M. *et al.* Stereotactic interstitial brachytherapy of malignant astrocytomas with remarks on post-implant CT appearance. *Neurosurgery* **23**: 348–54 (1988).

Three-dimensional Reconstruction of Neuroradiologic Data and Surgical Simulation

Cesare G. Giorgi, Ugo Cerchiari, Beatrice Alagna, and Davide S. Casolino

Introduction

In non-stereotactic planning of operative strategy, the surgeon's main difficulty is the lack of information on the geometric definition of the operative field, due to the few superficial anatomic landmarks available and the undetermined spatial orientation of neuroradiologic data within a geometric reference system. The amount of available data, poorly organizable within surgical landmarks, does not meet the surgeon's need of lesion localization and approach planning. As a result of the unique anatomic characteristics of the brain, contained in a rigid space and relatively unaffected by cardiac and respiratory movements, a notable spatial stability of anatomic information collected with neuroradiologic examination is encountered, both in diagnostic and operative phases. This spatial stability is maintained throughout stereotactic biopsies, functional procedures and interstitial radiotherapy, since no changes in preoperative anatomic volume are introduced in these cases during surgery. In open surgical procedures, parenchymal retraction and tissue removal often profoundly alter the preoperative geometry, and so this correspondence is lost.

In both situations, however, the surgeon can extract useful information from three-dimensional (3-D) processing of neuroradiologic data which, together with multimodal data derived from computed tomography (CT), magnetic resonance imaging (MRI), and angiography can be organized within an operative reference system. Anatomic data can be integrated with functional information, and the procedure can be planned with all possible data to hand. The high functional importance of encephalic structures justifies the introduction and continuous development of technologies to plan and monitor neurosurgical procedures.

Neuroradiologic examinations

The establishment of a reference system reproducible in both diagnostic and operative phases, within which images are orientated, forms the basis for surgical use of neuroradiologic information. This reference is made possible by the use of a stereotactic frame, onto which a localizer is mounted during the image acquisition phase.

With the introduction of CT, and subsequently of MRI, various techniques have been devised to establish the image plane within the reference of the stereotactic frame. Computation of target localization and of approach trajectories was originally performed on the same diagnostic consoles [1,2,3]. Later, dedicated graphic processors were introduced to handle images for surgery [4,5,6], not only because computational load was incompatible with normal diagnostic activity in radiologic departments, but also to allow wider flexibility.

Anatomic information used for surgical planning is derived from CT, MRI, and angiography, while planar X-rays and ultrasound imaging are used to monitor surgical progress. In contrast to radiologic departments, where images are mainly examined for their morphologic content, in surgery departments special attention is devoted to the quantitative aspect of information contained within the images, and in particular to their geometry.

Images available from current techniques are normally in digital form. When the acquisition geometry is known, neuroradiologic data can be correctly related to a reference system reproducible in the restitution phase. These procedures thus require frequent checking of CT acquisition geometry, and particularly of magnetic field uniformity and gradient linearity in MRI to minimize image distortion. Angiographic data, acquired in digital form with an image intensifier, are even more evidently deformed. Acquisition of angiographic images in a known reference system is successfully performed using a normal film which is subsequently digitized, employing instruments with a known acquisition geometry.

Similar considerations are valid for images obtained through ultrasound technology. The skull makes ultrasound unsuitable for preoperative acquisition phases, but valuable information for monitoring volumetric changes of cerebral anatomy can be obtained by this method during surgery.

Surgical procedures

Neurosurgical operations, with the exception of functional procedures, always aim to remove pathologic tissue in the most conservative way, saving as much healthy parenchyma surrounding the lesion as possible.

Information guiding neurosurgical procedures belongs to two categories: (1) strictly anatomic data, concerning the lesion volume and location, its morphologic characters, and the geometric coordinates of the lesion and surrounding structures; and (2) functional data, which characterize each morphologically-defined region and its relationship to other areas. In planning the removal of a deep-seated lesion, the surgeon considers both classes of data: functional information determines the risks of surgical approach, and guides the planning of the most appropriate trajectory, taking into account both the cortical and subcortical location of functions. Contemporary surgical techniques allow surgical approach to lesions with limited exposure of normal parenchyma, therefore mapping cortical functions becomes more and more important. It now becomes necessary, during surgical planning, to expand the classical knowledge of main cortical areas and major projection and association pathways by integrating data derived from other disciplines, such as epileptology and neuropsychology, as well as neurophysiologic and clinical data related to surgery, to constitute a functional model easily examined within a known reference system.

Classically, functional information is utilized in neuroablative or neuroaugmentative procedures carried on in the diencephalon to correct dysfunctions of the motor or sensory systems in man. In this class of operations functional information outweighs the importance of anatomic data, which is used mainly to scale a functional model in a geometric reference system, relative to the patient under scrutiny.

Procedures for morphologic data processing

Images from which geometric characters of the lesion and surrounding structures are assessed, derive from CT, MRI, and angiography, and are acquired within a surgical reference.

Data are collected under stereotactic conditions: images are framed within a known reference system using a localizer. CT and MRI images show different characteristics in normal and pathologic tissue: the anatomic detail is superior in MRI images, while spatial definition and geometry are superior in CT. Cerebral angiography, particularly indicated to localize vascular lesions, is by far the best method of revealing, in necessary detail, the position of vascular structures encountered along the surgical trajectory.

Considering in detail one of the proposed solutions for morphologic data processing for surgery, we will describe the method developed in the Neurosurgical Division of the Neurological Institute of Milan. The surgical workstation processes MRI and CT images, delivered from the radiologic department on magnetic tape. Images are recorded on a direct access file on a hard disk. The program allows for efficient handling of MRI and CT data, relative to the patient under scrutiny. On each image, corresponding to a section of the anatomic volume, landmarks produced by the intersection of the image plane with a localizer are visible. The surgeon chooses the most significant sequence of sections and establishes the structures from which he or she wants to extract the contours to obtain a 3-D representation. Data collection from images (position of localizer marks and contours of structures), can be carried out automatically, and subsequently edited by means of an interactive procedure. The position of landmarks and contours of borders between structures with high-contrast separation (e.g. ventricles, bone, cystic cavities) can be automatically extracted, while lesions with ill-defined borders, or located within regions of high functional importance, are better defined manually or via automatic contour-extracting algorithms, interactively editable by the surgeon.

Once the process of contour extraction of the lesion and of other structures of surgical relevance is completed for all available images, the program produces a representation of the selected structures, identified by different colors. These structures are presented on a monitor as 3-D objects with a "wireframe" representation, visualized from an arbitrary point of view. The picture also shows the frame of reference representing the actual stereotactic apparatus in use, together with trajectories of surgical tools. To further clarify the relative position of structure contours and stereotactic frame, CT and MRI sections are simultaneously shown, on the same images and from the same perspective (Fig. 5.1).

In order to obtain a stereoscopic representation of angiography congruent to the data of structures previously described, it is necessary to acquire a few angiographic projections from different known angles, so that the geometry of acquisition is identified with respect to the stereotactic frame [7]. These conditions allow for the coupling of each angiographic view with the representation of the "wireframe" contours, the outlines of the stereotactic frame and the surgical trajectory, as if they were all seen from the same angle of acquisition.

Angiographic pairs, completed with the geometric representation of the above mentioned objects, allow for a synoptic spatial perception of information of surgical interest. An additional feature is presented by the multiple acquisition of stereoscopic pairs: viewing contiguous angiographic frames in sequence, and thus examining the object from different angles, allows for more precise perception of the relative position of objects in depth.

The 3-D perception of the anatomic picture of surgical interest is simplified by the use of a stereoscopic monitor. This type of monitor presents stereoscopic images in interlaced frames. Images are separately addressed to the right and left eyes from an optical switch, driven by vertical synchronism. The optical switch is a circularly polarized screen, electrically driven, coupled with circularly polarized glasses.

Preoperative neuroradiologic information satisfies the surgical requirements in performing procedures like tissue biopsies or stereotactic positioning of radioactive sources for brachy-therapy: the surgeon selects the approach trajectory, checking its relationship with vessels and other healthy structures surrounding the lesion. He can estimate the tissue volume irradiated, or the concentration of a colloid isotope diluted in a cystic cavity.

Preoperative image reconstruction can also guide the microsurgical removal of deep-seated cerebral lesions, very often surrounded by regions of high functional importance, but here the surgeon must be prepared for the fact that surgical maneuvers will modify, to some extent, the original anatomic geometry. Techniques and surgical instrumentation have been developed to reach the lesion without dislocation of cerebral parenchyma, by using retractors coaxial with the chosen trajectory, mounted on the stereotactic frame [8]. Lesions suitable for this treatment are generally well defined with respect to the normal surrounding parenchyma by their color and texture, and therefore the surgeon can attain complete removal of the lesion using these guidelines, once the lesion

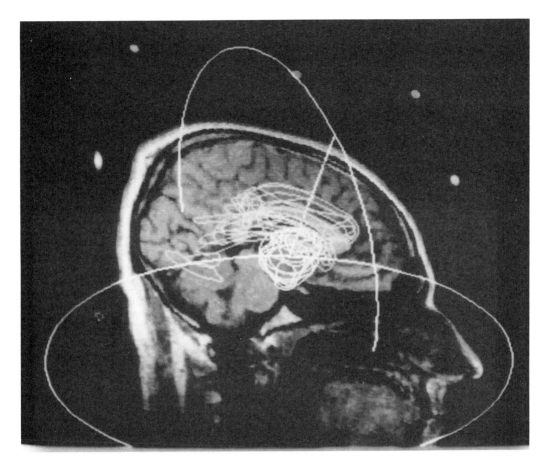

FIGURE 5.1 Three-dimensional representation of contours of tumor of the IIIrd ventricle, together with a sagittal MRI section, seen from an arbitrary perspective, with outlines of a given stereotactic frame and surgical trajectory.

has been stereotactically reached. In our experience lesions that were well defined with respect to the surrounding parenchyma have all been totally removed. The availability of a method that reconstructs in space the position and extent of a tumor's volume has always allowed for its removal through a small cortical incision, large enough to insert a retractor stereotactically, coaxial with the trajectory established in the planning phase. Nevertheless, although the possibility exists of performing a complete removal of a deep-seated lesion using adequate surgical instrumentation and guided by preoperative images, we believe that the theoretical completion of this methodology should incorporate some kind of intraoperative imaging device, capable of monitoring the approach to the lesion and its removal.

The solution of this problem can be ap-

proached at different levels of complexity. Solutions based on the development of MRI imaging instruments are under development, specially conceived for intraoperative applications and therefore characterized by simplified configuration and dimensions that make them suitable for intraoperative use [9]. Meanwhile, intermediate solutions providing intraoperative images with lower anatomic resolution are being explored, based on ultrasound technology.

Stereotactic use of ultrasound imaging offers advantages over conventional diagnostic applications: the probe can be mounted on the stereotactic frame in order to examine the volume included in the operative field. Changes in the visible lesion volume could be evaluated during the surgical phases, as well as the volume of the increasing operative cavity [10].

Procedures for functional data processing

Performing neurologic surgery not only involves dealing with the orientation of the anatomy of the surgical region, as described above, but also taking into account cerebral function localization. In order to do this, the surgeon needs to refer the functional information to a standard anatomy, and to use this data as a model, to be adapted to each patient undergoing surgery.

The problem of function localization has been historically raised by the procedures of functional stereotactic neurosurgery, and solved with the use of anatomic and functional atlases. The former, obtained through histologic techniques, are meant to be used following geometrical rules; the latter, containing general functional information, are not suitable for localizing an anatomic target with reasonable accuracy.

The main obstacle encountered in utilizing traditional atlases is represented by individual cerebral variability. Proposed solutions take into account scale factors along the three axes [11, 12,13] or structural contours modeled according to polar coordinates [14]. In our opinion these approaches do not completely fulfill the requirements, since scale factors of anatomic volumes vary three-dimensionally from point to point. This fact does not permit the matching of plain sections of different brains: points of a plain section of one brain will generally find their correspondent points on a curved surface in another brain. Moreover, having followed this approach, topological individual variability which cannot be solved even by curvilinear coordinates may be found. Function, as well as morphology, might in fact have a different topology in different individuals. For all these reasons it is necessary when performing functional procedures to guide the target localization with neurophysiologic data. The task we are now focusing on consists of finding a way to determine the set of curvilinear coordinates that allow for the best possible fit between the model and the individual case: this approach would solve the problem of labeling neuroanatomic images, reaching a precision unparalleled by other described methods.

To solve this problem a matching procedure has been developed that allows for the mapping of a 3-D MRI acquisition of a patient over another acquisition, obtained from a different patient, with the same imaging method [15]. The described method is cross-correlative and identifies corresponding local volumes. Two windows are opened and moved within both the volumes according to defined strategies. For every point in volume A, a corresponding point is searched for in volume B. These are the points that give the best cross-correlative value for the signal contained in the two windows around them.

The process of homologous points identification in the two volumes allows for the introduction of standard anatomic coordinates in different brains: in fact, on any brain defined in a Cartesian coordinate system, this frame of reference can be superimposed by the matching procedure on all other brains, addressing each point according to the curvilinear coordinate transformation. For example, the anterior commissure will have the same spatial coordinates in all brains.

The efficacy of this solution is largely due to the 3-D approach: previous attempts based on two-dimensional (2-D) methods failed to reach satisfactory correlation, mainly because plain sections of one volume correspond to curved surfaces in another, and 2-D windows do not carry sufficient information, due to the smaller pixel number [16].

The process of matching described above would allow for the superimposition of a 3-D model atlas onto any individual brain. The lack of an ideal model atlas (which would consist of a brain previously plotted using 3-D MRI technique and subsequently sectioned and stained) makes it necessary to run a matching algorithm between a 3-D MRI acquisition and a traditional stereotactic atlas. Since the process described is a cross-correlative one, the two data volumes need to carry the same kind of information. Tissue description in MR images is limited to white matter, gray matter and cerebrospinal fluid, and for this reason the matching process can only be performed at this level. MRI acquisition volumes need, therefore, to be segmented by identification of homogeneous regions to which a descriptive label is associated. Following this procedure, each voxel of the patient's volume is described by a vector whose three components allow the probability of belonging to one of the described tissues. If this can be obtained, the procedure can also be effective in matching MR image volumes with a corresponding anatomic atlas, since the match is performed taking into account the probability values of voxels, rather than their numeric values (Figs 5.2 and 5.3). This segmentative procedure can disclose geometrical information detailed enough to automatically generate a copy of a neuroanatomic atlas, adapted to the patient's geometry.

One of the most appealing applications of an atlas obtained through this method is the possibility of locating neurophysiologic and clinical observations in it, with a geometric dispersion due only to topological differences or to the diffuse localization of some functions, having solved inaccuracy due to the different curvilinear coordinates.

From what has been stated, it appears that the availability of a morphologic atlas, adapted to the patient's geometry, hinges upon the segmentation of an MRI acquisition into anatomic regions. Tissue characterization is only as good as the anatomic resolution of available 3-D MRI acquisition. Residual topological differences will be taken care of by an atlas whose segmentation takes into account these differences encountered in a large series of patients. Limits of regions described with this method will, of course, be "fuzzy," representing the probability of occurrence of observations. Processing MR images for segmentation involves problems related to the types of acquisition that have to be solved in the image preprocessing phase. Among these problems the most relevant are non-uniformity of gain within the image volume noise, and poor spatial resolution.

The quality of spatial resolution depends strongly on the acquisition time and is conse-

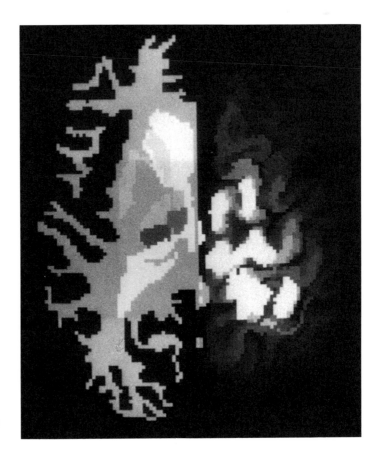

FIGURE 5.2 An example of a 3-D brain atlas, obtained by processing histologic sections with characterized substructures. Anatomic detail along the three axes is suitable for the process of matching with MRI image volumes.

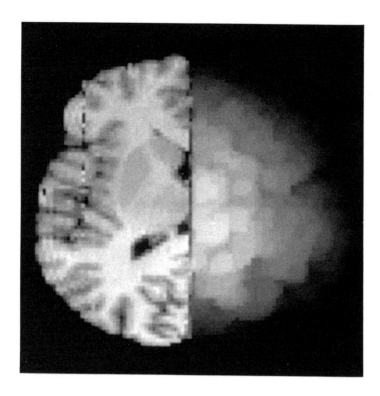

FIGURE 5.3 A flash 3-D MRI acquisition. Satisfactory anatomic resolution in a $128 \times 128 \times 128$ matrix is obtained with this technique in less than 15 minutes. Tissue characterization (segmentation), performed following the method described in the text, allows for the superimposition of a 3-D model atlas on individual MRI acquisitions.

quently affected by the volume of data that can reasonably be processed. The solution of the problem of noise has been achieved by a statistic filtering of the volume that reduces the signal scattering within the homogeneous areas of the image, by eliminating additional noise whose statistics are known [17]. Non-uniformity of gain, related to the field uniformity of MRI radiofrequency and acquisition coil, has been compensated for by modeling the function of gain of the acquisition coil with a polynom up to the fourth grade of the coordinates, with coefficients adaptively determined, starting from a cluster of initial coefficients. Correcting the values of signal with this gain function in the volume elements, the peaks of the histogram rise or fall as coefficients are varied, following the improvement or worsening of gain uniformity. The aim is to modify the original coefficients until the maximum height of the highest peak of the volume histogram is reached. This condition corresponds in the histogram to the highest possible dynamic (highest separation between peaks and their highest possible altitude).

The chosen segmentation approach does not aim to identify anatomic region borders since,

in principle, these are not closed 3-D objects, and their identification is only possible using local information where borders do exist. Borders are obviously two-dimensional, and their description rests upon a smaller amount of data than that available for 3-D tissue characterization.

Segmentation based on a single 3-D MRI acquisition can only be obtained using the value of local signal, possibly enforced by values of voxels surrounding the one under scrutiny. Therefore, besides the signal value, it has only been possible to introduce the standard deviation, calculated in a $3 \times 3 \times 3$ volume surrounding each voxel, as an additional parameter to obtain the segmentation. It has therefore been possible to represent graphically a 2-D histogram signal value/standard deviation, on which a cluster analysis can be performed. With this analysis the main cerebral tissues have been separated in a first approximation. To obtain a better representation of the segmented regions, additional computational procedures have been implemented.

The signal value of each image voxel of a volume acquired with MRI is composed of two entities: amplitude and phase. At present only amplitude has been employed, but it is likely that improvement of the actual result of segmentation procedures might be achieved by the use of spectroscopic information delivered by the phase.

Conclusions

Processing of neuroradiologic data from a surgical standpoint allows for their organization in a presentation which is useful for therapy planning. This concept not only applies to the convenience of organizing large amounts of data within a surgical frame of reference, but also introduces the possibility of merging functional information with morphology.

The traditional concept of the stereotactic brain atlas, utilized as a piece of morphologic information, to be integrated with available neuroradiologic data and to assist the surgeon in functional data organization, is now being substituted by a broader application. The atlas is becoming a powerful database for clinical and functional data, wrapped in its morphologic structure. Available computational resources now make it possible to use this information, interactively adapted to each patient's anatomy, and continuously upgraded following each procedure.

References

1 Apuzzo, M.L.J. & Sabshin, J.K. Computed tomographic guidance stereotaxis in the management of intracranial mass lesions. *Neurosurgery* **12**: 277–85 (1983).

2 Gildenberg, P.L., Kaufman, H.H. & Murthy, K.S.K. Calculation of stereotactic coordinates from the computed tomographic scan. *Neurosurgery* **10**: 580–6 (1982).

3 Mundinger, F. & Birg, W. CT-aided stereotaxy for functional neurosurgery and deep brain implants. *Acta Neurochir.* **56**: 245 (1981).

4 Peters, T.M., Clark, J.A. & Olivier, A. *et al.* Integrated stereotaxic imaging with CT, MR imaging and digital subtraction angiography. *Radiology* **161**: 821–6 (1986).

5 Giorgi, C., Casolino, D.S. & Franzini, A. *et al.* Computer assisted planning of stereotactic neurosurgical procedures. *Child's Nerv. Syst.* **5**: 299–302 (1989).

6 Kelly, P.J., Kall, B.A. & Goerss, S.J. Transposition of volumetric information derived from computed tomographic scanning into stereotactic space. *Surg. Neurol.* **21**: 465–71 (1984).

7 Giorgi, C., Cerchiari, U., Broggi G. & Passerini, A. 3-D reconstruction of cerebral angiography in stereotactic neurosurgery. *Acta Neurochir.* (suppl.) **39**: 13–14 (1987).

8 Kelly, P.J., Goerss, S.J. & Kall, B.A. The stereotaxic retractor in computer assisted stereotactic neurosurgery. *J. Neurosurg.* **69**: 301–6 (1988).

9 Abele, M.G. & Rusinek, H. *Generation of a Uniform Field in a Yokeless Permanent Magnet for NMR Clinical Applications.* Technical Report No. 19, New York University (1988).

10 Koivukangas, J. & Kelly, P.J. Application of ultrasound imaging to stereotactic brain tumor surgery. *Ann. Clin. Res.* **18**: 25–32 (1986).

11 Vries, J.K., McLinden, S., Banks, G. & Latchaw, R.E. Computerized three-dimensional stereotactic atlases. In: Lunsford, L.D. (ed.), *Modern Stereotactic Neurosurgery*, pp. 441–59. Boston: Martinus Nijhoff (1988).

12 Bertrand, G. & Olivier, A. Computer display of stereotactic brain maps and probe tracts. *Acta Neurochir. (Wien.)* **21**: 235–43 (1974).

13 Hardy, T. & Koch, J. Computer-assisted stereotactic surgery. *Appl. Neurophysiol.* **45**: 396–8 (1982).

14 Kall, B.A., Kelly, P.J., Goerss, S. & Frieder, G. Methodology and clinical experience with computed tomography and a computer resident stereotactic atlas. *Neurosurgery* **17**: 400–6 (1985).

15 Cerchiari, U., Del Panno, G., Giorgi, C. & Garibotto, G. 3-D correlation technique for anatomical volumes in functional stereotactic neurosurgery. In: Cappellini, V. (ed.) *Time-varying Image Processing and Moving Object Recognition.* Amsterdam: Elsevier North-Holland (1987).

16 Bajcsy, R., Lieberson, R. & Reivich, M. A computerized system for the elastic matching of deformed radiographic images to idealized atlas images. *J. Comput. Assist. Tomogr.* **4**: 618–25 (1983).

17 Borroni, M., Turrin, A., Cerchiari, U., Castellani, M.R., Gasparini, M.R. & Buraggi, G.L. Performance evaluation of some noise-smoothing techniques for Gamma-camera digital images. *J. Nucl. Med. Sci.* **29**: 245–51 (1985).

part II

Operating Room Environment

chapter 6

An Interactive Stereotactic Operating Suite

Stephan J. Goerss

Introduction

The effectiveness of a stereotactic system is dependent on the ease and availability of the database during a stereotactic procedure and how it is used with the stereotactic equipment. A stereotactic system needs to have a strong interconnection between the three phases of a procedure, so that there is an easy transition from one phase to the next. These three phases are: (1) data acquisition; (2) treatment planning; and (3) surgery — each phase has become increasingly intricate as more advanced technology is incorporated in stereotactic procedures. The transitions between each phase, as well as the actual events themselves, are more complex than their traditional stereotactic predecessors, and resulting in the use of computers and software as tools to compensate for this complexity.

Data acquisition has undergone the greatest transition incorporating computer generated images such as computed tomography (CT), magnetic resonance imaging (MRI) and digital subtraction angiography (DSA) into a patient's database. To utilize these studies, stereotactic frames have been modified or developed, with special reference devices for each modality to place reference marks onto each radiologic image [1–4]. These reference marks are then used to correlate the image to the stereotactic device.

In comparison to early stereotactic devices, the present day use of stereotactic frames remains nearly the same. Although the early systems did not have the availability of computer-generated images, they derived enough information from biplane radiographs to isolate the surgical target and determine a safe surgical trajectory. As with contemporary systems, a reference system incorporated into the device generated reference marks on the radiograph for correlating the location of a target within the device. Performing these procedures required access to X-ray equipment, leaving a choice of moving the procedure to the department of radiology or installing the required equipment in the operating room. For safety and convenience, anterior–posterior and lateral X-ray tubes were mounted into operating rooms and became a basic requirement for stereotactic operating rooms, allowing the surgeon to acquire, plan, and treat the patient in the operating suite in one session. The amount of data and the types of calculations were such that treatment planning could be completed with manual calculations. In many cases, calculations were nothing more than direct measurements on the radiographs which were corrected for magnification of the X-ray image.

Modern databases have expanded in the amount and type of information that is applied to stereotactic procedure, diversifying the types of procedure being completed under stereotactic conditions [5−8]. Multiple modalities are used, because a more complete and thorough surgical plan can be generated by complimentary information provided by each modality concerning the patient's anatomy and pathology. Using this approach does complicate the process of performing stereotactic procedures. Primarily, the surgeon has to digest the information being presented and formulate a practical surgical plan. This becomes much more difficult as the database multiplies. Surgical planning software packages have been developed to ease this process [9].

Incorporation of the additional databases has created practical issues on how to access and use this information. An advantage of traditional stereotactic procedure was that the source of the database was located in the operating room. At any point during a procedure, additional images could be acquired to monitor and document the procedure. Likewise, it would be desirable to repeat a CT scan intraoperatively, for example to confirm the location of a biopsy probe. Lundsford [10] described one approach to this problem by installing a CT scanner in the operating suite. This allowed the use of the scanner computer for treatment planning as well as the opportunity to repeat a scan at any time.

An alternative approach is to move the procedure to the diagnostic equipment. CT scanning suites have been the site for stereotactic biopsies. It does have the advantage of confirming the position of a biopsy probe with a CT image and using the CT computer for treatment planning, but is also has inherent drawbacks. Primarily, it leaves the surgeon exposed if a complication arises that cannot be attended to outside the operating room. It also limits the use of other modalities for the planning procedure.

The goal of combining the different modalities for more comprehensive surgical planning and treatment can best be reached by using a central surgical computer system dedicated to the purpose of stereotactic planning and treatment. The consolidation of information to a single site is advantageous because the surgeon has complete and uninterrupted access to the database at any time during the treatment planning or surgical procedure. The use of CT computers, although functional, generates conflicts from sharing equipment. Using the CT display console for treatment planning interrupts using the scanner while the treatment plan is being made. Likewise, a surgeon cannot access the computer while it is being used for its intended purpose. More importantly, these computers, located remotely from the operating area, are inaccessible to the surgeon to re-evaluate a surgical plan once a procedure has started.

At the end of the treatment planning session, the information needs to be configured in a form that can be used by the stereotactic equipment and is of value to the surgeon in the operating room. This goes beyond simply generating a three-dimensional (3-D) coordinate for a surgical target and a pair of angles for a trajectory. The computer needs to be available to the surgeon to interact with it during the surgical procedure, for review of the treatment plan or to alter the plan as the situation dictates. Furthermore, availability to a computer system allows for adding information, such as digital teleradiography, into the patient's database.

We have expanded the use of the computer beyond displaying graphics by interfacing specific devices used during a stereotactic procedure. The configuration of equipment described here has been incorporated into a stereotactic program because it has improved not only the accuracy and safety of performing surgery, but also the effective use of time and assistance provided for a surgeon during the actual procedure. The surgical system is centered around the computer, because the different facets of the procedure can then be controlled through one entity. An automated stereotactic positioner, which evolved from traditional stereotactic machines, can be activated by the surgeon through the computer to access different points in the head as he or she deems necessary. Using interactive devices such as the mouse or joystick, the surgeon can display a variety of images on the intraoperative monitors for the purpose of replaying the surgical plan or altering it. Also using the computer, digital teleradiographs can be added to the patient's database.

COMPASS™ system overview

The COMPASS™ Stereotactic System (Stereotactic Medical Systems Inc., New Hartford, NY) has evolved over the course of 10 years with the purpose of expanding the use of stereotaxy and surgical computer systems as neurosurgical tools. Figure 6.1 shows an isometric view of our operating room, including the COMPASS™ Stereotactic System. In essence, there are three staging areas represented in the diagram: (1) the treatment planning facility, which houses the computer system and is where the treatment plan is generated; (2) the control room adjacent to the operating room; this is used to review or generate a surgical plan; and (3) the stereotactic suite.

The treatment planning facility, located above surgery, houses a Sun 4/360 host computer (Sun Microsystems Inc., Milpitas, CA). In conjunction with this, a Vicom image processor (Vicom Inc., Fremont, CA) displays computer images and performs the graphics and image manipulations needed for treatment planning. Peripheral equipment to the Sun includes terminals and the ½ inch tape drive. The terminals provide access to the Sun from remote sites like surgery, where the software needs to be accessed. The tape drive is used to load diagnostic images from the different modalities

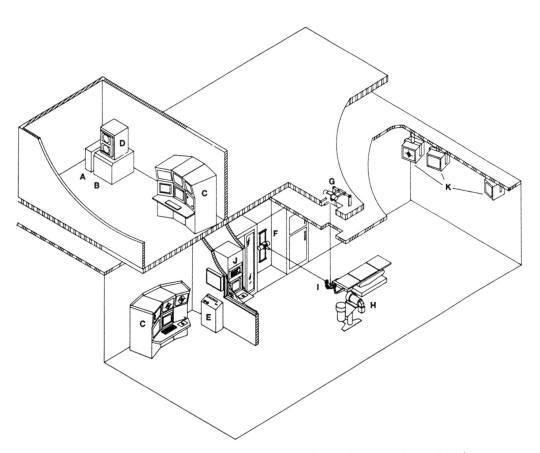

FIGURE 6.1 The physical layout of the stereotactic operating suite has three areas of operation. The treatment planning facility houses: the Sun computer (A); the Vicom image processor (B); a treatment-planning console (C); and a ½ inch tape drive (D). The control room adjacent to the operating room also has a treatment-planning console and X-ray controller (E). In the operating room is located the lateral X-ray tube (F); anterior–posterior X-ray tube (G); digital teleradiographic system (H); the COMPASS™ stereotactic positioner (I); the remote control console (J); and the computer display monitors (K).

onto the computer system as well as to archive patient data. From the data acquisition phase, images from CT, MRI, and DSA are loaded onto the system using ½ inch magnetic tapes and carried to the treatment planning facility, where independent programs read the images from the tape and transfer them onto the system disk.

Once stored on disk, the images are used by the COMPASS™ software package to calculate surgical targets, trajectories and tumor volumes during the treatment planning phase. Planning is performed at the treatment planning console, located adjacent to the computer room. This unit has three black-and-white monitors and a color monitor (Conrac Display Products Inc., Covina, CA) to display different combinations of images needed to plan a case. It also contains a computer terminal to access the computer and for inputting alphanumeric information.

A second unit is available in the control room adjacent to the operating room for replaying and revising surgical plans. Minor modifications are common once the surgical process has started. Once the patient is positioned in surgery, the surgeon may wish to change the trajectory, based on unforeseen circumstances. For example, the trajectory and target may be in conflict with the physical constraints of the stereotactic equipment. These changes can be easily made. This unit is also available for planning procedures intended to be completed in 1 day.

During the planning process, several conclusions are drawn after comparing the anatomy and pathology between the different modalities. First, an x, y, and z coordinate is calculated for the desired target, based on CT and, if applicable, MRI. This may be an intracranial lesion or a particular portion of anatomy such as the hippocampus [8].

After targeting, an optimal approach to the target is desired. Using DSA with the location of the target displayed, one can choose an avascular approach to the tumor determining the settings of the arc quadrant. The trajectory can also be displayed on CT and MRI images to determine if the path is violating essential brain tissue or to find at what level the trajectory intersects the boundaries of the lesion or anatomic feature.

In addition, a volume of the area of interest may be generated. Using CT and/or a variety of MRI sequences, one can outline a lesion or anatomic feature on every available image. The software will construct a volume from these contours and determine its location and orientation within the confines of the stereotactic positioner. Once completed, this volume is displayed as slices perpendicular to the trajectory. Each slice acts as a template for the tumor boundary at a particular depth in the surgical field.

The operating suite

The operating room has been renovated to lend itself to stereotactic procedures. The equipment installed is either portable or mounted in a location that is unobtrusive to other types of procedure. It is grouped into three categories:

1 The stereotactic instrumentation.
2 The teleradiography system.
3 The computer and graphics display monitors.
Each category, although capable of functioning independently, is linked with the others to perform a wide variety of procedures. The design is such that traditional as well as computer-assisted stereotactic procedures may be completed.

The automatic stereotactic system

At the heart of the operating room is the COMPASS™ stereotactic positioner. It is categorized as an arc-centered stereotactic system, as it positions the surgical target at the center of an arc-quadrant by moving the patient's head with respect to the arc. The advantage of moving the head with respect to the arc is that the alignment between the arc-quadrant and the two X-ray tubes remains constant throughout the procedure. Procedures with multiple targets, as in the case of implanting ^{192}Ir, do not require realignment of the X-ray tubes for each position.

The COMPASS™ stereotactic positioner has four major components (Fig. 6.2).

1 The stereotactic headholder.
2 The 160 mm arc-quadrant.
3 The 3-D slide.
4 The remote control console.
Together, these components function to access

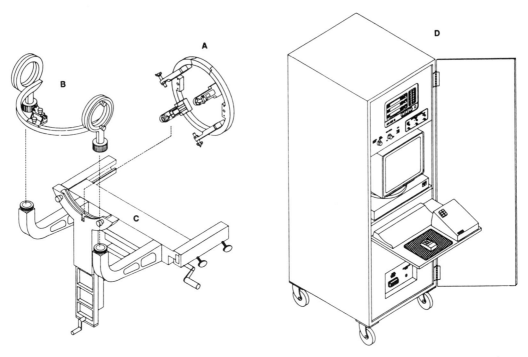

FIGURE 6.2 The basic components of the COMPASS™ slide are: the headholder (A); the 160 mm arc-quadrant (B); the 3-D slide (C); and the remote control console (D).

any point in the cranium and allow for a multitude of trajectories to the target.

The unit has seven degrees of freedom. The first three are supplied by the 3-D positioner and move the head linearly in the *x, y,* and *z* axes. Another is the depth to which the surgical probe is inserted. These four are responsible for accessing the target.

The next two, termed the arc and collar angles, are the angular settings of the arc-quadrant determining the trajectory to the target. These settings alter the approach of the surgical probe to the target. Adjusting these angles will allow the surgeon to select an optimal approach to the target that is avascular and passes through the least essential brain matter.

The last degree of freedom is a rotation of the headholder on the 3-D positioner. This feature, known as "patient orientation," allows the patient to be positioned in a variety of rotations during surgery, giving increased flexibility to the trajectory to the surgical target. Rotations in increments of 90° allow for supine, left, or right decubitus and prone positioning of the patient. Typically, rotations of 90° are used because they ease perception between the diag-

nostic images and the stereotactic instrumentation. However, the face of the basering is engraved with tic marks every 5°, allowing for intermediate rotations. This may improve ease of the surgical approach by bringing the lesion to a position where it can be easily reached. This feature may also be used to centralize the target in the arc. A rotation of 45°, for instance, will reduce the *x* value of a lateral target and center it in the arc-quadrant.

The stereotactic headholder

The headholder functions to immobilize the patient's head during the data acquisition process and during surgery, keeping the data in identical orientation for both portions of the procedure. In addition, the face of the basering serves as a constant reference plane for the 3-D matrix into which the patient's data is placed. It is to this surface that all the localization devices for the different modalities are attached, thus setting the correlation between the data sources.

An important feature of the headholder is its ability to be removed and reapplied in the original position. This has several advantages for computer-assisted stereotactic procedures. First, utilizing CT, MRI, and DSA requires several hours per patient to complete the diagnostic studies. Additional time is required to load the data onto the surgical computer system. Only when this is completed can the surgeon prepare a surgical plan. Scheduling of all the different studies, and trying to synchronize this with the surgical schedule, is at best difficult, and in many cases results in idle time for the operating room and surgeon while waiting for the acquisition of data. The ability to reapply the headholder allows the data to be acquired in one session, the surgical plan to be developed in a second, and surgery to be completed in timely fashion after the first two. An effective use of time is generated if two or three patients are undergoing stereotactic procedures planned from previously collected data. While these procedures are being completed, data on additional patients is being collected for the next surgical session.

Another advantage is that the same database may be used for subsequent procedures. For instance, results from a stereotactic biopsy may indicate the need for a stereotactic resection. The original database may be applied to the second procedure, eliminating the need for a second set of diagnostic studies.

Finally, this stereotactic system and the equipment supplying the database rely heavily on technology which is susceptible to breakdown. This requires postponement of the procedure until the situation is resolved. A single use application would result in the loss of any information acquired prior to the breakdown. The ability to reapply the headholder allows continuation from the stopping point. For instance, this could avert unnecessarily repeating an angiogram if the trouble occurred after the study and before the completion of the data acquisition process or surgical procedure.

The different components of the stereotactic headholder (Fig. 6.3) are as follows:

1 The basering with a removable mouth section.

2 A set of four vertical supports.

3 The vertical support bases.

4 A set of four locking collets.

5 Four plastic sleeves.

6 A set of four carbon fiber fixation pins.

The basering is a round aluminum ring with a removable portion called the mouth piece. The mouth piece, which attaches to the basering with two thumb screws, improves access to the oral area for the purpose of intubation, or for emergency access should the occasion arise during any portion of the stereotactic process. Each diagnostic machine has an adaptation plate which grips the basering, holding the patient in proper position during the procedure. In similar fashion, the basering attaches to the 3-D positioner during a surgical procedure.

Assembly of the headholder (Fig. 6.3) first requires the attachment of the vertical support bases to the basering with two 10-32 × 1 inch hex socket cap screws. There are a variety of attachment positions, allowing orientation in the way that best accommodates the patient. This feature is used to avoid previous craniotomies or to better accommodate small children. The position of the base is recorded, referring to the letter engraved on the face of the basering. Recording these positions is essential in order to reassemble the headholder for subsequent applications.

The vertical supports, molded from a nylon and carbon fiber composite, extend up from the face of the basering, offsetting the basering from the surgical field. The base of each vertical support has two tapered tabs which insert into the holes of the vertical support base. From the back of the vertical support bases, two ¼ inch-20 × ⅝ inch hex socket cap screws are screwed into the tapped tabs locking them into place.

Four collets, molded from Delrin, insert into keyed tapered holes located at the tops of the vertical supports. A Delrin nut screws onto the back of each collet, holding it in place. Through the center of each collet is a ⅜ inch hole for passing the plastic sleeve. Tightening of the nut draws the collet into the vertical support, collapsing the four jaws onto the plastic sleeve. Since the collet will grip the sleeve anywhere along the shaft, the sleeve can be adjusted to fit the individual patient.

A hollow plastic sleeve, also molded from Delrin, is advanced through the collet until it is against the scalp, suspending the headholder. A carbon fiber fixation pin passes through the center of the sleeve. The back end of the sleeve

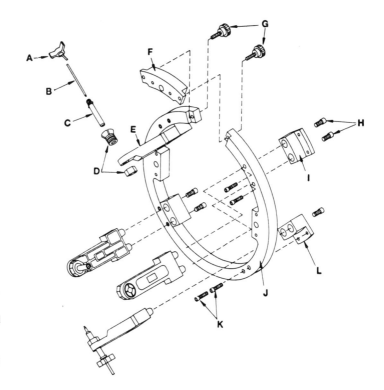

FIGURE 6.3 An exploded view of the headholder demonstrates the individual components as well as the assembly of the unit: locking cap for the plastic sleeve (A); carbon fiber pin (B); plastic sleeve (C); collet and nut (D); vertical support (E); removable mouth piece (F); thumbscrews for the mouth piece (G); vertical support screws (H); vertical support bases (I); basering (J); vertical support base screws (K); and vertical support base (L).

is designed as a pin vice for clamping onto the pin. A locking cap screws onto the back end of the sleeve, tightening the four jaws of the pin vice onto the fixation pin to lock it into place.

The fixation pin is molded of carbon fiber. The pin has a 9/64 inch (3.57 mm) diameter shaft identical to the diameter of the hole through the plastic sleeve. The tip of the pin has a 7/64 inch (2.77 mm) diameter × 4 mm flange that fits into the hole in the skull made during the application process. Resting the flange against the skull's surface allows the pin to be replaced reproducibly.

Application of the headholder

Once the headholder is assembled, a set of ear and nose bars is attached to the basering laterally and anteriorly, respectively. These bars aid in centering the headholder around the patient during the application process. Once completed, they are removed from the headholder.

The patient's head is suspended off the end of a gurney and supported by a modified microphone stand which has a cup to cradle the head. The assembled headholder is slipped over the head and the earbars are inserted into the

external auditory canals. These slide in a lateral direction to center left and right. The nose bar is brought to the forehead and centered over the bridge of the nose. This centers the headframe in the anterior–posterior direction as well as the front to back tilt of the headholder.

Once the headholder is oriented correctly, the plastic sleeves are advanced to the scalp and the collets are tightened. The scalp is infiltrated with a 50/50 mixture of 1 : 200 of 1% Xylocaine with epinephrine and 0.5% bupivacaine. A drill guide/tissue punch is advanced through the sleeve and pressed through the scalp, removing a core of tissue. A 7/64 inch (2.77 mm) drill bit with a pre-set depth stop is advanced until the depth stop rests against the back of the drill guide. This creates the correct depth hole to receive the flanged fixation pin.

Upon removing the drill and drill guide, a fixation pin is placed through the plastic sleeve and tapped into place. The pin is advanced until the flange is flush against the skull. The locking cap is screwed onto the sleeve to lock the fixation pin in place. This process is repeated for each vertical support.

With the headholder secured into place, a set of micrometers is attached to each vertical support. The shaft of each micrometer head is advanced to the back end of a fixation pin. This process measures the distance each fixation pin is extended from the skull: this distance is recorded in case a reapplication is required, regardless of whether the procedure is intended to be completed in 1 day.

Reapplying the headholder Reapplication is possible because the fixation pins can be inserted into the holes created during the application process. Once the headholder is reassembled and positioned over the patient's head, the pins are passed through the collets and tapped into the original twist drill holes, followed by passing the plastic sleeves over them and through the collets. After this, the locking caps are loosely applied and the collets are slightly tightened. At this point, the headholder is attached to the skull, but it can be slightly adjusted. The micrometer attachments are mounted onto each vertical support. Each micrometer is set to the original setting from the application procedure, thus resetting the fixation pin to the original depth. Upon completion, the collets and caps are thoroughly tightened.

The 160 mm arc-quadrant

The 160 mm arc-quadrant (Fig. 6.4), more commonly called the arc, is used to direct surgical instruments along a multitude of vectors to access a surgical target. The approach to the target is determined by the settings of the collar and arc angles, which together form an imaginary sphere. The collar angle is a rotation of the 160 mm radius arc about the horizontal axis and has a range of −30 to 120°. A value of 0° will project a probe along the axial plane of a patient and a value of 90° will project a horizontal path. The position of the arc car, located on the arc, determines the arc angle. It has a range of ± 60° with 0° being centered on the arc. The arc car is the component that holds a guide along a vector normal to this sphere, thus projecting a path through its center.

The advantage to this approach is that the instrumentation always projects a path through the focus, regardless of the arc and collar settings. This flexibility allows the surgeon to choose the optimal approach to the target to

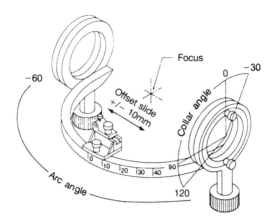

FIGURE 6.4 The arc-quadrant directs instruments to the target located at the focus. Altering the arc and collar angles will change the approach to the target, but will not affect accessing it. The collar angle has a range of −30° to +120°, whereas the arc angle range is ±60°. The offset slide allows for parallel trajectories by changing the laterality of the probe.

avoid vessels and important anatomic structures. Once the patient is positioned in the arc, it is easy to conceptualize the location of the target and, using one's experience, to select an appropriate trajectory, even without the aid of the software package. Although a seemingly small point, this feature eases the use of the equipment because one can simply use the arc to point to the target. This helps to reduce dependency on the computer, because one can visualize the target location and trajectory, thus confirming that the information provided by the treatment-planning software is correct.

A feature on the arc car worth mentioning is the offset slide. This is the portion of the arc car that actually holds the guide tube. It has the ability to slide left and right on the arc car, resulting in trajectories parallel to the normal vector. This feature was retained from the Todd−Wells machine because it is very useful for functional procedures where parallel electrode paths are regularly required for mapping out the thalamic nuclei.

Locating the focus of the arc requires some simple arithmetic. To position a probe at the focus, one needs to determine the distance from the back of the guide tube to the arc car. This distance, known as the extension, will vary depending on the proximity of the skull to the arc. One distance that remains constant is the distance from the proximal face of the arc car to the focus, which is 135 mm. To insert the probe to the focus one simply adds the extension to 135 mm. Measuring this combined length from the tip of a probe will position the tip at the focus. In cases such as biopsies, where serial biopsies are taken at various levels along the trajectory, the starting distance needs to be subtracted from the overall value.

In addition to the arc car is the stereotactic retractor mount (Fig. 6.5). Like the arc car, its position on the 160 mm arc determines the arc angle. The purpose of this unit is to direct retractor tubes along vectors normal to the center of the arc in the same manner as the arc car directs the guide tubes. With the retractor system are two tubes 140 mm long. One has an inner diameter of 20 mm and the other 30 mm. Each retractor tube has a Delrin collet to hold it into the retractor mount. A ¼ inch-20 nylon thumb screw on the mount base tightens onto the collet, locking the retractor tube into place.

The retractor tube maintains an open channel to the bottom of the surgical field. To start the resection, a cortical incision is made and the appropriate size of tube is inserted. Using a Sharplan 1100 CO_2 laser (Sharplan Inc., Tel Aviv, Israel), the surgeon, working through

the tube, extends the depth of the incision. A dilator, whose leading edge is shaped like the bow of a ship, is inserted through the tube to spread the incision while the retractor tube is advanced. Advancement of the retractor tube requires a repetitive sequence of incision and advancement.

The depth to which the retractor is advanced is important because it maintains the relationship between the surgical field and the software reconstruction of the tumor. The range of the tumor reconstruction is provided in millimeter distances from the target point along the trajectory. Measurement of the length of retractor extending beyond the retractor mount will determine its position along the viewline. Each retractor tube is engraved with three lines at the proximal end, representing the 0, +5, and +10 levels. When the zero mark is flush with the retractor mount, the tube is at the zero level. Any distance between the zero level and the retractor mount represents the negative level of the tube.

The COMPASS™ automated stereotactic positioner

The COMPASS™ stereotactic positioner is a 3-D slide which maintains a specific relationship between the arc-quadrant and the patient's head secured in a headholder. Each element attaches to the 3-D positioner, as seen in Fig. 6.6.

From the face of the base plate extend two arms used to suspend the arc-quadrant. The legs of the arc have tapered tabs which insert into receptacles at the end of these arms. Captive nuts of the arc screw down over the receptacles, securing the arc in place and setting the location of the focus with respect to the slide.

To the underside of the base plate attaches a 3-D dovetail slide, to which the headholder is secured. The x axis moves the headholder left and right, the y axis up and down, and the z axis in and out, adjusting its position with respect to the arc-quadrant. In doing so, different points are brought to the focus. The setting for each axis is read by the mechanical scales mounted to each axis. The value of these settings determines the coordinate of the point located at the focus.

Determination of the coordinates of the surgical target are made either with the COMPASS™

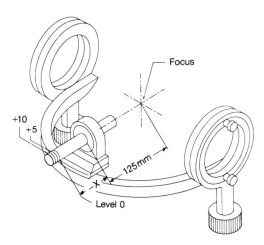

FIGURE 6.5 The retractor maintains an open channel to the tumor volume through which the surgeon can work. Measuring from the zero line to the retractor car (−X) will determine the depths of the surgical field proximal to the focus. Graduations at the end of the tube give the depths distal to the focus. These depths are entered into the computer to display the appropriate volume cross-section.

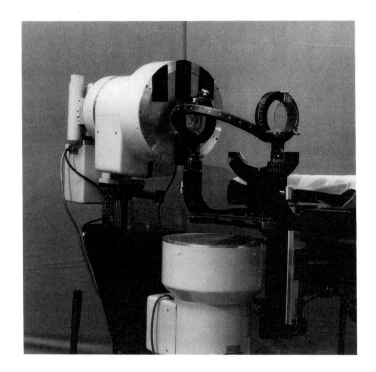

FIGURE 6.6 The 160 mm arc mounts onto the extension arms of the 3-D slide. The slide moves the headholder with respect to the stationary arc. Anterior-posterior and lateral reticules mark the location of the focus on teleradiographs. A set of image intensifiers, mounted onto a portable trolley, replace conventional film by providing the video source to generate digital teleradiographs.

surgical planning software or through calculations derived from biplane teleradiographs. A more detailed discussion of this process will follow.

The COMPASS™ stereotactic positioner evolved through many revisions, beginning with modifications made to a Todd–Wells stereotactic machine. This unit, originally designed for functional procedures, lent itself readily to biopsies and single point targets, where positioning of the 3-D slide could be completed prior to locking the patient in place. However, as software developments allowed for quantitative volumetric resections of tumor, intraoperative adjustments became necessary. This was very difficult once the scales and slides were covered with sterile drapes. One had to literally use a flashlight to accomplish a translation. For these reasons, when the COMPASS™ positioner was developed, each axis was equipped with linear encoders and stepper motors to allow positioning from a remote site.

The linear encoders are a portion of the Acu-Rite III digital display system (Acu-Rite Inc., Jamestown, NY). The encoders are glass scales with etched tic marks that are electronically counted by a reading head as it passes over the

scale. A conversion of these counts generates a remote digital display of the slide's position in addition to the mechanical scales. Being located remotely allows the slide's position to be monitored easily during surgery. In addition, the Acu-Rite III system is interfaced to the surgical computer forming a portion of the automated positioning system.

Stepper motors (Compumotor Division, Parker Hannifin Corporation, Rohnert Park, CA) are attached to each axis with a motor mount containing a 70 : 1 gear reduction. The purpose of this is twofold: (1) to reduce the physical size and weight of the motor, the gearbox compensates for the low torque of the smaller sized motors; (2) it mechanically limits the maximum velocity of the translation. This safety feature, added for automated positioning, prevents the slide translating faster than the surgeon can react. The gear ratio was calculated to provide a comfortable translation speed when the motors are running at maximum speed. Activation of the motors may be accomplished by one of two methods. The first method is by remote control via the control rack. Each axis is equipped with a set of push-button switches to activate the motors, one for the positive direction and the other for the negative direction.

Using this method, one simply depresses the desired direction to move each axis.

The other method is to have the computer position the target automatically. This method, to be discussed in further detail later, relies on the computer to determine the amount and direction each axis needs to be moved.

An earlier version of the 3-D slide was built onto a hydraulic industrial table, because it provided a solid base to keep the arc orthogonal to the X-ray tubes and the height could be adjusted to a comfortable working height. It was deemed unlikely, at this point in time, that tilting the head or the other articulations of a standard operating table would be of much value: on the contrary, it was believed that the added articulations would hinder X-ray collimation. This inflexibility did create problems with proper patient positioning for craniotomies. Since the head could not be elevated properly, the experience of brain swelling was not uncommon.

The development of a reliable X-ray alignment system alleviated the problems of obtaining precise collimation. The system, to be described later on, does not require a rigid mount for the stereotactic positioner to obtain good alignment. It had the ability to adjust for changes in the alignment intraoperatively. Because of this, the COMPASS™ positioner was designed to mount onto the arm rails of a standard operating table. In doing so, one could elevate the unit to a comfortable working height and raise the patient's head. For craniotomies, the table is positioned in a fashion that is optimal for the patient and the surgeon.

In addition to having the positioner mounted onto the operating table, a portable floorstand was fabricated onto which it could mount. The base of this unit has a large "O" ring a vacuum port. By using the room's vacuum system, the stand can be secured to the floor. Due to the latex flooring in our operating rooms, a metal plate was installed into the floor to prevent the vacuum from lifting the flooring.

The need for a floorstand is twofold. First, for functional procedures where precise X-ray alignment is essential, the floorstand provides a more secure base to maintain such alignment. If the operating table is used, operating room personnel leaning on the table could inadver-

tently corrupt the alignment without it being noticed.

The second use for the floorstand is for posterior fossa procedures where normal placement of the headholder would obstruct the surgical field. To access lesions in this area, the headholder is inverted to the patient so that it is suspended above (superior to) the head. In doing so, the basering is removed from the inferior portion of the head, leaving clear access to the region of interest. This is known as the "inverted position." From a mechanical standpoint, the patient is simply rotated 180° from the "normal" placement. For the 3-D positioner to deal with this situation requires the unit to be mounted onto the portable floorstand, and the two are rotated 180° to the operating table. In this fashion, the headholder, arc, and 3-D positioner maintain exactly the same orientation to each other. The only changes are anatomic, where left and right as well as superior and inferior are reversed.

The remote control console

To house all the electronic equipment for the motors and digital display system, a remote control rack is permanently installed into the operating room (Fig. 6.7). At the top of the unit is the Acu-Rite III counter for the digital display of the slide's position, at a level that is easily seen from most portions of the room.

Below this is the motor control section. A rotary switch determines whether the motors are to be activated automatically or remotely. Adjacent to this switch are three sets of two push-button switches used to activate the motors. This panel also has a speed control for setting the velocity of the motors when they are being operated remotely.

At the base of the unit are three Compumotor 2100-4 indexers. These circuit boards translate commands from a computer to drive the motors a certain number of steps in a given direction, at a given velocity. Also located in the base are the drives for each motor, which receive electrical pulses from either the indexers or the drives and amplify them to the motors.

In addition to this equipment, the rack also houses equipment to interface with the computer. First, there is a terminal to initiate the

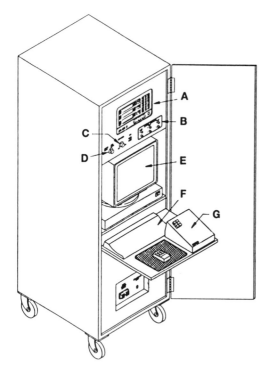

FIGURE 6.7 The remote control console built into the operating room houses the Acu-Rite III digital display (A). Three sets of push button switches (B) activate each motor in the + or − directions. Rotation of the potentiometer (C) determines the speed of translations when operating in the remote mode. Switch (D) determines whether the motors are to be activated remotely or automatically. The terminal (E) and keyboard (F) activate and interact with the surgical programs. The Vicom mouse and controller (G) are used to make menu selection from the surgical computer program.

software and to input certain information. There is a mouse device used to interact with the program. This includes six function buttons whose functions vary with the section of code in the program. Primarily, these are used to display various slices of tumor volume cross-sections. However, there is sufficient equipment to run any portion of the surgical software package as if it were being run at the treatment planning console. From this station, it is possible to select new targets, display old targets, review trajectories, or anything else that would provide information improving the outcome of the procedure.

Positioning a surgical target

Primarily, the COMPASS™ system relies on the computer software to calculate the x, y, and z values of points selected on CT or MR images depicting the area of interest. Using this approach, one need only to match the position of the slide to the calculated values.

The COMPASS™ positioner does, in fact, allow for the more traditional approach to stereotaxy by determining surgical targets from biplane teleradiographs. The 160 mm arc is equipped with a set of lateral X-ray reticules to mark the location of the focus on the lateral images. Likewise, an anterior−posterior reticule is attached to the arc extension arms to locate the focus in the anterior−posterior plane. This approach does assume proper alignment between the X-ray tubes and the stereotactic positioner, as described in the section on teleradiography.

To determine a target using traditional methods requires a biplane acquisition with a known setting of the 3-D slide. This could be a ventriculogram, for instance, used in planning a thalamotomy. The x, y, and z values for the slide's position need to be recorded at the time of the ventriculogram. Once the location of the target is mapped out on the X-ray images, the distance from the focus for both the y and z axes are measured from the lateral projection. Likewise, the distance between the target and focus is measured for the x axis from the anterior−posterior projection. These measurements are corrected for image magnification and applied to the starting position to determine the coordinate value of the surgical target.

Once the target is selected, the COMPASS™ automated positioner may be operated either manually, remotely, or automatically to access the target. Manual operation is the backup mode and ensures that the unit can be used in the event of power failure or technical difficulties. This method of operation requires the motors to be disengaged from the leadscrews, which are then turned with handcranks to translate the slide. The mechanical scales become the sole means of reading the position of each axis. A surgical target is easily accessed by simply turning the leadscrew until the mechanical scale of each axis reads the value of the calculated target coordinate.

Regardless of the method of operation, the mechanical scales generate the absolute value of the coordinate located at the focus of the arc, and should be checked prior to the start of the case. Both the remote and automatic operation of the positioner require a synchronization between the Acu-Rite III digital counter and the mechanical scales before the start of the case. This is accomplished by adjusting each mechanical scale to zero, followed by setting each axis of the digital counter to zero by depressing the *zero reset* button on the digital counter. This being completed correctly will result in the display having the same value as the mechanical scales.

Remote positioning of the COMPASS™ stereotactic positioner requires using the remote control panel of the remote control rack to activate the motors in lieu of using a handcrank. Depressing the push button switches for each axis will drive each axis in either the positive or negative direction until the desired coordinate is displayed on the digital display. A speed control knob is used to adjust the speed of translation. As with manual positioning, each axis needs to be set to the coordinate calculated during the treatment planning session.

Using the COMPASS™ stereotactic positioner in the automated mode requires the coordination of several pieces of equipment. The system has been designed as a closed loop system, meaning a dual method for confirming proper positioning of the slide. The foundation of the system is the array of stepper motors. One revolution requires 25 000 individual steps. Calculating for the pitch of the leadscrew and the gear ratio requires 1.1 million steps to advance the slide 1 mm. To calculate the number of steps that need to be applied, one must first know the present location of each axis and the desired position for the target. The software accesses the Acu-Rite III counter via an RS-232 communication port to determine the starting position of the 3-D slide. This position is compared with the final target position. The distance required to move each axis is calculated and translated into the appropriate number of steps. The velocity at which each axis will translate will be a percentage of the maximum velocity, based on a percentage of the longest move. In this fashion, each axis will begin and stop simultaneously. This is an important feature in that it emulates the method of translation made in the software package when accessing different portions of a large tumor.

At this point, the software addresses indexers for each motor conveying the number of steps each motor must take and the velocity at which to take them. A pause in the software will keep the motors dormant until the surgeon depresses a footswitch to activate the motor. If the footswitch remains depressed until completion of the move, the motors will automatically stop. If, at any point during translation, the footswitch is released, the translation is automatically terminated. Once the motors have stopped, the digital counter is always read to determine if the move has been completed correctly or not. If further translations are required, the process is repeated until the proper position is reached.

The process of starting and stopping during a translation is very common during a craniotomy. The surgeon, watching the move under direct vision, may opt to stop moving, to continue resecting or to deal with some bleeding that has started. This is done very simply by releasing the footswitch when the slide needs to be stopped and depressing it when it is time to resume translation.

In a automated system, one must deal with the problem of backlash of the leadscrew. This is a situation caused by mechanical gap between the teeth of the leadscrew and nut. When reversing the direction of rotation of the leadscrew, there is a small amount of rotation of the leadscrew which occurs before the slide actually begins to translate. Backlash does not affect positioning in a manual mode because one simply turns the leadscrew until the position is correct with regards to the mechanical scales. For this reason, linear encoders were chosen because, like mechanical scales, they are unaffected by backlash. They are mounted onto the slide independently of the driving mechanism and show only the relationship between the rail and car for a given axis. To position the slide remotely, one depresses the correct push buttons until the correct coordinate is displayed on the Acu-Rite III counter. Both approaches provide an absolute position between the rail and car.

However, it is very important in an automated system to keep track of backlash and therefore the last direction each axis has travelled. The sequence of events to move the slide requires the computer to determine the distance between the present position of the slide and the desired position. The number of steps each motor needs to take is determined, and if a change in direction occurs, an additional number of steps will be added to compensate for backlash.

The stereotactic operating suite

In order for the software to be completely useful intraoperatively, the computer has to be easily accessed in the operating suite, and therefore a certain amount of equipment requires to be installed in the operating area. In our particular situation, the treatment planning center is located remotely, one floor above the operating suites. To allow the software to be used more effectively and efficiently, a secondary treatment planning console was installed between the two stereotactic operating suites. This console is the center of operations for the two stereotactic operating suites as it is used to control the events happening in each room

The computer is also accessible directly from inside the operating suite. To accomplish this, several pieces of equipment were installed, primarily equipment contained in the remote control console, such as a computer terminal and a Vicom mouse to interact with the software. From this station, it is possible to use any portion of the COMPASS™ software package.

To view the computer images, each stereotactic suite is equipped with two 23-inch Conrac black and white monitors and a 19-inch Conrac color monitor. From these monitors, a surgeon is able to view the active surgical target, a CT or MRI trajectory, digital angiograms and cross-sections of tumor volumes. The importance of this is not only the information displayed, but also the availability of the information during the surgery. In some instances, the surgical plan needs to be altered as the procedure progresses. The surgeon needs to be able to modify or review the surgical plan as the case progresses.

Interaction with the computer program was always an issue with the architecture of the program. Our original program was a very structured one, since the flow of the program was predetermined by the question posed in software that required answers to be entered in via a terminal. As such, it was impossible for the surgeon to control the computer directly or to access information once the procedure began. This major drawback in the program brought about the latest version of software, which is a menu-based program. This approach provides several advantages. First, the surgeon is able to approach the software in a number of different ways. Secondly, using the software requires the user only to learn how to use a mouse to point a cursor on the display monitor to choose different menu selections. It was thought that this approach would also be advantageous in the surgical setting because the mouse could be draped, allowing the surgeon to continue to communicate with the computer directly during a procedure. Practically, however, the mouse is not easy to use under sterile conditions. Draping of the mouse makes it very clumsy to use as the drapes tend to be obstructive.

To overcome this, a joystick (Fig. 6.8) was fabricated to emulate the Vicom mouse. This unit attaches to the extension arm of the slide, suspending it in a position that is convenient to the surgeon. This unit has three function buttons identical to the Vicom mouse, giving it the same capabilities. The joystick is easily draped and functions well under these conditions.

Fixed tube teleradiography

The design of the operating suite is such that it can support conventional and computer-assisted stereotaxy. It has fixed X-ray tubes that truly render the room a stereotactic suite. The tubes are mounted orthogonal to each other, 4 m from the isocenter, maintaining the criteria of traditional settings for the purpose of reducing image magnification. At this distance, the X-ray beams are traveling close to parallel as they pass through the head. As a result, the magnification factor remains nearly constant throughout the patient's head. This is an important

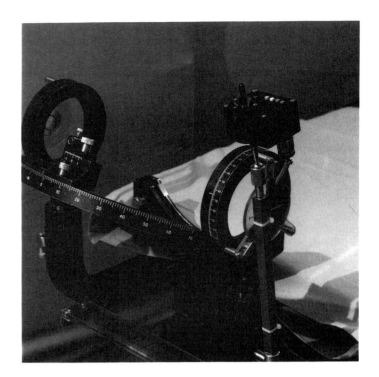

FIGURE 6.8 A custom joystick mounts onto the positioner, allowing the surgeon to interact with the software intraoperatively.

point if measurements are to made from the radiographs, as in functional procedures.

Proper alignment of the X-ray tubes is essential to accurately project the location of the focus on the radiograph. The criterion for alignment is to superimpose the isocenter and focus in such a manner that the positioner is orthogonal to each X-ray tube.

The majority of stereotactic procedures performed with the COMPASS™ system are completed with the unit attached to a standard operating table. Precise placement of the table for X-ray collimation is difficult, owing to the bulky nature of the operating table. A simplified process is to move the tubes. This is accomplished by mounting each tube on a 2-D slide. The slides provide the capability for linear translations, but cannot insure the tubes are orthogonal. This correction is handled differently for each tube. For the vertical tube, the tilts of the operating table are adjusted to make the positioner orthogonal. For the horizontal tube, there are two tilt adjustments, one for left/right and one for up/down. By themselves, the 2-D slides cannot perform the alignment. The necessary tool is a custom laser collimator (Fig. 6.9). This collimator has a laser mounted

perpendicular to the long axis of the collimating tube. The beam reflects off a mirror inside and is reflected out through the center of the aperture. Prior to installation, the mirror is adjusted until the laser beam is coaxial to the long axis of the collimating tube. Next, the collimator is mounted and adjusted until the laser beam projects directly into the center of the X-ray field. At this point, the laser and central beam are considered coaxial.

Alignment of the vertical tube is accomplished by first leveling the operating stereotactic positioner, using the tilt adjustments on the operating table. The arc-quadrant is then set to a collar and arc angle of zero degrees. This places the hole in the offset slide directly over the focus. Next, the laser beam is moved to the hole by translating the vertical tube. With everything correct, the central beam is projecting a path through the hole, focus and the center of the X-ray reticle.

In addition to the horizontal X-ray tube setup, a mirror mounted onto the lateral X-ray reticle and orthogonal to the focus is required. By moving the laser beam onto the mirror, and using the tilt adjustments of the horizontal setup, one can reflect the laser beam to its source.

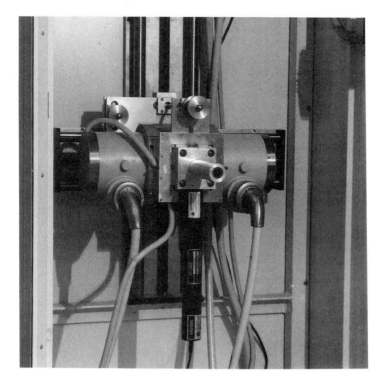

FIGURE 6.9 A custom laser collimator, attached to the X-ray tube, projects a helium–neon (HeNe) laser beam coaxial to the central X-ray beam to align the X-ray tube with the positioner. The X-ray tube is mounted on a 2-D slide in order to position the tube with respect to the stereotactic positioner. Notice the two adjustment knobs above the tube. These serve to tilt the tube up/down and left/right until it is orthogonal to the stereotactic positioner.

This insures the tube is orthogonal to the positioner. Once orthogonal, a linear translation will point the laser beam to the center of the reticule.

Historically, the intraoperative X-rays were the only source of information to derive the surgical target and were a necessity. Since many procedures are being planned without the use of this database, it is being omitted from stereotactic procedures altogether. However, the use of intraoperative X-rays is still a useful tool, even for computer-assisted procedures. The process of acquiring data, planning targets and trajectories, and finally applying the information to the stereotactic positioner, requires a multitude of very precise steps and calculations. A mistake, at any point, may create an error in positioning of the patient. The computer is only a tool to assist the surgeon. Human interaction can introduce errors into the system. A safe approach to use is a method independent of the computer to verify that the procedure is progressing correctly. Teleradiography can be used for such purposes by evaluating the location of the focus on the radiographs to anatomic landmarks. An experienced surgeon is able to tell if the target is in the correct location.

The COMPASS™ system requires some measuring and addition to determine how far to advance the surgical probe. Radiographs are able to confirm that this has been completed correctly. In addition to being a safety system, documentation of a procedure provides other information that may be useful in future procedures. For instance, having documented biopsy sites, one could correlate the location with pathology to help map the boundaries of a tumor.

Documenting each biopsy site, although prudent, is time-consuming and exposes the patient to additional radiation. A teleradiographic image intensifier system was constructed to overcome these drawbacks. An overview of the system comprises a set of circuit boards, the video acquisition digitizer/video acquisition processor (VAD/VAP), installed into the Vicom. The function of these boards is to accept a standard video signal and process it into a digital image. For this application, the video output from a pair of image intensifiers is sent to the VAD/VAP to generate digital teleradiographs.

For this system, a pair of image intensifiers (Precise Optics, Bay Shore, NY) are mounted orthogonally onto a portable cart and are positioned to the COMPASS™ positioner in lieu of X-ray films. Minor modifications of the X-ray equipment were required to synchronize the output of X-rays with image acquisition. To do this, a remote trigger switch was fabricated to activate the acquisition process when the X-ray exposure button is depressed.

This system was designed not to produce fluoroscopy, but rather single exposures as with film. Two distinct advantages are the availability of images in under 15 s and an eight-fold reduction of the radiation delivered. A typical exposure for a lateral projection, using film, is 400 mA at 80 KVp for 0.8 s. A similar exposure using the intensifiers requires only 50 mA at 80 KVp for 0.5 s. Our experience is that documenting a procedure requires an average of four sets of radiographs. Standard film techniques, which take an average of 7 minutes per set to present the images, require nearly 30 minutes of operating room time. In contrast, less than 1 minute of operating room time was spent with digital teleradiography.

The use of digital teleradiography does have limitations for functional procedures which require successive radiographs to be overlaid to compare positioning. It is not currently possible to provide this feature using digital teleradiography, but future work in this area may make this feasible.

The intramicroscope graphic display

Computer monitors in the operating room are useful and effective tools for displaying information in the patient's database. One type of image used extensively in volumetric resections is cross-sections of tumor volumes. These images provide a template of tumor boundaries as the surgeon works to resect a tumor. To be useful in a quantitative sense, a method is needed to correlate the surgical field to the computer display. The first attempt was an interactive laser micromanipulator. This device controlled the positions of both a CO_2 laser and a cursor on the slice image. The cursor was calibrated to the position of the laser in order to represent the location of the laser in the tumor volume. Perfect alignment of the laser was required to maintain calibration and, in the end, this approach was not very practical.

The next approach was to display cross-sections of a tumor along with a graphical representation of the retractor tube. The surgeon would use the retractor display as a guide in locating the edges of the tumor. This approach, although successful, continually caused the surgeon to divert his eyes from the surgical field to interpret the images.

This situation led to the development of the intramicroscope display. This device projects a scaled image of the tumor into the surgical microscope to be overlaid on the surgical field (Fig. 6.10). The image then becomes a template of the tumor boundary and guides the surgeon during the resection.

To accomplish this, a new beam splitter for the Zeiss microscope was fabricated. The left side was unaltered, allowing attachment of an assistant arm. A video monitor was mounted on the right side of the beam splitter. For the right side, the beam splitter was rotated 180°, bringing an image from the side port to the surgeon's eye. On this monitor is a display of tumor cross-sections. The monitor arm has a zoom feature that allows the image to be scaled to real size. Preoperatively, the microscope is focused onto a metric rule. Using a computer image of the 2 cm retractor displayed on the monitor, the zoom is altered until the retractor encompasses a true 2 cm diameter.

The zoom feature allows the surgeon to alter the field magnification of the microscope and still maintain proper scaling of the intramicroscope graphics. Intraoperative changes are accomplished by focusing the retractor display over the true retractor and adjusting the image size to fit.

In addition to being used with the stereotactic retractor, the intramicroscope graphics may be used on cases where a trephine is placed over a superficial lesion. The surgical software allows for the selection of a 38.1 mm or 50.8 mm trephine display. This display is centered over the actual trephine, showing the relationship between tumor boundary and the trephine edges.

Discussion

From an equipment standpoint, there are two categories of stereotactic procedures, those with a single-point target and those with a volu-

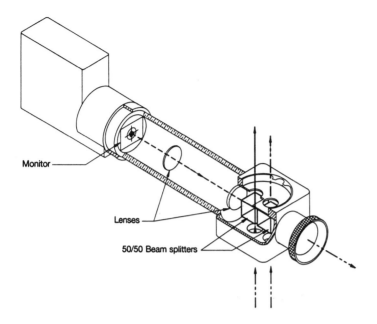

Monitor

Lenses

50/50 Beam splitters

FIGURE 6.10 The intramicroscope graphics mount onto a Zeiss surgical microscope to project a computer generated tumor cross-section to the surgeon. The scaled image appears superimposed over the surgical field and acts as a guide to the location of the tumor volume.

metric target. The single-point procedures possible with this system include biopsies, third ventriculostomies, cyst aspirations, ^{32}P installation, installing Ommaya reservoirs, electrode implants, implanting ^{192}Ir, and thalamotomies. Volumetric procedures are primarily craniotomies for the resection of intracranial lesions. However, selective removal of anatomic structures such as the amygdala or hippocampus is also possible.

From a mechanical standpoint, completion of these procedures is essentially the same once the treatment plan has been generated. For both categories of procedure, the surgical target is dialed in to the 3-D slide. For the majority of procedures, this target is in the center of an intracranial lesion. For procedures such as third ventriculostomies and hippocampectomies, an anatomic feature is used as the target. In either event, the slide is positioned to coordinates of the surgical target using one of the positioning methods.

The second step is to position the patient, with the headholder, onto the 3-D slide by inserting the basering into the headholder cradle. The patient orientation is set by rotating the basering until the number aligned with the tic mark matches the orientation of the planned surgical target. It is essential to confirm that the patient rotation matches the surgical plan to accurately access the desired target. Once pos-

itioned, the patient is prepared and draped in the usual fashion.

After draping, the process will vary depending on the individual procedure. For most procedures accessing a single point in space, the 160 mm arc-quadrant is secured to the extension arms and the X-ray tubes are collimated as previously described. Once the arc and collar angles are set to the predetermined values, the guide tube is advanced to the scalp. At this point, a set of X-rays are taken to confirm that the position of the patient is indeed correct. Once confirmed, a stab wound is made and the guide tube is advanced to the skull. Using a $\frac{7}{64}$ inch (2.77 mm) twist drill, a hole is made through the skull and the dura is opened with monopolar cautery and a coagulation probe.

At this point, the depth to which the desired instrument is to be inserted is calculated and inserted through the guide tube. Every essential feature of the target is documented using digital teleradiography. In a biopsy procedure, this would include each biopsy site. In other procedures, X-rays would document the final location of an electrode position, the tip of a needle for injecting ^{32}P, or the placement of a leukotome.

For point-in-space procedures, the computer is used to redisplay the treatment plan. This includes displaying the trajectory on CT, MRI, and DSA. Using the joystick or the Vicom mouse in the control rack, the surgeon can selectively display the portion of the surgical plan which would be most beneficial.

Volumetric procedures tend not to use the CT, MRI, and DSA images directly as in the single-point procedures. These procedures typically use information extracted from the database from the generation of a tumor volume. Cross-sections of the volume are displayed sequentially on the large graphic monitors with a representation of either a retractor tube or trephine opening. Using the joystick, the surgeon controls which level through the volume is displayed on the monitors and in the intra-microscope graphics display. The level displayed is determined as previously described.

Our experience has been that the 2 cm retractor is used on the majority of deep-seated lesions, even when the tumor boundaries extend beyond the limits of the tube [11]. To access these portions requires the head to be moved, bringing different portions of the lesion under the retractor tube. The amount and direction of this translation is determined with the aid of the computer and the graphics display in the operating room. Using the joystick, the surgeon selects the *translate* command from the software menu. This function generates a cursor on the monitor that is the size of the retractor tube being used. The surgeon will use the joystick to alter the location of the cursor until it is over the desired portion of the tumor cross-section. Once the cursor is positioned, a calculation is made to determine a new 3-D coordinate within the tumor volume which centers the desired section of tumor under the retractor tube.

Once the calculations are complete, the 3-D slide needs to be translated to match the new numbers. The method of translating the slide is the same as in positioning the original target value. In the manual mode, one would simply turn the handcranks until the mechanical scales show the appropriate values. This has the disadvantage of having the slide covered by surgical drapes. In the remote mode, the remote control buttons would be depressed until the digital display shows the correct values. The person assisting the surgeon with the translation would move each axis one at a time until the move was complete. The assistant would have

to stop and start at the command of the surgeon until the move was complete. In the automated mode, the surgeon only needs to depress the footswitch to start the movement. This approach has the least chance of positioning error introduced by human error. Because of the closed-loop positioning system, there is an automatic internal check to see if correct positioning has been obtained.

Conclusions

The use of computers for stereotactic procedures has been well established over the last 10 years, beginning with utilizing images that can only be generated with computing power. Since that time, great efforts have been made to develop treatment-planning software, with most of the effort being directed to the determination of a point in space. However, the planning and surgical software developed for this system greatly enhances the use and need for using the computer as a surgical tool, as it provides for a variety of procedures such as biopsies, volumetric craniotomies, third ventriculostomies, ^{32}P instillation, placement of ^{192}Ir sources, and cyst aspirations.

The layout of the stereotactic and computer equipment has made an environment conducive for using the computer as a neurosurgical tool. It is available and easy for the surgeon to access at any time during the last two phases of a stereotactic procedure. The surgeon is therefore more likely to use it because it is not disturbing his train of thought but increasing his confidence about the outcome of the procedure. In addition, using the computer does not increase the length of the procedure, and in some instances reduces it. For example, using the computer to generate digital teleradiographs maintains a safety factor in performing biopsies, while reducing operating time and cutting the radiation exposure of the patient. Efficient use of operating time is essential in any operating setting, and we have shown that computer-assisted stereotaxy can be effective.

The groundwork has been laid for using the computer as a surgical tool and applying a computer-assisted surgical plan. As technology and software improves, better and more detailed surgical plans will be simulated and applied in surgery and the computer will evolve into an essential surgical tool.

References

1 Brown, R.A. A stereotactic headframe for use with CT body scanners. *Invest. Radiol.* **14**: 300−4 (1979).

2 Goerss, S., Kelly, P.J., Kall, B.A. & Alker, G.J. Jr. A computed tomography stereotactic adaptation system. *Neurosurgery* **10**: 375−9 (1982).

3 Kelly, P.J., Alker, G.J., Kall, B.A. & Goerss, S.J. Method of computer tomography based stereotactic biopsies with arteriographic control. *Neurosurgery* **14**: 172−7 (1984).

4 Leksell, L. & Jernberg, B. Stereotaxis and tomography: a technical note. *Acta Neurochir. (Wien)* **52**: 1−7 (1980).

5 Kelly, P.J. Volumetric stereotactic resection of intra-axial brain mass lesions. *Mayo Clin. Proc.* **63**: 1186−98 (1988).

6 Kelly, P.J., Goerss, S., Kall, B.A. & Kispert, D. Computer tomography-based stereotactic third ventriculostomy: technical note. *Neurosurgery* **18**(6): 791−4 (1984).

7 Kelly, P.J., Kall, B.A. & Goerss, S. Computer assisted simulations for the stereotactic placement of interstitial radionuclide sources into computer tomography-defined tumor volumes. *Neurosurgery* **14**: 442−8 (1984).

8 Kelly, P.J., Sharbrough, F.W., Kall, B.A. *et al.* Magnetic resonance imaging-based computer-assisted stereotactic resection of the hippocampus and amygdala in patients with temporal lobe epilepsy. *Mayo Clin. Proc.* **62**: 103−8 (1987).

9 Kall, B.A. The impact of computer and imaging technology on stereotactic surgery. *Appl. Neurophysiol.* **50**: 9−22 (1987).

10 Lundsford, L.D. A dedicated CT system for the stereotactic operating room. *Appl. Neurophysiol.* **45**: 374−8 (1982).

11 Kelly, P.J., Goerss, S.J. & Kall, B.A. The stereotactic retractor in computer-assisted stereotaxic microsurgery. *J. Neurosurg.* **69**: 301−6 (1988).

part III

Functional Neurosurgery

A

Computer-based Stereotactic Atlases

Computer Three-dimensional Stereotactic Anatomic Reconstructions of the Human Brainstem

Farhad Afshar, E. Dykes, John G. Holman, and M. John Cookson

Introduction

The brainstem, perhaps more than any other part of the central nervous system, is tightly packed with nuclei and tracts whose configurations and relationships to each other vary at every millimeter from the midbrain to the cervicomedullary junction.

The classic neuroanatomic approach in studying these regions of the brain is based on the production of sequential transverse, horizontal and sagittal sections of varying thickness, and then at representative levels to relate particular structures to adjacent visible nuclei and tracts. From such studies, two-dimensional (2-D) atlases are constructed in one or more planes [1-8].

The rapid progress in neuroimaging techniques, such as computed tomography (CT) and magnetic resonance imaging (MRI), and their application to integrated stereotactic procedures, now enable all regions of the brainstem to be reached for tumor biopsy, interstitial irradiation [9], cysts, abscesses, and hematoma evacuation [10,11]. Such procedures increasingly require a precise knowledge of both the position and variability of structures through which a catheter, cannula, or electrode may be passed [12].

The ability to reconstruct these complex and variable anatomic structures in three-dimensional (3-D) format can both improve target site delineation and allow predetermined choices for the optimal and safest trajectory of the cannula or electrode.

The techniques of computer-assisted 3-D reconstruction of the brainstem, described below, enable structures to be rotated and viewed from any given direction, allowing better elucidation of a particular feature or features.

This chapter will deal primarily with techniques whereby data from a specific 2-D stereotactic atlas, produced by Afshar *et al.* [1,13] for the human brainstem and cerebellar nuclei, with variability studies of the major tracts and nuclei, has been regenerated using 3-D computer-based recording techniques. The latest techniques for the application of microcomputer-based reconstruction systems to produce realistic 3-D shaded images from serial sections will be discussed in detail.

During the past 100 years, physical models made of solid sheets of wood, plastic or wax have been used to build 3-D models. Augustine [14] described a lucite plate model with 3-D reconstruction of neuronal populations, drawing sections to scale on transparent sheets and assembling these into stacks for viewing. In recent years the use of computer graphic systems has enabled a more versatile approach.

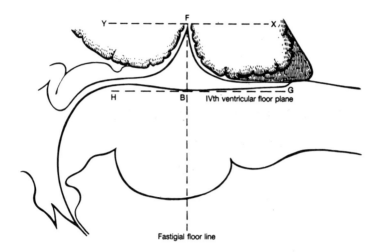

FIGURE 7.1 Sagittal section of brainstem to show reference points and planes for measurement of brainstem structures. F = fastigium; F−B = fastigial floor line. All transverse sections are related to the fastigial floor plane. Measurements caudal to the F−B line are designated as negative and those rostral as positive. H−B−G = IVth ventricular floor plane; Y−F−X = line passing through the fastigium and parallel to the IVth ventricular floor plane.

The 2-D stereotactic atlas — database for 3-D reconstruction

In stereotactic surgery, the localization of the target and subsequent electrode placement utilize a stereotactic brain atlas, together with microelectrode recordings [15] and electrophysiologic stimulation [16,17] using low voltage currents.

Criteria for optimal accuracy must further take into account the variability of nuclei or tracts, using measurements from well defined internal reference points and planes whose own inherent variability is known. The database for all our 3-D computer reconstructions of the human brainstem is based on the stereotactic atlas of Afshar *et al.* [1].

In this study the authors utilized autopsied human cadavers in which the brainstem was fixed *in situ* within the posterior fossa, using the Corsellis technique [18]. Specific measures to minimize shrinkage and distortion were undertaken and the techniques used have been detailed in earlier publications [19−25]. Reference points and planes with the least inherent variability for measuring structures within the brainstem were chosen. These reference points were chosen to be at the midpoint between the rostral mesencephalon and the cervicomedullary junction and have been found to be readily demonstrable radiologically, using air ventriculography, reconstructed CT scanning, or with sagittal magnetic resonance (MR) studies.

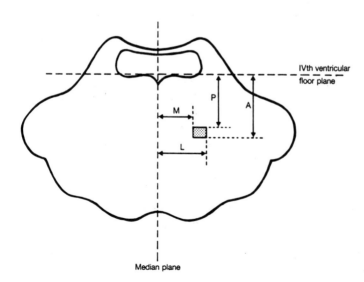

FIGURE 7.2 Anterior and posterior measurements of structures rostral to the −15 mm level are measured from the IVth ventricular floor plane. A = anterior, L = lateral; M = medial; P = posterior.

For the purposes of the original 2-D atlas, the plane of section for the 1 mm transverse slices (shown in Fig, 7.1) was based on the fastigium of the IVth ventricle (F) and the point B on the IVth ventricular floor opposite to the point F. The line HBG is a tangent to the IVth ventricular floor and forms a second plane of reference from which anterior—posterior measurements of structures in the brainstem and pons are made. Medial and lateral borders of structures are measured from the midline of the brainstem (Fig. 7.2), and rostral and caudal measurements of each nucleus and tract are related to the fastigial—IVth ventricular line, FB (Fig. 7.1). With structures more than 15 mm caudal to the fastigium, the anterior—posterior measurements of structures were taken from the posterior surface of the medulla (Fig. 7.3).

Using such techniques, all the major nuclei and tracts within the brainstem were precisely mapped and variability tables of each structure at every 1 mm calculated. This information has been presented as both probability table and computer graphic display printouts. From the wealth of anatomic statistical data a composite atlas of 1 mm sections in the transverse plane was drawn (Fig. 7.4), from the upper mesencephalon to the cervicomedullary junction. Each of the structures drawn is based on calculations of means from the data obtained from 70% or more of the specimens.

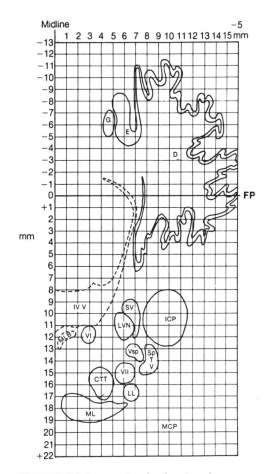

FIGURE 7.4 Stereotaxic atlas drawing of hemi-brainstem transverse section, 5 mm caudal to the fastigial level. CTT = central tegmental tract; D = dentate nucleus; E = emboliform nucleus; G = globose nucleus; ICP = inferior cerebellar peduncle; LL = lateral lemniscus; LVN = lateral vestibular nucleus; MCP = middle cerebellar peduncle; ML = medial lemniscus; MLB = medial longitudinal bundle; SpTV = spinal tract of V; SV = superior vestibular nucleus; IV V = fourth ventricle; Vsp = spinal nucleus of V; VI = VI nerve nucleus; VII = VII nerve nucleus. The drawings in heavy outline are based on statistical data and indicate structures are present in 70% or more of the specimens studied. Note that one of the reference lines in this example uses the fastigial plane (FP), as cerebellar nuclei are incorporated. For brainstem structure the IVth ventricular floor line is more frequently used.

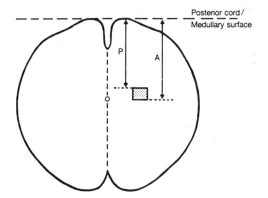

FIGURE 7.3 Anterior and posterior measurements of structures caudal to −15 mm level are measured from the posterior medullary surface. A = anterior; P = posterior.

Conversion of 2-D data to 3-D format

Two techniques have been used for acquisition of 2-D data to produce 3-D reconstructions.

Initially each transverse section of the original atlas was photographed and produced as a positive on 35 mm photographic film. Each slide was then digitized on an $x-y$ plotting microscope [26]. A total of 54 sections at 1-mm intervals were thus digitized. On each section positions of two or more reference grid points were also digitized. In order to enable correct orientation of one section to its adjacent section, these fixed reference points common to all sections were used in the x and y plane. A second method used involved the acquisition of data from a digitizing tablet. The points were recorded and displayed on the screen of a computer by a program which uses the GEM graphics package and the IBM EGA display board. This program allows editing to be performed on the current slice being processed. Individual points, sets of points or a whole section of data can be deleted and replaced. The data recorded include two reference points per section, the z value of the section and pairs of x, y coordinates. Each structure is treated individually to produce a separate data file. The contours are scaled and orientated to the correct alignment and size relative to each other. Each individual structure is then represented in an internally consistent fashion.

Multiple structures forming a single field of view, however, need to be related to a common coordinate system. A further program scales and orientates the structures which are to be displayed together, relative to an appropriate origin and coordinate axes. Points are digitized in a clockwise direction for external surfaces and in a counter-clockwise direction for internal surfaces.

The original programs used to produce the 3-D reconstructions were written in FORTRAN and run on a CDC 6600 computer at the University of London Computer Centre (ULCC). This used several microfilm plotting subroutines then available from the library of subroutines for microfilm plotting (DF Film), also available at ULCC. The initial 3-D reconstructed views were based on the programs of Kimura *et al.* [27]. With minor modifications, we were able to generate 3-D displays of the brainstem sections with and without a hidden line removal technique. The latter technique enables visualization of structures through overlapping struc-

tures (Fig. 7.5). Where a hidden line removal technique is used, those structures which underly a structure from the viewing position are not drawn, and this improves the 3-D quality of the regenerated structures (Fig. 7.6). Programs for these techniques now exist for both large computers [28–30] and microcomputers [31–3]. With the available data, rotation through any of three coordinates is possible and allows viewing of specific structures from any direction. Its value is readily appreciated in the example given. A further program was written to view reconstructed structures as stereopairs in any given orientation. Each image is reconstructed such that the interocular angle is 6°. The use of stereo-spectacles enables true 3-D views of specific nuclei and tracts throughout their course within the brainstem, and is particularly useful in pre-planning optimal trajectories in stereotactic or open surgical procedures to the brainstem. These programs suffered serious limitations, being based on large mainframe systems, with no possibility of on-line user interaction with the image generation process.

More serious were fundamental limitations of reconstructions based on the drawings. In

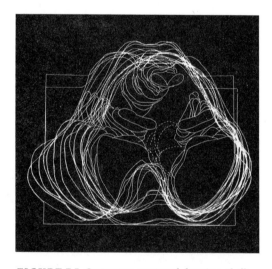

FIGURE 7.5 Computer generated drawing of all sections rostral to the fastigium containing the periaqueductal gray dorsally, the medial lemniscus within the tegmentum, and the corticospinal tracts anteriorly. In this reconstruction, no hidden line removal technique has been applied, enabling tracts to be visualized through overlapping structures.

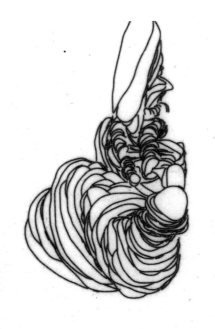

FIGURE 7.6 Computer generated drawing of eight hemi-brainstem structures using hidden line removal technique and viewed from caudal to rostral. The structures included in this reconstruction include the corticospinal tract anteriorly, the central tegmental tract and the superior cerebellar peduncle posteriorly, with its rostral and medial configuration.

Choice of computer display technology

Two methods are commonly used for the display of medical imaging data. One method is typically used for data originating from scanning techniques such as CT, positron emission tomography (PET), or MRI. Each image from the scanner is a 2-D picture of a slice of finite thickness consisting of 3-D cuboid volume elements — "voxels." The manipulation and display of voxel data requires large amounts of random access memory (RAM) and disc space, and is inevitably slow. The second technique is to display the surface as a mesh of "tiles" or "patches." Storing the data in a surface representation can be more compact, and is a more natural method to use for data which are generated as a set of contours. An additional bonus of the latter technique is that producing realistically rendered surfaces on voxel-based systems is computationally expensive, and less feasible to do within a reasonable time on a basic computer system such as the IBM PC. The images presented here typically took a few minutes each to produce.

The computer display system

The reconstruction and display programs are written in Microsoft C for the IBM PC. The display boards used can be the IBM VGA, Real World Graphics PC4000, and IO Systems PLUTO. The PLUTO and PC4000 boards have resolutions of 768 × 576 pixels each and support 256 simultaneous colors or shades from a range of approximately 16.7 million. To allow realistic shading, a maximum of seven colors is allowed to be specified at one time, permitting the use of at least 32 shades per color. All the illustrations shown here (Figs 7.7–7.10) were produced at a resolution of 768 × 576 pixels. The program to produce the 3-D reconstructions was written by Cookson, Holman, and Dykes [16,34].

The corrected x, y, and z coordinates generated by the digitizing process are then inputted to a program which processes the serial sections to produce a 3-D model of each individual structure. A triangulation algorithm is used to reconstruct the surfaces between adjacent

the reconstructions produced, the reconstruction of the surface connecting the contours was left to the imagination of the viewer. If the contours overlapped from the chosen viewpoint, and the object was structurally simple, the illusion of three-dimensionality could be maintained and the image was relatively easy to interpret. Difficulties arose when the field of view was more complex or if the contours did not overlap significantly. When several objects were present, confusion arose over which contours belonged to which object. These difficulties were due to the lack of adequate depth and shape cues.

The development of microcomputer technology and good quality computer graphics lead to the possibility of producing a microcomputer-based 3-D reconstruction system that will allow user interaction, leading ultimately to a system capable of interactive treatment planning for preoperative use.

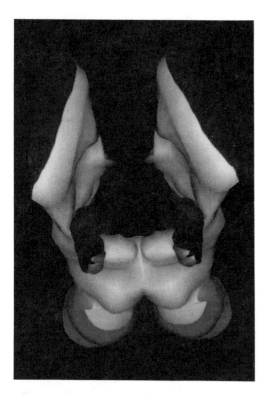

FIGURE 7.7 Computer generated 3-D
reconstruction in solid outlines and shaded images
after smoothing techniques have been applied.
Ordinarily this is displayed as a color graphic which is
shown here in grayscale. Superior and cerebellar
peduncle, central tegmental tract, and red nucleus
are each indicated by a separate color. Structures
viewed from caudal to rostral, counter-clockwise tilt
of 15° about the *x* axis.

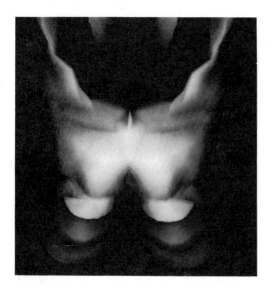

FIGURE 7.8 Structures as in Fig. 7.7. Counter-
clockwise tilt of 90° about the *x* axis.

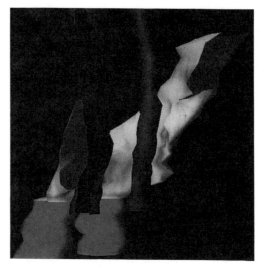

FIGURE 7.9 Structures as in Fig. 7.8. Central
tegmental tract on one side. Superior cerebellar
peduncle to enable a view within these solid
structures.

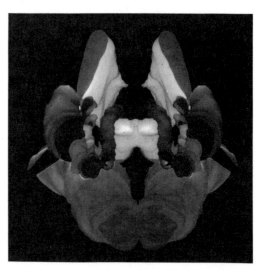

FIGURE 7.10 Brainstem structures as viewed in
Fig. 7.7 are usually depicted in color (shown here in
black and white). The trigeminal nerve can be seen
extending laterally. Also note the inferior cerebellar
peduncle, descending spinal tract of V, and superior
vestibular nucleus.

contours in the form of strips of triangles. At each step in the triangulation of a pair of contours, a new triangle is added to the strip so far constructed by incorporating the next point from one of these contours.

Decisions as to the relationships between features in sequential sections often requires higher-level knowledge of the nature of the structures being modeled. For this reason, although triangulation can be performed automatically, provision is made for optimal human intervention. Screen display is provided for points from each pair of adjacent sections and an editing facility enables one to indicate the correct alignment of features between sections. Where objects branch and join, an extra section is interpolated in order to maintain continuity. For two objects of roughly circular cross-section joining into a single object, the form of the joining section is an approximate "figure of eight." Similar constructions can be made for more complex objects.

The surface-modeling program produces two output files for each structure. A file of triangle information contains an index of the vertices making up each triangle and the corresponding triangle normals. A file of vertex information contains the 3-D position of each vertex and the estimated surface normal vector at that vertex. The normal at a vertex is estimated by averaging normals of triangles sharing the vertex. This representation of the surface model is permanent and is used by the image generation program to display images as required.

Image generation

The image generation program produces shaded images from the data created by the surface-modeling program. To choose a view, the user specifies the target point within the object to appear at the centre of the image and then describes the position of the observer relative to the target.

The user may also define, on the screen upon which the image is to be generated, the magnification of the image and the size and shape of the viewpoint. The triangles making up the surface model are transformed to take account of these viewing parameters, and mapped into the 2-D display screen, using a perspective projection for maximum realism. The position of the front and back planes of the view volume can be specified. Clipping is applied to remove triangles and parts of triangles which fall outside the "view volume" determined by the parameters.

An optional "cutting plane" can be placed between the front and back clipping planes to cut off all parts of the current object closer to the viewpoint. Unlike the clipping planes, whose positions are fixed, the cutting plane can be removed or its position varied, for different objects. A cutting plane can be moved through a scene, which slices the object so that those parts closer to the observer than the plane are not displayed. The plane can be removed, and structures displayed subsequently can be drawn in their entirety. For hidden-surface removal, a depth-buffer algorithm is used to suppress the display of parts of an object that would be obscured from the chosen viewpoint by other parts closer to the observer [35].

For a realistic shaded image, the color and intensity of each pixel in the image must be chosen to simulate the effect of light falling upon the corresponding point of the object's surface. Each object is displayed with shades taken from a color scale determined by the illumination conditions and the surface characteristics of the object.

The user defines the field illumination parameters by setting the position of a single point source of white light and the intensity of this incident light source relative to that of the ambient illumination. The diffuse reflection characteristics of the surface are chosen by describing the appearance of the object, when illuminated by diffuse white light, in terms of its hue saturation and value. The user can also specify parameters which determine the specular reflection characteristics. The "degree of highlighting" determines the maximum intensity of the highlights, while the "degree of shine" alters their size. Thus, the shinier the object, the smaller the highlights. An effect of transparency can also be achieved by displaying an object as a fine mesh of pixels, through which underlying objects can be seen. Additionally, a "window" can be "cut" in the surface of an enclosing object to view enclosed structures.

A smoothing technique described by Gouraud [36] was used to avoid the faceted appearance that would result from an exact representation of the surface model. The shades of the vertices of each triangle are calculated from the calculations of the vertex normals produced during surface reconstructions. The shades of other pixels in the image of the triangle are then derived by linear interpolation from these vertex shades.

Once the triangulated representation is stored on disk in the machine, the generation of new views can be produced quickly. In particular, contours or unshaded wireframe images of triangles can be displayed very rapidly, allowing rapid identification of a suitable viewpoint from which a full shaded image can be produced.

Future developments

Improvements in the surface-modeling software are under active development. These improvements include techniques for easy and realistic joining of branched structures. This is possible with the existing programs, but slow.

The representation of the surface of an object by triangular tiles has allowed a further application of the program. The surface area of an object is estimated by running the area of all the triangles making up the surface model. The program can also produce estimates of volumes, and could produce centers of mass, moments, etc. This will have a major impact on the future developments of planning stereotactic−CT integrated interstitial brachytherapy for the treatment of malignant brain tumors. Simultaneous display will be possible for the isodose contours of radioactive materials and model structures.

The estimates of statistical variability in the dimensions of structures can be increased by the modeling program suite. In particular, structures can be dilated or transformed to provide surfaces of special treatment-planning value. Dilation of a structure by 2.5 times the standard error of the mean will provide a surface enclosing the 99% confidence limits of the extents of the structure.

If a structure is to be avoided during the passage of a cannula or electrode, such a representation should be invaluable. Equally, where it is essential to reach the center of a chosen target, contraction of the nearer surface provides a high level of confidence in the accuracy of the location of the target.

The system described in this paper is highly optimized in terms of speed. Time-critical segments of code have been translated from C to ASSEMBLER. It would be possible to improve speed several-fold by using a faster processor, several of which are available. However, the most promising prospect is the use of machines with highly parallel architectures, so that processing could be transformed quickly enough to allow animation and the exploitation of kinetic-depth effects for even better depth cues. A particularly interesting possibility is the use of the Intel i860 chip in an add-on board in the PC, which would allow real-time manipulations.

References

1 Afshar, E., Watkins, E.S. & Yap, J.C. *Stereotaxic Atlas of the Human Brainstem and Cerebellar Nuclei.* New York: Raven Press (1978).

2 Andrew, J. & Watkins, E.S. *A Stereotaxic Atlas of the Human Thalamus and Adjacent Structures.* Baltimore: Williams & Wilkins (1969).

3 Delmas, A. & Pertusit, B. *Topometric Cranioencephalique chez l'Homme.* Paris: Masson et Cie (1959).

4 Schaltenbrand, G. & Bailey, P. *Introduction to Stereotaxis with an Atlas of the Human Brain,* Vols I, II and III. Stuttgart: Thieme Verlag (1959).

5 Schaltenbrand, G. & Wahren, W. *Atlas for Stereotaxy of the Human Brain,* 2nd edn. Stuttgart: Thieme Verlag (1977).

6 Spiegel, E.A. & Wycis, H.T. *Stereoencephalotomy.* New York: Grune & Stratton (1952).

7 Van Buren, J.M. & MacCubbin, R.A. An outline atlas of the human basal ganglia with estimation of anatomical variants. *J. Neurosurg.* 19: 811−39 (1962).

8 Talairach, J., David, M. & Tournoux, P. *Atlas de l'Anatomie Stereotaxique.* Paris: Masson et Cie (1957).

9 Gutin, P.H., Phillips, T.L. & Hosobuchi, Y. Permanent and removal implants for the brachytherapy of brain tumours. *Int. J. Radiat. Oncol. Biol. Phys.* 7: 1371−81 (1981).

10 Bosh, D.A. & Beute, G.N. Successful stereotaxic evacuation of an acute pontomedullary haematoma. *J. Neurosurg.* 62: 153−6 (1985).

11 Hondo, H., Matsumoto, K., Tomida, K. & Shichijo, F. CT-controlled stereotactic aspiration in hypertensive brain haemorrhage. *Appl. Neurophysiol.* 50: 233−6 (1987).

12 McComas, A.J., Wilson, P., Martin-Rodriguez, J., Wallace, C. & Henkinson, H. Properties of somatosensory neurons in the human thalamus. *J. Neurol. Neurosurg. Psych.* **33**: 716−7 (1970).

13 Afshar, F. *A Stereotaxic Atlas of the Human Brainstem.* Doctoral thesis, University of London (1977).

14 Augustine, J.R. A lucite plate method for 3-dimensional reconstruction of neuronal populations. *J. Neurosci. Meth.* **4**: 63−71 (1981).

15 Tasker, R.R., Organ, L.W. & Hawrylshyn, P.A. The thalamus and midbrain of man. Springfield IL: Charles Thomas (1982).

16 Holman, J.G., Cookson, M.J. & Dykes, E. Applications of microcomputer-based reconstruction system to produce realistic three-dimensional images from serial sections. *Med. Inf.* **14**(2): 173−84 (1989).

17 Ohye, C., Fukamachi, A. & Narabayashi, H. Spontaneous and evoked activity of sensory neurones and their organisation in the human thalamus. *J. Neurol.* **203**: 219−34 (1972).

18 Corsellis, J.A.N. Individual variation in the size of the tentorial opening. *J. Neurol. Neurosurg. Psych.* **21**: 279−83 (1958).

19 Afshar, F. Variability study of human brain stem structures. *J. Neurol. Neurosurg. Psych.* **37**: 1278, (1974).

20 Afshar, F. & Dykes, E. A three-dimensional reconstruction of the human brainstem. *J. Neurosurg.* **57**: 491−5 (1982).

21 Afshar, F., Dykes, E. & Watkins, E.S. Three-dimensional stereotaxic anatomy of the human trigeminal nerve nuclear complex. *Appl. Neurophysiol.* **46**: 147−53 (1983).

22 Afshar, F., Dykes, E. & Mason, J. Three-dimensional visualisation of the trigeminal nuclear complex. *J. Anat.* **136**: 636 (1983).

23 Afshar, F. & Dykes, E. Computer generated three-dimensional visualisation of the trigeminal nuclear complex. *Surg. Neurol.* **22**: 189−96 (1984).

24 Afshar, F. Practical techniques in the study of stereotactic neuroanatomy. In: Crockard, H.A., Hayward, R., & Hoff, J.T. (eds.) *Neurosurgery. The Scientific Basis of Clinical Practice*, pp. 70−89. Oxford: Blackwell Scientific Publications (1985).

25 Afshar, F. Three-dimensional colour-coded computer graphic display of the anatomical data for the guidance of stereotaxic surgery. *Neurosurgery: State of the Art Reviews* **2**(1): 149−63 (1987).

26 Dykes, E. & Clement, J.G. The construction and application of an x−y co-ordinate plotting microscope. *J. Dent. Res. (D)* **59**: 1800 (1980).

27 Kimura, O., Dykes, E. & Fearnhead, R.W. The relationship between the surface area of enamel crowns of human teeth and that of dentine−enamel junction. *Arch. Oral Biol.* **22**: 677−83 (1977).

28 Cahan, L.D. & Trombka, B.T. Computer graphics − three-dimensional construction of thalamic anatomy from serial sections. *Comput. Progr. Biomed.* **5**: 91−8 (1975).

29 Johnson, E.M. & Capowski, J.J. A system of three-dimensional reconstruction of biological structures. *Comput. Biomed. Res.* **16**: 79−87 (1983).

30 Dykes, E. & Afshar, F. Computer generated three-dimensional reconstructions from serial sections. *Acta Stereologica* **1**: 297−304 (1982).

31 Vanden Burghe, W., Aerto, P., Claeys, H. & Verraes, W. A microcomputer based graphical reconstruction technique for serial sectioned objects with hidden line removal. *Anat. Rec.* **215**: 84−91 (1986).

32 Gras, H. A "hidden line" algorithm for 3D reconstruction from serial sections − an extension of the NEUREC program package for a microcomputer. *Comput. Progr. Biomed.* **18**: 217−26 (1984).

33 Zyola, M.J., Jones, R.A. & Hogan, P.G. Surface reconstruction from planar contours. *Comput. Graph.* **11**: 393−408 (1987).

34 Cookson, M.J., Dykes, E., Holman, J.G. & Gray, A. A microcomputer based system for generating realistic 3D shaded images reconstructed from serial sections. *Eur. J. Cell Biol.* **48** (Suppl. 25): 69−72 (1989).

35 Foley, J.D. & van Dam, A. *Fundamentals of Interactive Computer Graphics.* Reading, MA: Addison-Wesley (1982)

36 Gouraud, H. Continuous shading of curved surfaces. *IEEE Trans. Comput.* **20**(6): 723−8 (1971).

chapter 8

Microcomputer Management of Stereotactic Atlas Data

Joseph H. Goodman and Gary L. Rea

Introduction

Stereotactic procedures directed at subcortical central nervous system tissue such as thalamic nuclei require an understanding of the three-dimensional (3-D) geometry of the target and its surroundings. Target regions have been mapped in stereotactic atlases, which use normal anatomic structures as reference points to establish geometric relationships of areas immediately adjacent to those structures. Traditionally, stereotactic procedures have been carried out with intraoperative ventriculography to identify those reference points so that they may be correlated with atlas data. This has been necessary because the variation of external landmarks makes them unsuitable for accurately identifying small deep structures. Brains vary morphologically from individual to individual [1], as does the structure of each hemisphere of the same brain, so that, even with the use of internal landmarks adjacent to the thalamus, accurate localization of thalamic nuclei is difficult if mapping is based on only a few histologic preparations. Localization of an anatomic target is best achieved by knowing that target's probability of being present at given distances from identifiable landmarks, and atlases based on variability studies provide the best source of this information. Computerized statistical analysis of data, collected from a sample large enough to establish normal vari-

ability of CNS structures, is available in atlas form, and the logical extension of working with this data is to employ computers to use it in the operative setting.

Basic computer concepts and terminology

Computer-aided design (CAD) uses computer hardware and software to store and retrieve data and to perform the repetitive and complicated calculations necessary to provide graphic solutions to design problems. Evolving to meet the needs of engineers and architects, CAD programs can, through input/output functions of a library of subroutines, precisely create, manipulate, and display drawing elements in 3-D space [2]. Components of CAD systems include the computer-based system, a database, the program library, and a communications subsystem. Subroutines included in professionally written programs are straightforward and enable the user to work with points and lines, create polylines, and use on-screen dimensioning capabilities. The utility of this technology for stereotactic surgery is obvious.

When use of this technology was initiated to store and retrieve information contained in the atlases, data acquisition methods and graphic routines thought necessary for stereotactic surgery were approached through custom programming on a minicomputer, using

FORTRAN as the programming language. It soon became apparent that commercially available products, such as CAD software and personal computers, had all the features necessary to manipulate graphic data for our purposes, and AUTOCAD (Autodesk Inc., Sausalito, CA) was selected to carry on the project. This program, capable of 3-D data display and accessible with only a basic familiarity with the commands, makes possible the writing of custom menus specifically for surgical purposes. The program creates "entities," i.e. lines, text, points, and polylines, that can be depicted on a Cartesian coordinate system. These entities can be assigned colors and linetypes and can be layered (an extremely useful subroutine allowing components of the drawing file to be turned on or off in the display process). Three-dimensional reconstructions are made by assigning elevations to entities according to distances from established reference planes of the drawing file. The entities can be manipulated using the various editing features, including the ability to erase, move, copy, drag, and rotate drawing entities, as well as to change the dimensions and aspect ratios of each drawing. Other features available for depicting 3-D digitized images include extrusion and hidden line suppression.

Stereotactic atlas data derived from variability studies

Thalamic atlas

In 1969, a comprehensive atlas of thalamic structures, as well as the adjacent cerebrum, midbrain, and upper portion of the pons, was published by Andrew and Watkins [3]. This work was prepared using cadaver specimens that were fixed *in situ* within the cadaveric skull to reduce distortion. Measurements to establish the shrinkage artifact during the fixation process were also performed. The brains used in this study were bisected, and distance relationships between the anterior commissure (AC), posterior commissure (PC), and the posterior inferior margin of the foramen of Monro (FM) were established. It was found that using the foramen of Monro as a fixed point on the FM−PC line from which to compare relationships between these three landmarks minimized the apparent scatter between points. Thus the FM−PC line was chosen as the reference plane for the atlas.

Histologic sections were prepared from 1-mm sections obtained at right angles to the FM−PC line, beginning at the foramen of Monro and extending through the pulvinar. Structures of interest were identified according to histologic criteria, and scaled measurements of the boundaries were made as follows. The most medial and lateral extents of the borders were taken and related to the midline. The most superior and inferior borders were measured in relation to the FM−PC plane. The anterior and posterior limits of each structure were taken from the posterior margin of the foramen of Monro in relation to the FM−PC plane. Structures included in the study are outlined in Table 8.1. Computer analysis was used to establish the mean values of the medial, lateral, superior, and inferior boundaries, and also to establish the standard deviations and standard errors of the mean of the boundaries. These data allowed determination of the mean position of the anterior and posterior boundaries in the sagittal plane. Frequency distribution curves for each structure were also determined. This stat-

---

TABLE 8.1 Structures measured in the thalamus and adjacent areas

Centromedianum	Dorsalis superficialis
Nucleus ruber	Medial geniculate body
Ventrocaudalis internus	Lateral geniculate body
Nucleus subthalamicus	Mamillothalamic tract
Zona incerta	Corpus mamillare
Lateral thalamic mass	Globus pallidus
Nucleus medialis	Amygdalum
Anterior nucleus	Substantia nigra

istical data was used to prepare line drawings of a model thalamus in both the coronal and sagittal planes.

Cerebellar atlas

A complementary atlas to the thalamic variability study has been compiled and published by Afshar *et al.* [4]. This investigation of cerebellar and brainstem structures used the same methods as the original study and further delineated sites potentially useful as stereotactic targets. Nuclei and tracts studied in this atlas are listed in Table 8.2. A large number of specimens were precisely measured and subjected to statistical analysis to establish the probability of locating known structures in reference to internal landmarks that could be visualized by neuroimaging techniques. Reference planes for measurement of structures within the brainstem and cerebellum included a tangent through the floor of the IVth ventricle for the horizontal plane, a perpendicular line through the fastigium from the floor of the IVth ventricle, and the midline of the brainstem. This three-axis orientation was in keeping with traditional stereotactic techniques, employing radiographic identification of ventricular landmarks with positive contrast ventriculography. The goal of this atlas was to identify and localize targets thought at the time to have potential in the treatment of the spasticity of cerebral palsy and other disturbances of muscle tone and posture. It was believed that precise localization of these structures might also be useful for treating certain pain syndromes, such as those mediated by the trigeminal and spinothalamic systems.

Computerization of atlas data

Data collected and compiled in these two atlases is quite extensive, and the statistical analysis presented in the texts further adds to the information available for applications to surgical procedures. Although the original intent of both publications was to provide structural maps for use in surgery, these atlases also present precisely a wealth of anatomic data that may be useful to students of anatomy and physiology.

Microcomputers can manage large quantities of data, and systems capable of performing the input/output functions necessary to handle stereotactic atlas information are now both available and reliable. The cost-effectiveness of using a microcomputer for this purpose can be judged by comparing capabilities of the newer generation microprocessors, storage devices, and software developments with what is needed to establish a mini- or mainframe system to accomplish the same result. Basic hardware to computerize this information includes a microcomputer with sufficient random access memory to accommodate the necessary operating system and graphic software. Hard

---

TABLE 8.2 Structures measured in the brainstem

Nuclei	Tracts
XIIth nerve nucleus	Spinothalamic tract
Red nucleus	Medial lemniscus
Substantia nigra	Lateral lemniscus
Locus ceruleus	Central tegmental tract
Vth motor nucleus	Vth spinal tract
Principal sensory and Vth spinal nucleus	Inferior cerebellar peduncle
Superior vestibular nucleus	Superior cerebellar peduncle
Lateral vestibular nucleus	Corticospinal tract
Medial vestibular nucleus	
Inferior vestibular nucleus	
VIth nerve nucleus	
VIIth nerve nucleus	
Nucleus and tractus solitarius	
Inferior olivary nucleus	
Gracile nucleus	
Cuneate nucleus	

disk drives exceeding 20 Mbytes are standard on most systems currently in use, and are more than sufficient to store data entered from the text. Data input by alphanumeric keyboard and by digitizing pad allows both tabular and graphic information entry. Tape drives, image processors, optical storage devices, and hard copy output devices can further enable a personal system to meet specific task requirements.

A system designed to manipulate atlas data is currently in use. An IBM-AT microcomputer (IBM Corporation, Boca Raton, FL) with 2.6 Mbyte random access memory, 30 Mbyte fixed-disk drive, and a high resolution graphic display in combination with a transparent digitizing pad (Scriptel Corporation, Columbus, OH) can be used to enter graphic data from line drawing formats and to incorporate X-rays into the data management process. Display output is converted to hard copy graphics with a six-pen, color graphics plotter (Hewlett-Packard, Palo Alto, CA). Scaled drawings plotted on transparency film are a convenient method of transporting data to operative X-rays.

More elaborate methods of incorporating imaged data into the computer display have been investigated: pictures have been loaded with a frame grabber; computed tomography (CT) and magnetic resonance imaging (MRI) images have been downloaded from the original tapes; and contour maps based on pixel grayscale have been generated. Quite acceptable displays can be obtained, with full centering and windowing capabilities. These techniques can significantly reduce some of the potential sources of measurement error, but they also increase the complexity of the system. Therefore, the decision to include full imaging and graphics capability into a microcomputer should be made on the basis of what such a system is expected to accomplish, and also with an understanding of what is required to manage the increased complexity of its associated hardware and software.

Construction of a drawing database file from the atlas

Statistical atlas data are depicted relative to the FM−PC line in several ways. Measurements of each border of the individual structures at a known distance from FM, the number of structures observed, the standard deviations, and standard error of the mean are presented as tables. Frequency distribution charts and probability tables, calculated to show the chance of establishing structural relationships at given coordinates, are also available. Representative histologic sections and line drawings, compiled from the statistical data, provide graphic depiction of the data in both coronal and sagittal views. A coronal line drawing from the atlas, 16 mm posterior to FM, is shown in Fig. 8.1.

These line drawings, entered into a database file as polylines, can be processed by subroutines within the program at the user's discretion. Because each drawing entity is a separate file with an assigned elevation relative to the foramen of Monro, all of the program's subroutines

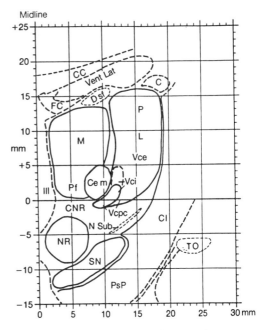

FIGURE 8.1 Contours of a thalamic section 16 mm posterior to the foramen of Monro, as derived from statistical data collected in the Andrew and Watkins atlas [3]. Significant structures are outlined on a Cartesian plane with the FM−PC line serving as the 0,0 coordinate. Atlas drawings are at 5 × real scale and can be manually digitized from a calibrated digitizing pad for entry into a drawing database file. C = caudate; CC; = corpus callosum; Cem = centrum medianum; FC = fornix; NSub = nucleus subthalamicus; NR = nucleus ruber; M = medial nucleus; PsP = pes pedunculi; TO = optic tract; Vce = ventralis caudalis externus; Vci = ventralis caudalis internus; Vent Lat = lateral ventricle.

are available for 3-D, interactive graphic manipulation.

Comparison of the coronal section 16 mm posterior to FM adjacent to a sagittal section 10 mm from the midline is shown in Fig. 8.2. This plot demonstrates how coronal and sagittal maps can be compared, to identify particular nuclei and their borders graphically by editing polylines and coding regions of interest. Windowing commands that outline areas for editing subroutines (such as *zoom*, *hatch*, and *copy*) aid in selective display and are useful for

instructional purposes (Fig. 8.3). Combining both imaging and graphics capabilities allows display of both atlas data and neurodiagnostic images such as MRI scans. Overlays to establish anterior–posterior, superior–inferior, and right–left coordinates can then be generated from image-derived graphics of the patient's contours for surgical planning. On-screen display of a computer-generated graphic from the drawing file database on a sagittal MR image is shown in Fig. 8.4. This requires scaling the drawing to coincide with the image scale.

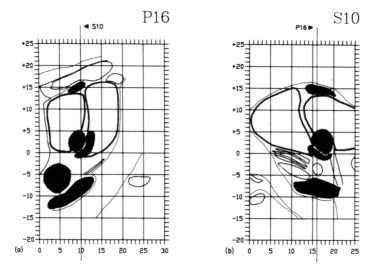

FIGURE 8.2 CAD subroutine-processed drawing files allow entities contained in the database to be displayed in whatever combinations are desired, and also provide a method of graphic enhancement to emphasize certain structures and their relationships. An example of (a) a coronal section 16 mm posterior to FM, plotted next to (b) a sagittal section 10 mm lateral to the midline as it appears by plotting output display, is shown.

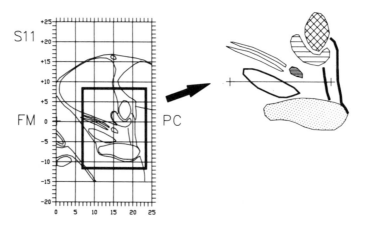

FIGURE 8.3 Certain commands, such as windowing, can be used for illustrative and instructional purposes. Areas outlined by this process can be subjected to editing features contained in the program library.

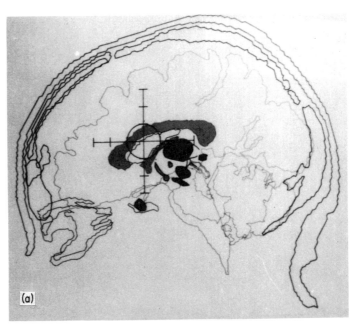

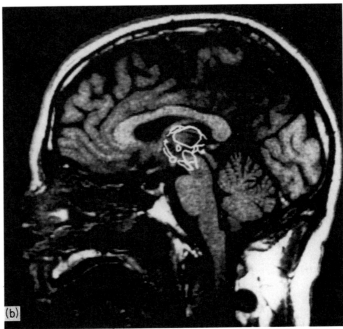

FIGURE 8.4 Microcomputer image display of a sagittal T1-weighted MRI scan can be used to show anatomic structures. Entities in a drawing file can be manipulated with a series of transformations within the program and inserted in the correct anatomic location on the image. Further graphic manipulation of the image by contouring algorithms allows creation of a graphic overlay for correlation with a lateral operative radiograph, so that anterior–posterior and superior–inferior frame adjustments can be determined.

Drawing insertion at FM, and rotation to align with the FM–PC line, accurately align sagittal thalamic boundaries with the patient's profile, as demonstrated by the image. This also demonstrates how graphic subroutines that enhance intracranial structures such as the corpus callosum may be included in the working drawing file. This combination is geometrically more precise in the lateral projection than in the coronal, because of differences in the axis tilts that occur in anterior–posterior views of the image and drawing.

A coronal MR image with a superimposed thalamic contour 1 mm posterior to FM is shown in Fig. 8.5. This appears to accurately depict relationships relative to the midline. However, because of discrepancies between the FM–PC plane as it exists in the image, and the FM–PC

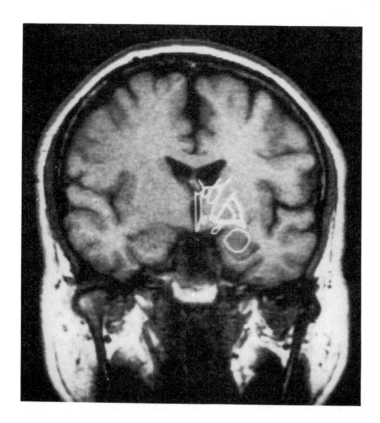

FIGURE 8.5 Insertion of thalamic contours in the coronal plane for establishing right−left or *y* coordinates is accomplished in the same manner as described in Fig. 8.4. Accurately establishing the vertical dimension in this situation requires reformatting the drawing file or using projective geometry to produce anatomically correct relationships.

plane of the drawing file, the geometric relationships are accurate only along the right−left axis. When a discrepancy exists between reference planes, techniques such as those described by Kelly [5] can be used to reformat atlas sections to achieve geometrically correct graphic depictions of the thalamic nuclei. The anterior−posterior projection can accurately depict midline relationships to determine the *y* coordinate in conjunction with *x* and *z* coordinates established from lateral views. Using orthogonal views in this manner allows accurate x_t, y_t, z_t target coordinates to be established, without having to modify the drawing files to correct for axis differences.

Correlation of atlas data with stereotactic radiographs

The basic requirement of stereotactic surgical procedures is to integrate 3-D data, i.e. *x*, *y*, and *z* coordinates, from multiple sources into a mutually concordant set that can be used for target selection. The various data sets to be integrated include atlas information, headframe coordinates, operative X-rays, images of appropriate ventricular landmarks, and the coordinates of the patient. Recently, computerization of stereotactic procedures has emphasized target determination of intracranial structures, using fiducial landmarks that are an integral part of the stereotactic apparatus. These markers, identified on scans done at the time of the procedure, are used to calculate targets and target trajectories; also, comparing fiducials from one imaging modality to the next makes integration of information from multiple sources possible.

The approach we have used for functional procedures directed at deep subcortical structures relies on orthogonal radiographs obtained with permanently installed, fixed-distance X-ray equipment using an 11 foot (3.35 m) tube-to-film distance. This reduces film magnification artifact to acceptable levels. Transfer of sagittal drawing contours onto an overlay scaled to real dimensions on a lateral operative ventriculogram is shown in Fig. 8.6. This illustration includes thalamic contours along with a grid

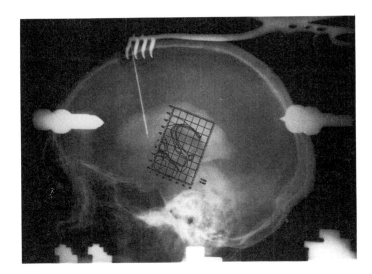

FIGURE 8.6 Atlas drawing files scaled to real size produce overlays that can be correlated with operative radiographs. Sagittal thalamic contours S14 and S16, as they exist in relation to the FM—PC line, are demonstrated.

inserted at FM, rotated to coincide with the FM—PC line, and scaled to real size. Although our studies comparing spatial differences between positive contrast ventriculograms and ventricular structure, as defined by MRI images, show only slight variance [6], we continue to use operative ventriculograms for target selection and confirmation of probe placement for a number of reasons: the author's training in traditional stereotactic techniques; the ease of obtaining consistent radiographs in an operative suite specifically designed for stereotactic procedures; lack of complete confidence that no shift of brain structures might occur with the introduction of air upon burr hole placement; the necessity of having a film copy of the probe at the target site for future reference; the elimination of the need to obtain a scan as part of the procedure; and finally, in the case of computer malfunction, the option of referring to the original text and carrying the procedure through to completion.

Considerations in computerized stereotactic data management

During the past two decades, imaging modalities have become available that allow visualization of deep brain structures. Both CT and MRI are proving to be useful for stereotactic procedures requiring target localization based on normal brain relationships. Transformation of atlas data

to a resident computer format for CT-guided target acquisition has been accomplished with acceptable accuracy [5,7]. Magnetic resonance images provide axial, coronal, and sagittal reconstructions capable of defining the ventricular system with excellent anatomic detail. The obvious landmarks as revealed by MRI technology are especially useful in improving the integration of target sites into a stereotactic coordinate system. Even though currently existing scans are prone to spatial distortions from chemical shifts, nonlinearity of the magnetic field, eddy currents, and the formatting process, the information is extremely valuable; and shortcomings in the quality of data obtained are correctable to some extent [8].

Recent advances in microcomputer technology, i.e. reliable hardware and "user-friendly" software, have made computerization of data required for stereotactic surgery available with a relatively modest commitment to equipment. To bring a microcomputer system on-line requires a working knowledge of computer basics to select a system to meet the user's needs. Becoming familiar with software commands and making the programs meet the requirements of the problems to be solved require a significant investment of time. With increasing computer literacy and device standardization, many problems involved with computerization of specialized personal applications will become less formidable. The combination of new generations of hardware that are better, smaller, faster, and more economical may eventually result in computer terminals providing data access as conveniently as textbook atlases do now.

Design and implementation of a computerized surgical application is an educational experience, and several points became apparent during the evolution of this project. Because of their availability, ease of operation, and adaptability, personal computers have a definite role as a tool in applications such as stereotactic surgery. The surgeon's understanding of complex 3-D relationships can be clearly enhanced by using the information and analysis made available through the computer's capabilities. However, computers cannot solve problems; they merely ease the burden of data management and repetitive calculations necessary for complex routines. Regardless of what we may hear of the future development of "artificial intelligence" and machines capable of mimicking the thought process, today's computers depend upon knowledgeable operators designing programs to meet specific application needs.

References

1 Brierley, J. & Beck, E. The significance in human stereotactic brain surgery of individual variation in the diencephalon and globus pallidus. *J. Neurol. Neurosurg. Psychiat.* **22**: 286–98 (1959).

2 Encarnação, J. & Schlechtendahl, E.G. History and basic components of CAD. In: Encarncão, J. & Hayes, P. (eds) *Computer-aided Design: Fundamentals and System Architectures*, pp. 10–33. Berlin: Springer-Verlag (1983).

3 Andrew, J. & Watkins, E.S. *A Stereotactic Atlas of the Human Thalamus and Adjacent Structures.* Baltimore: Williams and Wilkins (1969).

4 Afshar, E., Watkins, E.S. & Yap, J.C. *Stereotactic Atlas of the Human Brainstem and Cerebellar Nuclei.* New York: Raven Press (1978).

5 Kall, B.A., Kelly, P.J., Goerss, S. & Gideon, F. Methodology and clinical experience with computed tomography and a computer-resident stereotactic atlas. *Neurosurgery* **17**: 400–7 (1985).

6 Rea, G.L. & Goodman, J.H. Interactive computer graphic image analysis for functional neurosurgery. *Appl. Neurophysiol.* **50**: 274–7 (1989).

7 Hardy, T.L. Stereotactic CT atlases. In: Lunsford, L.D. (ed.) *Modern Stereotactic Surgery.* Boston: Martinus Nijhoff (1988).

8 Schad, L., Lott, L., Schmitt, F., Sturm, V. & Lorenz, W.J. Correction of spatial distortion in MR imaging: a prerequisite for accurate stereotaxy. *J. Comput. Assist. Tomogr.* **11**(3): 499–505 (1987).

9

Computer Rendering of Stereotactic Atlas Data and Whole-brain Mapping with Computed Tomography and Magnetic Resonance Imaging

Tyrone L. Hardy, Laura Brynildson, and Bruce Bronson

Introduction

Since the mid-1970s, computerized digital imaging such as computed tomography (CT) and magnetic resonance imaging (MRI), have been developed and used with the stereotactic technique. Advancements in the general design and performance of computers have been the basis upon which this imaging technology has developed and improved. This has led to the development of some additional new imaging technologies, including various radioisotope scanning techniques for metabolic and perfusion imaging, and digital subtraction angiography (DSA), which are also being used with stereotaxy. The development of various stereotactic frames, for example, the BRW/CRW [1, 2], Leksell [3–6], Riechert, Mundinger and co-workers [7–10], Kelly [11], Patil [12], Laitinen [13], and others [14], have paralleled the development of these imaging technologies and have thereby greatly increased the diversity and efficacy of stereotactic neurosurgical procedures (for review, see Bosch [22] and Lunsford [14]).

As a result of these technological advancements, the stereotactic technique has expanded from its earlier use, primarily in the treatment of dyskinesias and pain syndromes, to include the treatment of seizure disorders, aneurysms, brain tumors, and many other neuropathologic conditions. In recent years there has also been a significant increase in the number and variety of stereotactic surgical techniques and instrumentation. Stereotactic open craniotomy, stereotactically controlled microsurgery, brachytherapy, and radiosurgery have been added to the neurosurgeon's armamentarium and arc being increasingly employed.

The major advantage of various computer imaging technologies is that they allow the surgeon to "see" certain brain structures or lesions and to aid in planning stereotactic surgical procedures. Unfortunately the images acquired by these various scanning technologies are not standardized in a common format and, until recently, no method for comparing and using images from various scanning modalities in a single system has been available.

We have sought to solve this problem by the development of a system we call CASS (computer-assisted stereotactic surgery) (trademark of MIDCO, Albuquerque, NM, patent pending) (Fig. 9.1a). This system is a complex integration of various hardware components in a software environment, which provides the surgeon with a means of acquiring digital images from virtually any scanner, e.g. CT, MRI, DSA, positron emission tomography (PET), and various other isotope and imaging devices (Fig. 9.1b). These images are stored in the system in a common format independent of the original scanning device. CASS is therefore a peripheral image processing system, designed specifically

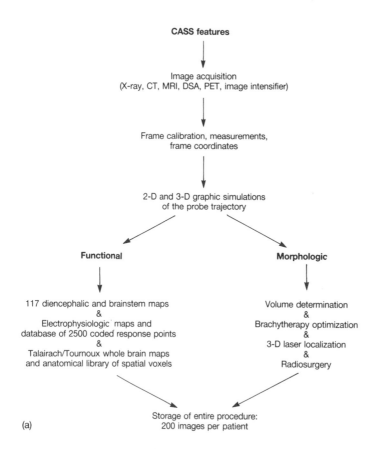

CASS features

↓

Image acquisition
(X-ray, CT, MRI, DSA, PET, image intensifier)

↓

Frame calibration, measurements,
frame coordinates

↓

2-D and 3-D graphic simulations
of the probe trajectory

Functional

↓

117 diencephalic and brainstem maps
&
Electrophysiologic maps and
database of 2500 coded response points
&
Talairach/Tournoux whole brain maps
and anatomical library of spatial voxels

Morphologic

↓

Volume determination
&
Brachytherapy optimization
&
3-D laser localization
&
Radiosurgery

Storage of entire procedure:
200 images per patient

(a)

FIGURE 9.1 (a) Flowchart of CASS system organization. (b) Example of display of image library showing images from multiple image sources acquired into the system.

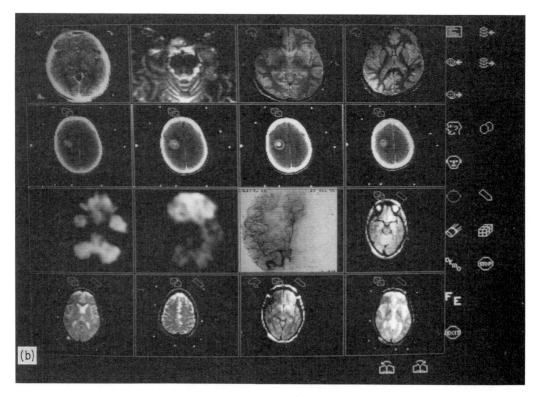

(b)

for stereotactic surgery. This chapter will focus primarily on the use of CASS for functional stereotaxy in relation to computer rendering of stereotactic atlas maps with CT and MRI images. Some additional features of CASS will also be reviewed.

Historical background

Early development

In the early 1970s, prior to the advent of CT/MRI stereotaxy, we developed and used, during a number of stereotactic procedures, a computer system that could display digitized diencephalic brain maps to the neurosurgeon during stereotactic thalamotomy for dyskinesias [15−18]. The software programs for the system operated in a computer which had a peripheral graphics display terminal that could be taken to the operating suite for interactive use by the neurosurgeon. Patient data for stereotactic coordinates was obtained from standard contrast ventriculograms and entered for use into the system. That system, as well as all subsequent versions, consists of the following important features:

1 The capacity to display scaled digitized diencephalic maps, which can be adjusted to the size of the patient's diencephalon as determined from measurements (e.g. intercommissural distance, thalamic height, and IIIrd ventricle width) taken from a preoperative stereotactic contrast ventriculogram. Since the target position for diencephalic subnuclear structures is generally determined by proportional extrapolation from standardized stereotactic atlas maps [19−21], this particular feature allows the atlas maps to be expanded or contracted to more closely fit a given patient's diencephalic measurements, thus increasing the accuracy of target position and size determination. The problems resulting from diencephalic anatomic differences between the atlas map and a given patient's actual brain dimensions were thereby considerably diminished.

2 The capacity to correct the complex three-dimensional (3-D) geometric problems inherent in a precise stereotactic technique, and to present an on-line graphic display of the position of stereotactic probes and electrodes superimposed on atlas map cross-sections of the human thalamus. The software functions of the computer system corrects for these many variables and, by graphic simulation, helps the surgeon to accurately envision the position of a probe or an electrode with respect to various subdivisions of the thalamus [22,23].

3 The system is able to store and selectively display the position of various coded electrophysiologic responses found during exploratory diencephalic stimulation and recording. This capability remains important because data gathered from various electrophysiologic methods (e.g. exploratory stimulation and recording about the intended target site) can be stored in a disk-based file, which can be interrogated to display selected response points from a large group of patients on a digitized map background. Data displayed in this manner can be used to more precisely determine presumed thalamic nuclear zones, and is useful in the mapping of the electrophysiologic topography of the diencephalon [15,16,22−28]. These early developmental capabilities remain essential features of the CASS system and have been used as a foundation for subsequent system development.

Recent developments and enhancements

The stereotactic brain maps of the diencephalon, with architectonics by Hassler [29], were digitized for use with the original system from the earlier Schaltenbrand and Bailey stereotactic atlas [20]. Software routines for modifying the computer displays of the brain maps were necessary to correct for deficiencies in anatomic sectioning (the horizontal atlas map sections vary 8° from the intercommissural plane), and for variations in the sizes of the atlas maps (the frontal atlas maps were considerably smaller than the horizontal maps). The coordinate system for the digitized atlas map sections were based, as those of the anatomic atlas maps, on a brain coordinate system constructed about the IIIrd ventricle core; that is, an intercommissural line bisected by a midcommissural line and a horizontal line representing the basal plane of the brain [20,21,30,31]. The diencephalic atlas maps by van Buren and Borke were also digitized for use in the system [31].

The brainstem and cerebellum maps of the newer Schaltenbrand and Wahren atlas [21] afforded an opportunity to expand our computer mapping capabilities to include these rhombencephalic structures. Incorporating these maps into our computer system required the development of a coordinate system that would allow the simultaneous display of diencephalic architectonics with that of the corresponding brainstem and cerebellum. Allowance was also required for variations in the angle of the junction of the diencephalon with the lower brainstem. For example, the angle of intersection will be closer to 90° in a patient with a brachiocephalic brain in which brainstem angulation is perpendicularly oriented. Both coordinate systems can be moved independently of each other; the size of the brain maps, including the brainstem length, can be readily varied to match the patient's anatomic dimensions, as determined from contrast ventriculograms or from currently available CT and MRI scans. As noted in previous publications [16, 32], this was accomplished by developing a method of intersecting an upper (diencephalic) coordinate system constructed about the IIIrd ventricle core, with a lower coordinate system constructed about the IVth ventricle. Adjustments for differences in brainstem sizes were achieved by a software subroutine that could be prompted to expand or contract the digitized maps.

Advancing computer technology has resulted in the development of high-resolution, color graphics raster display monitors that can interface with small computer systems. As a result, it became possible to modify our computer system so that it could use such a monitor to display CT images and also benefit from the addition of color graphics. The result was our first portable CT–CASS system [16,28,33], which could store, manipulate, and selectively display CT images in the operating room, independent of the CT scanner. Our previously digitized atlas maps could also be superimposed on CT sections of the diencephalon. This method of graphic operative simulation could serve as a valuable guide for using CT data in performing functional neurosurgery. The advantage of the CT–CASS system is that it avoids the extreme expense of a CT-dedicated stereotactic system or the cumbersome and cost-inefficient use of a non-dedicated CT scanner for performing stereotactic surgery. As opposed to these CT-controlled stereotactic techniques, most stereotactic surgeons are inclined by circumstance to use a CT-guided method, in which preoperative CT images are taken to the operating room for use during surgery. Our efforts, therefore, have been focused on improving this CT–CASS system, which is an enhanced CT-guided technique. We have recently expanded our computer system by the development of a multimodality image acquisition interface, so that image data from a number of imaging modalities can be acquired into the system. By the use of this newer image acquisition capability, along with improved stereotactic frames [1–9,11–14], which have localizer modules for various imaging modalities, we have been able to expand our system to use MRI and other image data for stereotaxy. CASS is also particularly useful in these other forms of image-guided stereotaxy, since it is not always practical or safe to perform stereotactic surgery in most radiology imaging suites.

Current hardware environment

The present hardware system (Medical Instrumentation and Diagnostics Corporation (MIDCO), Albuquerque, NM) is based on the Motorola (Phoenix, AZ) 68030 microprocessor and functions on a VME BUS (Motorola Mostek and Signetics) at a clock rate of 25 MHz with 8 Mbytes of on-board dynamic memory. The system has a hard disk drive sufficient in storage size to hold 200 CT, MRI, or other images. Images can be acquired into the system by either tape, camera, Ethernet, or a programmable digital image acquisition interface. These acquisition capabilities allow image acquisition from a number of imaging modalities (Fig. 9.1) for composite viewing within the same image display environment.

A high-speed image pipeline processor, with digital image processing of 16 "bit planes" of graphics overlay, is resident in the system. A 19 inch high-resolution color graphics video monitor is used for image display and graphics. The monitor has an infrared "touch screen" in a special bezel around the margins of the monitor screen, for ease of cursor functions and software menu manipulation through the use of icons. The user interrogates the system by pointing at either "path" or "processor" icons. By the use of this interface the system can be used in a sterile fashion during an operative procedure. No keyboards or joysticks are required in this type of user interface, and the user can easily move about in a system having a large software library with minimal confusion.

The system also has a 5¼ inch, 155 Mbyte streaming tape drive for archiving of surgical procedures, and a high resolution thermal hard copy unit which produces instant polaroid-like hard copies of screen images. This hardware system is small, portable, and has sufficient memory and speed to efficiently execute software commands. For 3-D imaging, an 80 MFLOPS (million floating point operations per second) parallel processor with 8 Mbytes of additional dynamic memory has been integrated into the system to enhance the computer's performance. This creates a system functioning at about 46 MIPS (million instruction points per second).

Software environment

The software for CASS is written in Kernighan and Ritchie C [34] under the UNIX System 5.3 operating system (Bell Laboratories, Blue Bell, PA). The software environment is structured on a multimodular, multidivisional icon-driven menu system, which currently consists of over 200 000 lines of code. The various software features of the system, which can be combined in various ways during the system's use, are separated into several major groupings. There is a separate menu system for *image acquisition, image manipulation, probe positioning, image building, brain atlas map positioning,* and a number of other processes which will be described subsequently.

The software routines are organized on a 16-bit plane hardware overlay format for graphic simulation and composite image display. Each bit plane has been assigned specific software functions. For example, CT/MR images require a minimum of 8-bit planes (2^8) to display the standard 256×256 grayscale matrix of the average scanner. This particular bit plane over-lay feature is analogous to stacked transparent cellophane planes upon which different data or images can be written. The information on these planes is overlaid and therefore viewed as a composite picture on the video monitor. Software routines allow data on each plane to be manipulated separately. Thus, this particular hardware–software format allows the independent manipulation of CT/MR images, brain maps, probes, electrodes, coordinate and map measurements, and coded electrophysiologic data points to produce various composite images for operative simulation during surgery.

Digital image guided functional stereotaxy

Most stereotactic surgeons regard the nucleus ventralis intermedius (VIM) [22,19,14] of the thalamus as the anatomic target site of choice for lesion production to treat dyskinesias. Others prefer to extend the lesion slightly into the dorsal subthalamic H-fields of Forel. The total target is small, approximately $6 \times 4 \times 4$ mm. It is bounded by anatomic areas with important functions, e.g. motor fibers in the internal capsule laterally; the sensory nucleus posteriorly; the mamillothalamic bundle anteromedially; and the subthalamic nucleus inferiorly. Therefore, lesion localization must be accurate and should not extend into these surrounding areas. Digital imaging techniques for localization, like CT and MRI scans, permit direct imaging of this target area, which could only be inferred from contrast encephalographic techniques. Although current CT and MRI scanning technology cannot discern specific thalamic nuclei, they can demonstrate the thalamocapsular border, which is the lateral limit of a thalamic lesion in VIM, and other major landmarks (e.g. the anterior commissure, the posterior commissure, and the IIIrd ventricle margins) necessary for determining the target area. At our institution we use the GE 9800 CT scanner (General Electric Corporation, WI) and the GE Signa MRI scanner for our stereotactic procedures.

CT-guided technique

In our CT-guided technique, the base frame of the stereotactic instrument is attached to the patient's head, and then contiguous, small-increment CT images are taken in the region of the thalamus. For adequate reformatting purposes, CT images taken in 1.5 mm increments in an area approximately 20−30 mm above the posterior clinoid process, will generally include both anterior and posterior commissures. Once images through the commissures are obtained, the thickness of the images can be increased. This will reduce scanning time and the radiation dose to the patient. The area of smaller contiguous cuts then can be bracketed (above and below) by 4−5 mm slices. These scans are then used to obtain a reformatted midsagittal CT scan.

The anterior and posterior commissures are identified on the midsagittal image, from which a scanner-generated reformatted horizontal CT image is next obtained. Latchaw *et al.* described a somewhat similar technique [35]. An image at this level is in the intercommissural plane and represents the maximal depth along the *z* ordinate. (A probe placed much below this level could damage the subthalamic nucleus.) This, along with other images parallel to the intercommissural plane, can be stored in CASS. The patient and the computer can then be transported to the operating room for surgery, leaving the CT scanner available for its regular use.

Alternatively, in another technique, the CT gantry can be angled at approximately 15° posterior−inferior to a line drawn from the angle formed by the junction of the base of the frontal fossa and the descending anterior wall of the frontal fossa and the superior tip of the posterior clinoid process. This technique has been devised as a modification and expansion of a method used by Kamm and Austin [36] for determination of the anterior and posterior commissural line from bony landmarks. We have tested this method on several occasions and have found that we can reliably locate the anterior and posterior commissures by angling the gantry, and the need for reformatting to obtain images parallel to the intercommissural plane is thus avoided (Fig. 9.2). This method has the advantage of potentially reducing any error in stereotactic frame fiducial positioning which may occur from reformatting, since the quality of the reformatted images is dependent on the slice thickness of the individual images used to create the reformatted images.

Regardless of the method used to obtain images in, and parallel to, the intercommissural plane, it is extremely important to note that a 3-D localization system, for example the BRW/CRW [1, 2] or the Kelly [11] localization system, where there are three arrays of fiducials to accurately indicate an image's plane within the stereotactic frame, is far superior to fiducial localization systems which employ fewer fiducials and thus only give localization in two dimensions. The latter localization systems generally require fixation of the stereotactic frame to the CT gantry and have a limited number of fiducials. Under such conditions, accurate 3-D localization is not possible if images are obtained with the CT gantry angled in such a manner that images are not perpendicular to the coordinate system of the stereotactic frame, or if similar reformatted images are obtained. In such cases the error along the anterior−posterior *y* ordinate and the *z* ordinate may be much greater than perceived, and care must be taken to rely a little more on stimulation and recording for target point determination. The less the image angulation and the distance of the target point from the center of such stereotactic frames, the less the potential for error.

In the operating room, the computer system's software for image enhancement and manipulation can be used to identify and further clarify the thalamo-capsular border, which is the lateral boundary of the intended target area of VIM for dyskinesia. In this regard, the computer's software routines for pixel analysis can sharpen the CT image, and, if desired, white matter and gray matter can be color-coded separately for even greater contrast. The software routines for diencephalic map manipulation can be used next to create composite CT scan/map overlay images (Fig. 9.2) that will show the relative position of thalamic nuclear divisions. Measurement subroutines allow "tentative" determination of the target coordinates.

The mediolateral *x* coordinate and the anterior−posterior *y* coordinate of the chosen target site can be determined very accurately by CT measurements; *z* coordinate determinations are not so accurate, because they are dependent

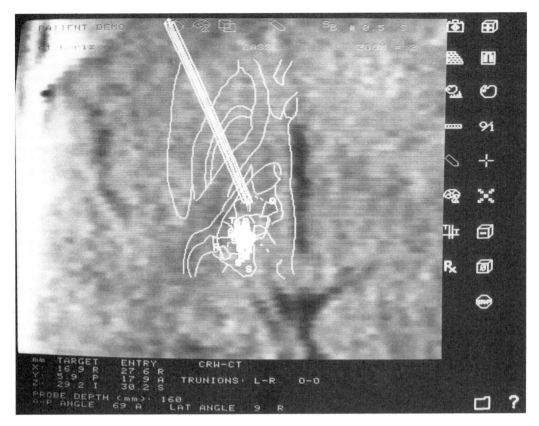

FIGURE 9.2 Use of the BRW/CRW stereotactic localization system for a functional procedure. A brain map is overlaid on a CT section through the intercommissural plane, and the map has electrophysiologic touch-evoked recording responses to hand, thumb, and finger, plotted in the region of ventralis caudalis. A probe's trajectory is simulated to an inferior ventralis intermedius target. In this method the probe's target position is indicated to the computer with the probe's entry point at a higher section to determine the probe's intended angle of trajectory. Note coordinates below. Icons for system's use are to the right. Image at this horizontal level was obtained by angling the CT gantry. Map is from Schaltenbrand and Bailey [20], at 0.5 mm superior to intercommissural plane.

on scan-slice thickness and, as noted above, the stereotactic fiducial localization method. To avoid damage to the subthalamic nucleus, with the attendant risk of hemiballism, care must be taken to ensure that the depth of a stereotactic probe tip does not extend along the z ordinate for more than 1 mm below the intercommissural plane. After the coordinate measurements for the intended target site are determined, a trajectory for the stereotactic probe can be simulated for evaluation and adjustment prior to its actual placement in the target area.

MRI technique

Stereotactic frame manufacturers have recently developed MRI-compatible localization systems

[1–9,11–14] which can accurately indicate frame coordinates taken from either frontal, sagittal, or horizontal images. This stereotactic localization capability has afforded us the opportunity to utilize MRI scans for the performance of functional stereotaxy. Our studies [37] indicate that current MRI scanners of 1.5 T (tesla), with appropriate calibration and slice thicknesses of 3 mm or less, are sufficiently accurate for functional stereotaxy. Previous studies by other authors, however, have indicated that scanners of less than 1.5 T may not be accurate enough for functional procedures [2,38,39]. With CASS we now almost exclusively use MRI for our functional stereotactic procedures because it has the advantage, as opposed to CT scanning, of full 3-D localization of the target point on frontal, sagittal, and horizontal images (Fig. 9.3). With proper scanning parameters, we feel accuracy with this 3-D localization technique is superior to CT scanning localization.

In the MRI technique, a midsagittal image is first taken to identify the anterior and posterior commissures in the mid-IIIrd ventricle plane. The scanner is then set so that oblique axial sections are obtained along the intercommissural plane. Oblique coronal scans can next be taken which are perpendicular to sections coplanar to the intercommissural plane. In effect, image sections are obtained through the thalamus in planes which closely correspond to the intracerebral coordinate system about the IIIrd ventricle core, which has been used as a standard for atlas map and target point referencing [20,30]. It is important for this technique to have a full 3-D stereotactic fiducial localization system like the BRW/CRW system [1,2], Leksell [4], or Kelly [11].

It has been our clinical experience that the following two scanning parameters (Table 9.1) can be used to acquire good quality images for functional procedures. In either technique the objective is to have enough contrast on midsagittal images to be able to adequately identify the anterior and posterior commissures, and to have enough contrast between white matter and gray matter on frontal and horizontal images to clearly distinguish white and gray matter zones for thalamocapsular border identification. In addition, the stereotactic frame fiducial indicators must also be clearly seen in any imaging technique, so that appropriate frame calibration and target point determination can be performed. It should also be noted at this point that care should be taken in positioning the stereotactic frame on the patient's head, such that images taken through the intercommissural plane do not include the stereotactic frame fixation pins, which will distort the MR images.

Inversion recovery T1-weighted technique using standard petroleum-filled MRI localizer fiducials*

In this technique the MRI petroleum- or oil-filled localizer fiducials, standard to many stereotactic frames [1−9,11−14], are used with the scanning parameters noted in Table 9.1 to produce high contrast T1-weighted inversion recovery images, which show the anterior and posterior commissures well on a midsagittal image, while also producing images having good white matter/gray matter contrast for identification of the thalamocapsular border on frontal and horizontal images (Figs 9.2, 9.4, 9.5). This technique can produce parasagittal images which adequately show the anterior commissure (Fig. 9.3b). Such is rarely the case by other scanning parameters. Localizer fiducials are also well shown by this technique. Care must be taken to adjust scanner parameters so that fiducial positions in relation to each other are not distorted by the imaging technique. Significant error can result in some cases due to improper scanning parameters.

T1- and T2-weighted technique using a special BRW/CRW MRI localizer

In this technique, an MRI localizer (manufactured by Radionics, Inc., Burlington, MA) is used which contains hollow core silastic bladders which are filled with normal saline. Scans taken with the parameters noted in Table 9.1 can produce images having fiducial indicators, which are well seen on both T1- and T2-

---

* See General Electric MRI Technical Manual.

FIGURE 9.3 (*opposite*) (a) Example of windowing capabilities with stereotactic probe simulation to a VIM target on sagittal, horizontal, and frontal MR images. Top left window is reserved for magnification of various views. Images acquired by the use of saline-filled fiducial localizers. Probe's position determined by indicating target point and angles to system. (b) Example of the use of the BRW/CRW system for a functional procedure with a sagittal MRI at 13 mm lateral to the mid-IIIrd ventricle and a map overlaid with touch-evoked responses to face plotted in the region of ventralis caudalis. Note probe's simulation to a target in the basal ventralis intermedius/dorsal subthalamic area. Map is from Schaltenbrand and Bailey [20], and has been touched up by artist for clarity.

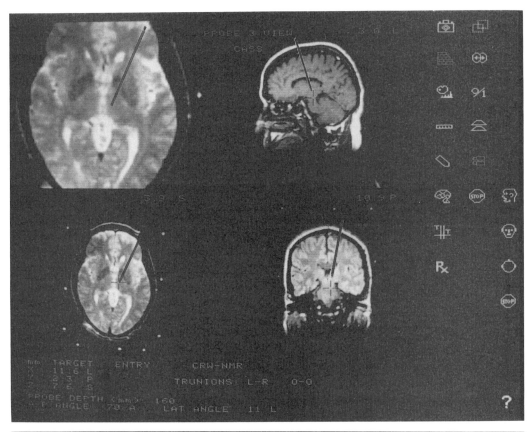

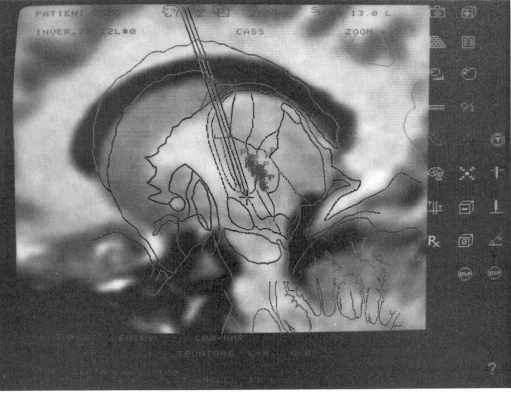

TABLE 9.1 MRI scanning parameters for functional procedures

Localizer	Pulse sequence	Image options	No. of echoes	Time interval/time(s) echo	Recovery time (s)	Field of view	Thick/space*	Start/end	Matrix†	No. of excitations
Inversion recovery T1-weighted technique										
Sagittal	PS	NF	1	0/20	300	32	3/0	L9−R9	128	2
Coronal	PS	NF	1	0/20	300	32	3/0	Prescribed	128	2
Axial	IR	NF	1	700/43	1800	32	3/0	Prescribed	256	1
Coronal	IR	NF	1	700/43	1800	32	3/0	Prescribed	256	1
Sagittal	IR	NF	1	700/43	1800	32	3/0	Prescribed	256	1
T1- and T2-weighted technique										
Sagittal	PS	SAT	1	0/20	600	32	3/2.5	L20−R20	256	1
Coronal	VEMP	F.Comp	2	40/80	2000	32	3/2.5	Prescribed	256	1
Axial	VEMP	F.Comp	2	40/80	2000	32	3/1.5	Prescribed	256	1
Sagittal	VEMP	F.Comp	2	40/80	2000	32	3/1.5	Prescribed	256	1

* Image slice thickness and space between slices.
† Number of pixels squared in image display.

PS, partial saturation equivalent; IR, inversion recovery; NF, no frequency; Prescribed, graphically prescribed image planes; L9−R9 (L20−R20), left to right 9 mm (20 mm); VEMP, variable echo multiplanar; F. Comp, flow compensation; SAT, saturation.

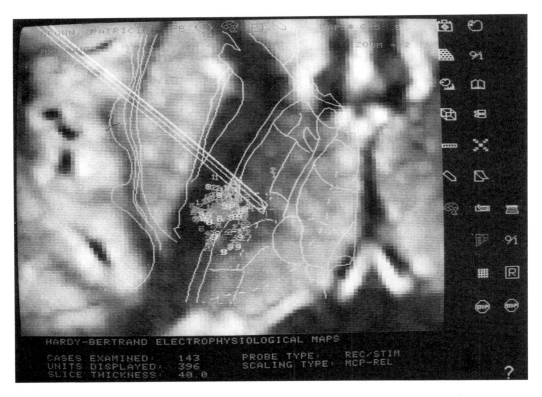

FIGURE 9.4 Horizontal MR image slightly above the intercommissural plane with a corresponding map superimposed. Electrophysiologic responses from stimulation in the internal capsule are plotted and the probe's trajectory toward ventralis intermedius is simulated, in this case for a patient with unilateral Parkinsonism. Map is from Schaltenbrand and Bailey [20], at 6.5 mm above the intercommissural plane.

weighted MR images. We have found that T1-weighted images give good localization of the anterior and posterior commissures on the midsagittal image, while the T2-weighted images give excellent white matter/gray matter contrast, necessary for distinguishing the thalamocapsular border. We feel that this fiducial indicator technique is superior to the above-noted petroleum-fiducial-filled technique, since it results in less fiducial positional distortion. If the standard petroleum filled fiducials are used, we find that they are poorly seen on T2-weighted images. In addition, scans should be taken with "flow compensation" to reduce the background noise, which can frequently obscure fiducial localization. The normal saline filled bladders in the fiducials are readily identifiable with the above scanning parameters, and are probably equal to the use of copper sulfate as advocated by others [11], with-

out the need for adjustment of concentration. In addition, these silastic bladders can also be filled with radioisotopes for radioisotope imaging localization.

Images obtained by either of the above-noted MRI techniques can then be taken with CASS to the operating room, where diencephalic anatomic maps can be overlaid on the corresponding MR image section for accurate determination of the target area in the thalamus (Figs 9.3 and 9.4). In the MRI technique, as in the CT technique, care must be used to avoid placement of the stereotactic probe tip along the *z* ordinate more than 1 mm below the intercommissural plane, so as to avoid damage to the subthalamic nucleus. We find that this limit can be more readily discerned on sagittal MR images, and is thus an additional advantage to the use of MRI imaging for functional stereotaxy.

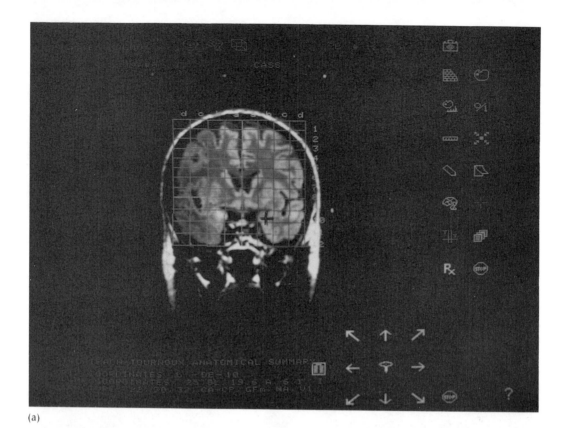

(a)

(b)

FIGURE 9.5 (a) Frontal, (b) sagittal, and (c) horizontal MR images with the BRW/CRW localization system and the Talairach/Tournoux whole brain mapping system in place. Below each map is a listing of the Talairach

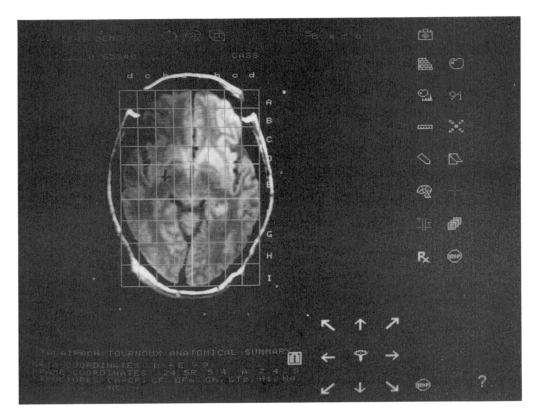

(c)

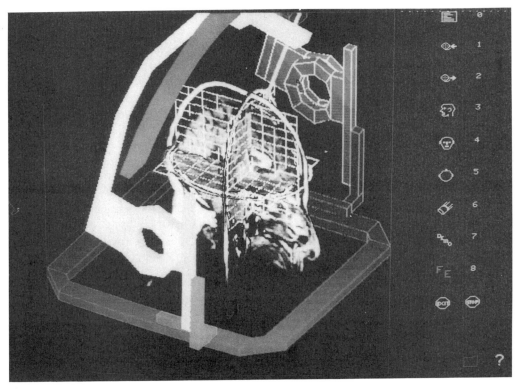

(d)

coordinates, the BRW/CRW frame coordinates and the structures represented by the voxel in which the cursor is placed. (a), (b), and (c) represent a 2-D version, and (d) represents a 3-D version.

Mapping techniques provided by the CASS system

Although the methods described herein for the use of coordinate measurements derived by CT or MR imaging greatly aid in increasing the accuracy of localizing a particular target structure for functional neurosurgery, it is important to remember that they do not completely eliminate error. The position of a diencephalic subdivision in any particular diseased brain cannot be exactly predicted by the surgeon [25]. The need for adequate anatomic target determination, and a neurophysiologic test to confirm that a probe or an electrode is positioned in the proposed therapeutic target site, has long been recognized as a necessary step in stereotactic surgery for dyskinesias, as well as for pain syndromes. We use an anatomic mapping technique, along with a stimulating and recording technique, to confirm the limits of the target area before placing a therapeutic lesion [15, 16,18,24–26,40,41].

Anatomic mapping system

The CASS System contains 117 diencephalic and brainstem maps (Table 9.2) in frontal, sagittal, and horizontal views. These maps are digitized directly from three standard and well known atlases: the Schaltenbrand and Bailey [20], Van Buren and Borke [31], and Schaltenbrand and Wahren [21] stereotactic atlases. Each map can be individually scaled and superimposed over any patient's brain image for specific mapping purposes. Atlas maps can be readily swapped between the different authors to compare thalamic and/or brainstem architectonics. Our mapping technique follows the Brierley and Beck principle [42] of thalamic

proportioning for nuclear localization. It is particularly useful in functional stereotactic procedures. In cases of dyskinesias, we have found that the placement of the probe in the target area is precise enough that a significant diminution or stoppage of a tremor is seen at the time the probe is positioned in the target.

In clinical use, CASS prompts the surgeon to choose an atlas section which closely corresponds to the level of the CT or MRI section through the thalamus. For horizontal images, the surgeon is then required to place a cursor identifying the anterior commissure, the posterior commissure, the wall of the IIIrd ventricle and the thalamocapsular border at the level of the intercommissural plane. An atlas map tailored to fit these parameters is then graphically overlaid on the image (Figs 9.2, 9.4). If MR images are used, a similar method is available to place maps on sagittal and frontal images (Fig. 9.3). Maps can also be tailored to fit additional co-planar image sections.

Electrophysiologic mapping system

As previously noted, a physiologic method for confirming the boundaries of an intended target site is a necessary requirement for accurate functional stereotaxy. The diencephalic microelectrode *recording* technique by Jasper and Bertrand [41], and a *stimulation* technique developed by Bertrand *et al.* [40], have been found to be good methods of obtaining discrete electrophysiologic response data points [15, 16,24–26] for confirming the target's position. We have used both techniques clinically, but now, as a result of the availability of our electrophysiologic database in CASS, we primarily use the stimulation technique in functional stereotactic procedures.

TABLE 9.2 Number of digitized atlas maps stored in CASS

Horizontal, frontal, and sagittal diencephalic maps:	
Schaltenbrand and Bailey atlas [20] (Hassler Architectonics)	49
Van Buren and Borke atlas [31]	28
Sagittal and cross-sectional brainstem and cerebellar maps:	
Schaltenbrand and Wahren [21]	40
Total	117

The microelectrode technique has a curved electrode with a 1−2 μm tip for obtaining unit cellular recordings from thalamic touch, pressure, joint, muscle, and other thalamic afferents (Table 9.3). Similarly, the stimulation technique (Table 9.4) uses a curved electrode with a 1-mm tip for obtaining discrete sensory and motor responses at low current levels (only responses at current levels below 0.9 mA have been used for electrophysiologic mapping). We have found that the use of curved recording and stimulating electrodes allows the sampling of a large thalamic area around the intended target site with minimal need to reposition the stereotactic probe.

The CASS system contains an extensive database of approximately 2500 electrophysiologic response points, compiled over a 28-year period. Data from 153 specially selected stereotactic functional procedures for dyskinesias and pain syndromes were used after the careful review of over 350 cases. This electrophysiologic mapping data system represents the meticulous selection of data, and the accurate

TABLE 9.3 Computer coding of recording unit responses

Attention units	A	
Non-evoked (rhythmic and non-rhythmic) units		1
Evoked responses		Evoked rhythmic (tremor synchronous)
Deep, unspecified units (including pressure)		
Face	B	2
Hand	C	3
Shoulder−arm	D	4
Leg	E	5
Joint units		
Wrist	F	6
Elbow	G	7
Knee	H	} 8
Ankle	I	
Muscle (or movement) units		
Tongue	J	} 9
Face	K	
Hand	L	} 0
Arm	M	
Leg	N	>
Touch units	Cells	Fibers
Tongue	O	*
Face	P	?
Thumb	Q	#
Index	R	$
Other fingers	S	&
Hand	T	%
Arm	U	+
Leg	V	<
Foot	W	~
Trunk	X	⌐
Bilateral (voluntary) movement units	Z	
Novelty units	Y	

Degree of certainty: 3, certain; 2, reasonably certain; 1, uncertain

TABLE 9.4 Computer coding of stimulation responses

Motor		Reliability	
Tongue	1		
Face	2	3 Good	≤ 1 V
Neck	3	2 Fair	1.1−1.9 V
Thumb	4	1 Poor	≥ 2 V
Fingers	5	*Note*: Each volt (average) 0.3 mA	
Hand	6		
Arm	7		
Leg	8		
Foot	9		
Trunk	0		
Eyeball	A		
Pupils	B		
No response	X		
Tremor increased	C		
Tremor decreased	D		
Sensation		Reliability	
Tingling			
Tongue	E	3 Good	≤ 0.5 V
Face	F	2 Fair	0.6−1.0 V
Hand	G	1 Poor	> 1.0 V
Leg	H		
Half of body and limbs	I		
Dizzy	J		
Nausea	K		
Noise	L		
Visual	M		
Pain			
Face	N	*Note*: All "X" responses have	
Arm	O	reliability of 1. Each volt	
Leg	P	(average) 0.3 mA	
Hot or cold			
Face	Q		
Arm	R		
Leg	S		
No response	X		
Sensation to mechanical stimulus	Y		
Opposite capsular or sensory border	Z		

3-D plotting of response points, found during exploratory diencephalic stimulation and recording with microelectrodes during the normal course of stereotactic thalamotomies for dyskinesias and depth electrode implantation for pain syndromes.

These response points can be selectively displayed according to the surgeon's area of interest or need (Figs 9.2, 9.3, 9.4). The CASS software routines have been developed to accurately store, sort, and selectively display electrophysiologic response point data as to their true spatial coordinates about a common origin. CASS also allows for response points to be sorted according to a number of additional parameters, which include diagnosis, various diencephalic measurements, subtypes according to various stimulation and recording responses

(Tables 9.2 and 9.3), and various scaling methods [15,16,24−26].

Response point mapping data can be scaled to a normalized thalamic size for averaging purposes, or scaled about a common origin of either the anterior commissure, the midcommissural point or the posterior commissure. This feature allows for variations in the groupings of response data, which differ according to intercommissural distance and the reference origin chosen. For example, we have found that the posterior commissure is a more reliable reference for target point determination than other reference points. This is possibly due to the fact that the target area for dyskinesias, VIM, is closest to the posterior commissure [15,26,42]. Our studies also indicate that the anterior border of ventralis caudalis (posterior border of ventralis intermedius) varies between 5 and 9 mm anterior to the posterior commissure, depending on intercommissural length [15,26,42]. We have used this measurement as an additional confirmation of an intended target site's position.

In practical use, the electrophysiologic mapping system is used to confirm or further identify the location and boundaries of an intended target area. For example, a CT or MR image has a corresponding anatomic atlas map superimposed on it to closely match the image section with an atlas map section. The electrophysiologic database is then interrogated to select electrophysiologic data according to the patient's diagnosis, intercommissural distance, IIIrd ventricle width, thalamic height, and the desired electrophysiologic response type contained within a specified sample thickness above and below the map area displayed. These data are then superimposed with the corresponding atlas map on the image section for composite viewing (Figs 9.2, 9.3, 9.4). For cases of dyskinesias, the thalamic zone within the overlaying atlas map's VIM region, and anterior to plotted touch-evoked recorded responses from the face or hand, or stimulation responses in the same body regions, would indicate the most statistically probable region of the intended target area. The lateral boundaries of the target can be determined by visual inspection of the thalamocapsular junction, as indicated by the CT or MR image slice, along with the atlas map

overlay and plotted motor responses to stimulation in the internal capsule (Fig. 9.4). We have found that the target for dyskinesis is generally 5−9 mm anterior to the posterior commissure with the probe tip at the intercommissural plane (26). Laterality varies according to the width of the IIIrd ventricle [43]. For "narrow IIIrd ventricles" (2−5 mm), the target is around 13−15 mm lateral to the mid-IIIrd ventricle plane, while for "large IIIrd ventricles" (6−16 mm), the target is around 15−18 mm lateral to the mid-IIIrd ventricle plane. These general parameters can be used as further confirmation of the target site.

An additional example of the use of this mapping system is the determination of the specific thalamic zone which represents a particular body area, for the placement of depth electrodes as treatment for a chronic pain syndrome. For example, plotted touch-evoked responses from the face would indicate the most statistically probable thalamic zone for placement of a depth electrode for chronic facial pain.

Talairach/Tournoux proportional voxel mapping system

With the gracious permission of Drs Talairach and Tournoux [30], and advice of Dr Mark Rayport (University of Ohio), we have added their whole-brain proportional voxel mapping method to the CASS system. In this system the whole brain is proportioned according to the standard Cartesian coordinate system about the IIIrd ventricle core, as has been previously mentioned in this chapter. Our method includes both a 2-D (Figs 9.5a, b, and c) and a 3-D (Fig. 9.5d) version of their mapping system, which allows the user to place a cursor on an MR image and rapidly determine the anatomic structures represented by the voxel indicated. If a stereotactic frame is also placed, then the stereotactic frame coordinates and the Talairach/Tournoux coordinates are displayed on the monitor screen. A search can also be instituted so that the user can request a certain anatomic structure, and it will be identified on all corresponding image sections. We have found this mapping method to be of use for the following:

1 Determining a stereotactic probe's anatomic trajectory through the brain during various stereotactic surgical procedures, and as an aid to preplanning a stereotactic surgical approach.

2 Depth electrode implantations for the study of seizure foci (also useful for button array placement for cortical electroencephalographic studies).

3 Identifying the anatomic sites of various responses obtained with electromagnetic encephalography.

In this technique a minimum of four MRI images are required to set up the proportional voxel method for the computer program's use. These include a midsagittal image, a horizontal image along the intercommissural plane, and frontal (coronal) images perpendicular to the intercommissural plane through both the anterior and posterior commissures. From these images the central coordinate planes about the IIIrd ventricle core can be identified for use by the computer, as well as the superior, anterior, posterior, and inferior margins of the brain as seen on these various sections. The computer then proportions the brain into voxels according to the Talairach/Tournoux coordinate system.

Additional features of CASS which can be used with brain mapping

The image manipulation feature of the CASS system

This feature provides for the manipulation of stored images and consists of routines that enhance, contrast, and color the grayscales of the images. Included in the submenus of this larger menu are routines (Fig. 9.6) for:

1 Pixel analysis of the entire image, including edge detection, ramping, windowing, histogram, and colorization.

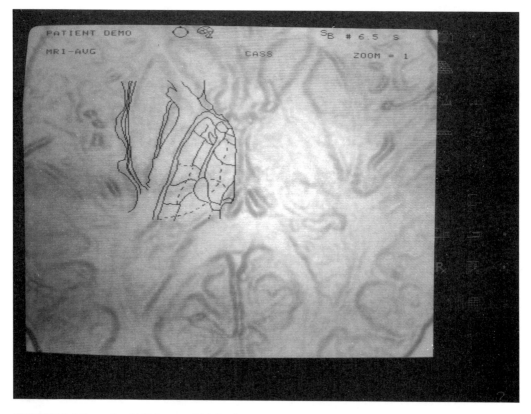

FIGURE 9.6 Example of MR image which has been averaged to infinity and passed through a special edge detection routine which draws boundaries around subnuclear divisions of the thalamus. Compare the anatomic map, which is overlaid on the left, with the nuclear areas indicated by this special technique, on the right.

2 Reduction and enlargement of specific areas of interest in an image.

3 Contrasting, smoothing, and sharpening of images.

4 Image comparison and image editing.

Stereotactic frame calibration and probe positioning feature of the CASS system

This feature provides a method for determining the placement of a surgical probe within the brain, and is designed to work in conjunction with any stereotactic frame. According to the stereotactic frame design, in this routine the fiducial indicators are marked by cursor positioning on the initial image of a series of images acquired into the system. All subsequent images acquired along a given ordinate are automatically calibrated. In the calibration procedure each image is checked by the computer for uniformity of fiducial positioning within acceptable tolerances. The image slice level is determined, and automatically named according to its spatial position within stereotactic frame space. Once calibration is completed, the coordinates of any point in the stereotactic frame can be rapidly determined.

By the use of associated submenus, the probe's position can be rapidly determined and simulated by any of three methods. In the first method, a target point and then an entry point on corresponding CT or MRI slices are chosen, and the computer then computes the probe's trajectory and the target point and entry point frame coordinates (see Fig. 9.2). In the second method, the surgeon selects the target point on a given image slice and then enters the probe's angles of approach. The computer then determines the frame target coordinates and simulates the probe's trajectory according to the angles entered (Fig. 9.3). The third method (Fig. 9.3) is a 3-D method of probe positioning, whereby a probe's position can be interactively updated in separate windows, and the target point and trajectory changed while the probe's position is simultaneously viewed on frontal, sagittal, and horizontal images in the same display. This method results in a reduction of error in target point determination, since variability due to scan slice thickness along any given ordinate is reduced by comparable determi-

nation of a target point's ordinate position in an opposing scan slice. In all methods CASS presents the graphical simulation of the probe in the brain, along with the display of the probe's intersection with various scanner image planes.

The image-building feature of the CASS system

This feature provides the surgeon with several methods of enhancing the conceptualization of an intended procedure or of image comparison. Included in *image-building* are routines for transforming and aligning images using size and positional algorithms, transparent viewing of images for comparison of different scan techniques, and routines for various 3-D simulations of the probe. The features included in the *image-building* menu are:

1 *Perspective view* for viewing the probe through stacked images with maps superimposed on each image slice (Fig. 9.7).

2 *3-view* to simultaneously see the probe in various combinations of sagittal, frontal, and horizontal (Fig. 9.3).

3 *Flicker-frame-overlay* for transparent viewing of two images in relation to each other and translation of data from one imaging modality to another (Fig. 9.8).

4 *3-D simulation* with the capability of embedding 3-D graphics in the image (Figs 9.5d and 9.9).

5 *3-D whole-brain rendering* and surface peeling and transparency (Fig. 9.10).

Other major CASS features

Complex volumetric determination

CASS is able to perform complex volumetric determination, by the use of multiple polygons constructed about tumor segments which are displayed on several CT or MRI slices. The calculations are performed by an accurate pixel-fill technique within a 2-D (CT) or 3-D (MRI) calibrated frame reference system. Multiple polygons can be drawn on differing image sections and incrementally totaled. The polygons constructed about the suspected tumor margins can then be rapidly transferred to a 3-D matrix for viewing in a 3-D display and for brachytherapy or external beam radiation therapy optimization (Fig. 9.9).

3-D radiation therapy optimization

In this method, wireframe simulation of the tumor margins is integrated with actual MR or CT images, to give a visual 3-D rendering of the tumor within the stereotactic frame (Fig. 9.9). The wireframe simulations of the tumor boundaries can be further rendered in such a manner as to simulate a "shell" form of the tumor, and a special transparency technique is used to give a visual simulation of the tumor shell above and below a given image slice. Image slices can also be stacked in various manners and reformatted for perspective. Radio-isotope seeds or beam arcs can then be simulated within the tumor (Fig. 9.9), as well as their selected surrounding therapeutic isodose zones. By rendering the tumor margins in both wireframe and "shell" form, the user can get an index of how certain isodose zones fit within the confines of the tumor margins. This is used as a visual optimization technique, in which the surgeon can incrementally simulate isotope or beam arcs for tumor dosimetry optimization.

Future features of the CASS system

We are currently completing the development of a full 3-D angiographic simulation technique with the use of either DSA or MR imaging data. Such 3-D imaging also allows full transparency. In addition, a 3-D laser localization apparatus has been developed, which can be simulated in three dimensions with our CASS system for whole-brain mapping localization, tumor positioning, and volume determination. These, as well as some other techniques involving stereotactic ultrasonography and robotics, will be presented in subsequent publications.

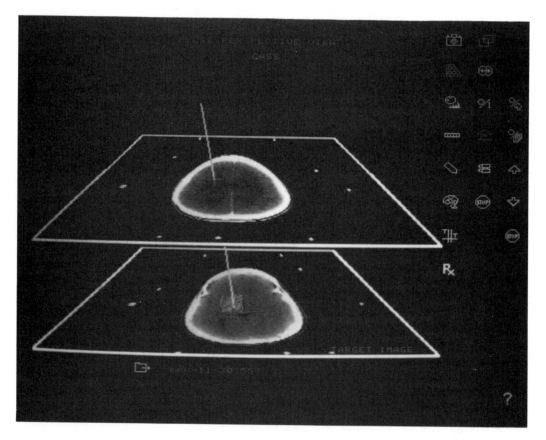

FIGURE 9.7 Example of probe perspective view, showing CT images at the top near probe entry point, and lower image at probe's target with maps superimposed on lower image.

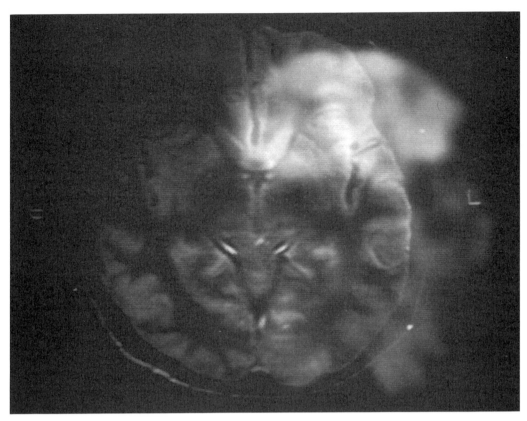

(a)

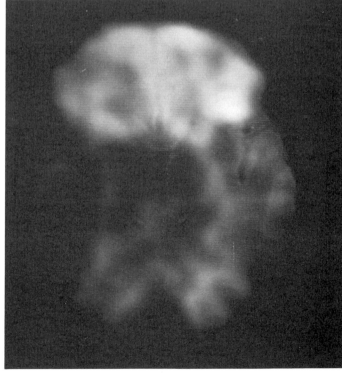

FIGURE 9.8 Flicker-frame overlay technique in which a PET image (*right*) is being transformed and overlaid on an MR image. In (a), images are shown side-by-side in the same display, and in (b) are superimposed. Areas of interest in one system can be marked and transposed to another. Note hypometabolic right temporal lobe. This method is useful in conjunction with Talairach/ Tournoux mapping for seizure focus identification.

(b)

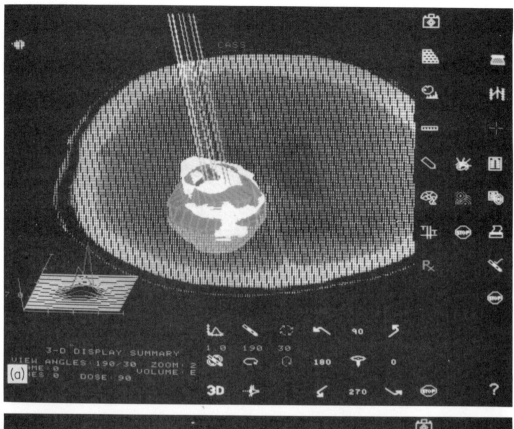

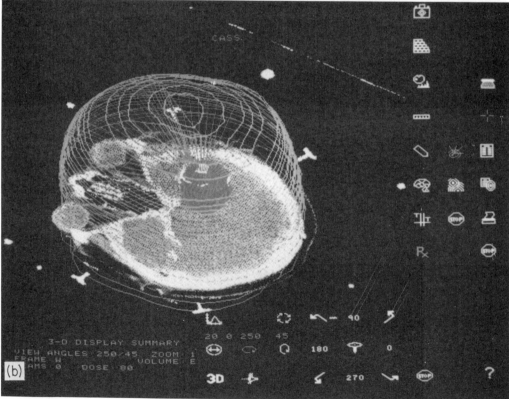

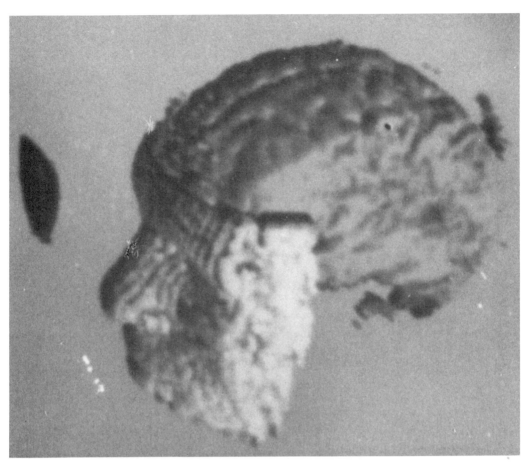

FIGURE 9.10 Whole-brain rendering by a specially designed "ray-tracing" technique, using a reduced data set of 32 MR images. Whole-brain rendering showing skin and bone of face in place. By this technique various structures and portions of structures can be removed, or left in place, or rendered in transparency form to see underlying structures. This technique can be used in conjunction with brainstem and Talairach/Tournoux mapping to better define certain anatomic structures.

References

1 Brown, R.A. A stereotactic head frame for use with CT body scanners. *Invest. Radiol.* **14**: 300–4 (1979).

2 Cosman, E., Heilbrun, M.P. & Wells, T. Jr. Magnetic resonance stereotaxy. In: Apuzzo, M. (ed.) *Surgery In and Around the Brain Stem and the Third Ventricle.* Berlin-Heidelberg: Springer-Verlag (1986).

3 Leksell, L. A stereotaxic apparatus for intra-cerebral surgery. *Acta Chir. Scand.* **99**: 220–33 (1949).

4 Leksell, L. *Stereotaxis and Radiosurgery: An Operative System*, pp. 69. Springfield, IL: Thomas (1971).

5 Leksell, L. & Jernberg, B. Stereotaxis and tomography: a technical note with 6 figures. *Acta Neurochir. (Wien)* **52**: 1–7 (1980).

6 Leksell, L., Leksell, D. & Schwebel, J. Stereotaxis and nuclear magnetic resonance. Technical Note.

FIGURE 9.9 (*opposite*) (a) An example of 3-D brachytherapy optimization technique, in which tumor volume and dosimetry zones are shown in relationship to each other. Graphic simulation of tumor volume and dose zones are presented in relation to actual CT (MR) imaging for anatomic correlation. (b) Example of 3-D radiosurgery optimization technique, in which tumor volume and dosimetry zones are shown in relationship to each other. Graphic simulation of tumor volume, dose zones, skull contours, and beam arcs are presented in relation to actual CT (MR) imaging for anatomic correlation.

J. Neurol. Neurosurg. Psychiatr. **48**: 14−18 (1985).

7 Birg, W. & Mundinger, F. Computer programs for stereotaxic neurosurgery. *Confin. Neurol.* **36**: 326−33 (1974).

8 Birg, W. & Mundinger, F. Calculation of the position of a side-protruding electrode tip in stereotactic brain operations using a stereotactic apparatus with polar coordinates. *Acta Neurochir. (Wien)* **32**: 83−7 (1975).

9 Birg, W., Mundinger, F. & Klar, M. A computer program system for stereotaxic neurosurgery. *Acta Neurochir. (Wien)* (suppl.) **24**: 99−108 (1977).

10 Riechert, T. & Spuler, H. Instrumentation of stereotaxy. In: Schaltenbrand, G. & Walker, A.E. (eds) *Stereotaxy of the Human Brain*, pp. 350−60. New York: Thieme-Stratton (1962).

11 Kelly, P.J., Goerss, S.J. & Kall, B.A. Modification of Todd−Wells system for imaging data acquisition. In: Lunsford, L.D. (ed.) *Modern Stereotactic Neurosurgery*, pp. 79−97. Boston: Nijhoff (1987).

12 Patil, A.A. The Patil system. In: Lunsford, L.D. (ed.) *Modern Stereotactic Neurosurgery*, pp. 117−125. Boston: Nijhoff (1987).

13 Laitinen, L.V. A new stereoencephalotome. *Zentralbl. Neurochir.* **32**: 67−73 (1971).

14 Lunsford, L.D. (ed.) *Modern Stereotactic Neurosurgery*. Boston: Nijhoff (1988).

15 Hardy, T.L. Computer display of the electrophysiological topography of the human diencephalon during stereotaxic surgery. Master's Thesis, McGill University, Montreal, Canada (1975).

16 Hardy, T.L. Stereotactic CT atlases. In: Lunsford, L.D. (ed.) *Modern Stereotactic Neurosurgery*, pp. 425−9. Boston: Nijhoff (1988).

17 Thompson, C.J. & Bertrand, G. A computer program to aid the neurosurgeon to locate probes used during stereotaxic surgery on deep cerebral structures. *Comput. Programs Biomed.* **2**: 265−76 (1972).

18 Thompson, C.J., Hardy, T.L. & Bertrand, G. A system for anatomical and functional mapping of the human thalamus. *Comput. Biomed. Res.* **19**: 9−24 (1977).

19 Guiot, G. & Derome, P. The principles of stereotaxic thalamotomy. In: Kahn E.J., *et al.* (eds.) *Correlative Neurosurgery*, 2nd edn, pp. 376−401. Springfield, IL: Macmillan (1969).

20 Schaltenbrand, G. & Bailey, P. *Introduction to Stereotaxis with an Atlas of the Human Brain*. New York, Stuttgart: Thieme (1959).

21 Schaltenbrand, G. & Wahren, W. *Atlas for Stereotaxy of the Human Brain*, 2nd edn. Stuttgart: Thieme (1977).

22 Hardy, T.L. A method for calculation of rotational angulation in stereotactic surgery. *Surg. Neurol.* **13**: 437−9 (1980).

23 Hardy, T.L. & Koch, J. CASS: a program for computer assisted stereotaxic surgery. In: Heffernan, H.G. (ed.) *Proceedings of the 5th Annual Symposium on Computer Application in Medical Care, Washington, DC.*, pp. 1116−26. (1981).

24 Bosch, D.A. *Stereotactic Techniques in Clinical Neurosurgery*. Vienna: Springer-Verlag (1986).

25 Hardy, T.L. A method for MRI and CT mapping of diencephalic somatotopography. *Stereotact. Funct. Neurosurg.* **52**: 242−9 (1989).

26 Hardy, T.L. Bertrand, G. & Thompson, C.J. The position and organization of motor fibers in the internal capsule. *Appl. Neurophysiol.* **42**: 160−70 (1979).

27 Hardy, T.L., Bertrand, G. & Thompson, C.J. Touch-evoked thalamic cellular activity: the variable position of the anterior border of somesthetic SI thalamus and somatotopography. *Appl. Neurophysiol.* **44**: 302−13 (1981).

28 Hardy, T.L., Koch, J. & Lassiter, A. Computer graphics with computerized tomography for functional neurosurgery. *Appl. Neurophysiol.* **46**: 217−26 (1983).

29 Hassler, R. Anatomy of the thalamus. In: Schaltenbrand, G. & Bailey, P. (eds) *Introduction to Stereotaxy with an Atlas of the Human Brain*, Vol. 1, pp. 230−90. Stuttgart: Thieme (1959).

30 Talairach, J. & Tournoux, P. *Co-planar Stereotaxic Atlas of Human Brain. 3-Dimensional Proportional System: An Approach to Cerebral Imaging*. New York: Thieme (1988).

31 Van Buren, J.M. & Borke, R.C. *Variations and Connections of the Human Thalamus*, Vols 1 and 2. New York: Springer (1972).

32 Hardy, T.L. & Koch, J. Computer-assisted stereotactic surgery. *Appl. Neurophysiol.* **45**: 396−8 (1982).

33 Hardy, T.L., Lassiter, A. & Koch, J. A portable computerized tomographic method for tumor biopsy. *Acta Neurochir. (Wien)* (suppl.) **33**: 444 (1983).

34 Kernighan, B.W. & Ritchie, D.M. *The C Programming Language*. Englewood Cliffs, NJ: Prentice-Hall (1978).

35 Latchaw, R.S., Lunsford, L.D. & Kennedy, W.H. Reformatted imaging to define the intercommissural line for CT-guided stereotaxic functional neurosurgery. *Am. J. Neuroradiol.* **6**: 429−33 (1985).

36 Kamm, R.F. & Austin, G. The use of bony landmarks of the skull for localization of the anterior−posterior commissural line. *J. Neurosurg.* **22**: 576−80 (1965).

37 Brynildson, L.R.D., Hardy, T.L., Bronson, B., *et al.* A method for flicker frame overlay. *Abstract and Poster Presentation at the Annual American Association of Neurological Surgeons Meeting, Washington DC.* April 1989.

38 Peters, T.M., Clark, J., Olivier, A., Marchand, E., Mawko, G., Dieumegarde, M., Muresan, L. & Ethier, R. Integrated stereotaxic imaging with CT, MR imaging, and digital subtraction angiography. *Radiology* **161**: 821−6 (1986).

39 Villemure, J.G., Marchand, E., Peters, T., Leroux, G. & Olivier, A. Magnetic resonance imaging stereotaxy: recognition and utilization of the commissures. *Appl. Neurophysiol.* **50**: 57−62 (1987).

40 Bertrand, G., Blundell, J. & Musella, R. Stimulation during stereotactic operations for dyskinesias. *J. Neurosurg.* **24**: 419−23 (1966).

41 Jasper, H.H. & Bertrand, G. Thalamic units involved in somatic sensation and voluntary and involuntary movements in man. In: Purpura, D.P. & Yahr, M.D. (eds) *The Thalamus*, pp. 365−90. New York: University of Columbia Press (1966).

42 Brierley, J.B. & Beck, E. The significance in human stereotactic brain surgery of individual variation in the diencephalon and globus pallidus. *J. Neurol. Neurosurg. Psychiatr.* **22**: 287−98 (1959).

43 Hardy, T.L., Bertrand, G. & Thompson, C.J. Position of the medial internal capsular border in relation to third ventricular width. *Appl. Neurophysiol.* **42**: 234−47 (1979).

chapter 10

Computer-assisted Stereotactic Functional Neurosurgery

Bruce A. Kall

Introduction

Computer-assisted stereotactic functional neurosurgical procedures may be performed in selected patients with medically intractable parkinsonian tremor and rigidity. New stereotactic techniques using precise digital imaging, stereotactic localization and computer-resident stereotactic atlases provide useful three-dimensional (3-D) information to plan the procedure. These allow the surgeon to localize the thalamic lesion precisely for each patient, thereby reducing the risk associated with these procedures.

Important subcortical structures vary spatially from patient to patient in relationship to midline radiologic reference points [1-3]. This variability increases the further the target is from the midline [2]. Recently, computed tomography (CT) and magnetic resonance imaging (MRI) have been used to visualize the configuration of the IIIrd ventricle and the thalamus for functional stereotactic procedures. Large gray matter structures such as the thalamus, and fiber pathways such as the internal capsule, can be visualized on these images. Nevertheless, small subcortical nuclei usually accessed for functional target sites are indistinguishable.

This chapter describes our experiences with two techniques for planning nucleus ventralis intermedius/ventralis oralis posterior (VIM/VOP) (VL) thalamotomy procedures: (1) a computer-resident stereotactic atlas overlaid onto radiologic examinations [4]; and (2) a new CT/MRI multimodality technique for determining the target point. Final frame settings for the actual surgical target were determined by stereotactic ventriculography modified by microelectrode recordings, and were compared to the computer-generated techniques. Acceptable results were noted from these two computer-based techniques when compared to the ventriculography/electrode recording method.

Stereotactic computer system

The computer and imaging platform utilized for these techniques is a Sun 4/300 Series computer, tightly coupled with a Vicom VME image processing system, described in detail in Chapter 16. The display device is a multimodality, multiscreen workstation that houses three independent grayscale monitors as well as one color monitor. All software is written in a combination of PASCAL, C, and FORTRAN, and utilizes a stand-up menu system and mouse graphical user interface (GUI). The system uses a variety of specialized data structures to store the relevant information.

Stereotactic localization technique

The stereotactic localization technique employs the COMPASS™ Stereotactic System (Stereotactic Medical Systems Inc., New Hartford, NY and Rochester, MN) and is described extensively in Chapters 6, 16, and 22. Briefly, a multi-modality headframe is rigidly applied to the patient's head before diagnostic imaging attached with a carbon fiber pin fixation system. A micrometer-based reapplication technique is employed so that the headframe may be applied for the preoperative studies, removed, and re-applied on the day of surgery.

The patient undergoes CT and MR imaging on General Electric 9800 and 1.5T Signa^R systems respectively. A modality-compatible localization device attaches to the headframe during each study, and allows the computer to relate every point on every image into the stereotactic coordinate system of the COMPASS™ stereotactic positioner regardless of slice thickness, angulation, and plane of section. 5-mm thick contrast-enhancing CT slices, overlapping every 3 mm, are collected from CT with a 35 cm field of view. MRI imaging is performed with a 24 cm field of view in three series: (1) sagittal, with TE20-TR500, 4 mm thick, 0 mm skipped; (2) transverse, with TE30/80-TR2000, 4 mm thick, 1 mm skipped; and (3) transverse, with IR 170-TR2000, 5 mm thick, 1 mm skipped. These images are then transferred to the operative computer system using magnetic tapes.

Stereotactic atlas technique

Stereotactic atlases provide a standard definition of subcortical structures, from which 3-D stereotactic coordinates may be calculated in spatial relationship to anatomic landmarks. The spatial limits of the structures delimited in the atlas are only accurate for the brain specimens used in the anatomic study undertaken to produce the atlas; therefore, these unmodified "maps" do not reflect the actual anatomic geometry of an individual patient undergoing surgery.

Geometric modifications of atlas maps conforming to landmarks on an individual's CT and/or MR images are mathematically complex and do not conform to strict concatenations of rectangular rotations, scaling, and translation transformations. We have developed a computer-based polar warping mechanism [4], whereby a graphic transformation from atlas to CT and MRI is accomplished by geometrically

manipulating sectors of digitized atlas brain sections within corresponding anatomic boundaries on the individual patient's diagnostic images. The stereotactic coordinates of any subnuclei identified on the atlas-labeled images may then be related to the stereotactic frame for surgical intervention.

Atlas database

We utilize the Schaltenbrand and Wahren stereotactic atlas [5] for these procedures. This atlas is composed of a series of photographs of sample human brains sliced in relationship to planes (AC−PC) drawn between the anterior commissure (AC) and the posterior commissure (PC). The coronal sections are cut parallel to a perpendicular erected from the midpoint of AC−PC, while the sagittal sections are parallel to the midline. The horizontal sections are parallel to a 7° oblique line through the midpoint of AC−PC. Each photograph has an associated acetate overlay that delineates substructures on that image. Each photograph also has coordinate markers and a centimeter scale that define its relationship and distance from the AC−PC plane, the intercommissural plane, and the midline. Our technique uses the slices from the horizontal and sagittal atlas series, which were both cut from the different halves of the same brain specimen.

Each substructure, defined by histologic groups, was manually traced on each photograph on which it appeared, categorized by tissue type (white or gray matter), delineated into anatomic sectors (e.g. thalamus), and cross-referenced with its full anatomic name and abbreviation. The numbering mechanism employed also allows substructures to be grouped by structures as well as by plane of section and level within that plane. The original page and frame numbers from the atlas itself can also be used as reference for displaying images.

Atlas labeling technique

The CT transverse images are utilized to create a sagittal midline reconstruction. The anterior and posterior commissures are then identified, the midpoint identified, and CT sections are produced 7° oblique to this plane. Alternatively, the General Electric Signa[R] software can be used on the scanner to set up the MRI acquisition directly from this oblique plane. These images correspond to the horizontal microscopic sections from the atlas. An image is required at a distance from AC−PC corresponding to an atlas section for this technique.

The CT or MRI oblique image is magnified on the computer screen to zoom in on the area of interest. The CT- or MRI-defined boundary of the anatomic sector corresponding to the atlas is then outlined by the surgeon, using the mouse. Specifically, the surgeon outlines the thalamic sector on the oblique slice corresponding to the horizontal zero-level atlas section, bounded medially by the lateral wall of the IIIrd ventricle, laterally by the medial wall of the internal capsule, and posteriorly by the superior colliculus.

The software then geometrically compares the sector outlines from the radiologic and atlas-traced sectors. A series of polar warping vectors are then calculated, which transform the atlas-derived sector configuration into the radiologic-defined sector configuration [4]. All

substructures from the atlas within this transformed sector may then be geometrically warped onto the CT or MRI section (Fig. 10.1). This warping, however, may not display the substructures in shapes that are readily distinguishable because of the transformation. Annotation of substructures' names directly onto the CT or MRI sections would result in a cluttered picture. Therefore, an interactive substructure identification mechanism was developed.

The physician enters the anatomic name or abbreviation and the software will automatically place the cursor within the substructure of interest. Alternatively, the surgeon may place the cursor within any substructures on the annotated image and the computer will display the anatomic name and abbreviation.

In order to determine the stereotactic coordinates of the desired anatomic subnuclei, the individual substructure of interest may be warped to fit within the transformed sector. The surgeon places the cursor within the substructure and the 3-D stereotactic coordinates are then calculated to place this point within the focus of the COMPASS™ positioner. More

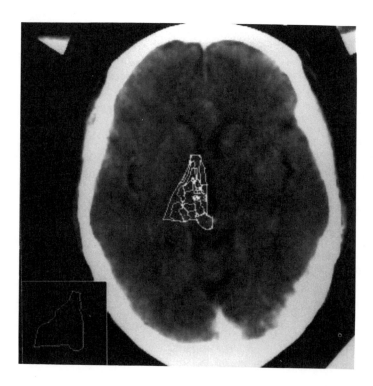

FIGURE 10.1 Obliquely reconstructed CT slice reconstructed parallel to AC−PC plane. The surgeon has identified the outline of the thalamic sector and the software has warped the atlas substructures to fit within this boundary. The configuration outline of the sector from the atlas appears in the inset at the lower left corner.

than one target may be identified within the substructure to measure its size.

Multimodality technique

This new technique utilizes axial CT as well as sagittal and transverse MR images. The surgeon selects the midline MR images that best demonstrate the intercommissural plane and thalamus. These images are then displayed on the computer screens. The surgeon selects AC and PC on the midline image (Fig. 10.2), and the software connects these two points, measures the length of the connecting line, identifies its midpoint and draws a perpendicular emanating from it. This drawing is simultaneously displayed onto a lateral sagittal slice exhibiting the floor of the lateral ventricle and

body of the thalamus (Fig. 10.3). The surgeon selects the top of the thalamus, and the height of the thalamus is then determined on this image.

The software then displays a drawing of the subnuclei divisions of the lateral ventral nuclear masses of the thalamus, utilizing a technique proposed by Guiot. This is displayed on the midline slice exhibiting AC–PC (Fig. 10.4). The surgeon selects a target point on this sagittal MRI image, 2.5 mm above the AC–PC line, in the posterior portion of VOP, 1 mm anterior to the junction of VOP and VIM (Fig. 10.4). The stereotactic coordinates of this point are then calculated.

The software then automatically finds the closest CT axial slice corresponding to this point. It then searches this image and identifies the

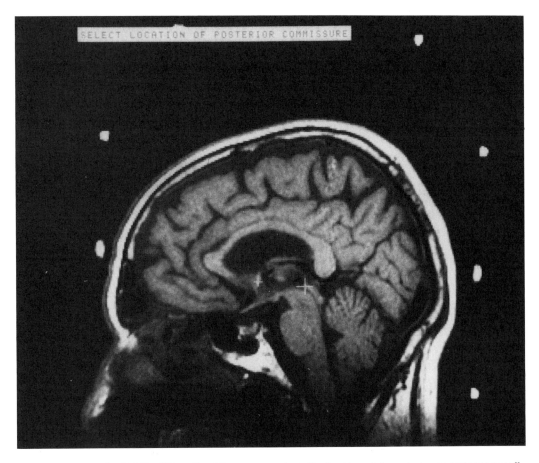

FIGURE 10.2 Sagittal MRI midline slice. The surgeon selects the location of the anterior commissure (small cursor) and posterior commissure (large cursor).

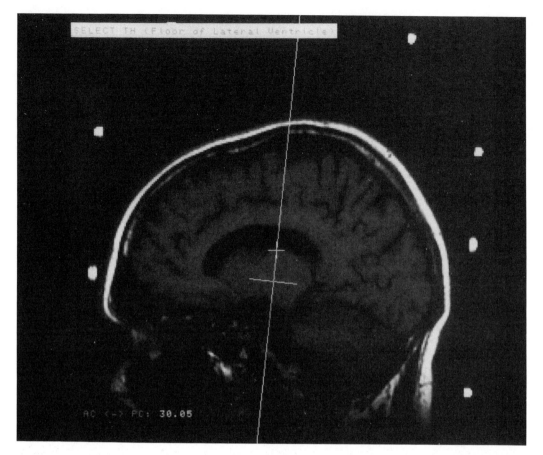

FIGURE 10.3 The AC–PC plane (horizontal line) is translated onto the lateral sagittal MRI slice exhibiting the floor of the lateral ventricle and body of the thalamus. The software draws a perpendicular from the midpoint of AC–PC and the surgeon selects the superior aspect of the thalamus (cursor). The height of the thalamus is determined from this image.

closest correlated point (adjusted for image angulation and thickness) and annotates this point. A line is drawn parallel to the midline through this point. The surgeon then identifies a point on this line on the lateral wall of the IIIrd ventricle as a constant reference point (Fig. 10.5) and a point 11.5 mm lateral to this point on the line is identified. Stereotactic co-ordinates are calculated for this lateral point (Fig. 10.6). This coordinate is then cross-correlated to the closest transverse MRI slice by the same techniques as for MRI to CT. The software identifies this correlated point, draws a line perpendicular to the midline and identifies the reference point 11.5 mm lateral to the ipsi-lateral wall of the IIIrd ventricle. The physician

then selects a point on this image in the mid-lateral portion of VOP to utilize as the proposed surgical target (Fig. 10.7).

Stereotactic ventriculography and microelectrode recording

In spite of the availability of stereotactic CT and MRI, we have continued to employ positive contrast ventriculography for stereotactic thal-amotomy. Thus, all computer-resident atlas and multimodality generated stereotactic coordi-nates can be compared to the actual target coordinates generated from positive contrast ventriculography modified by microelectrode recording. The stereotactic ventriculogram is

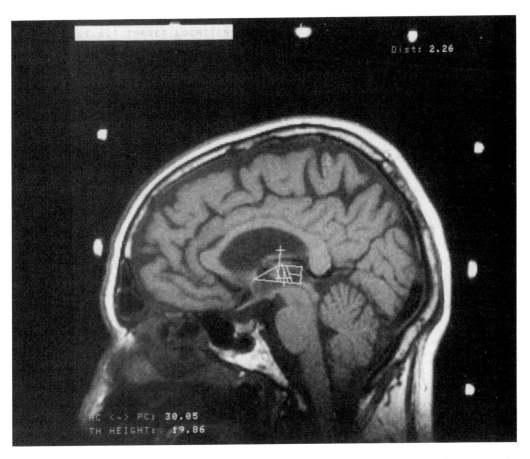

FIGURE 10.4 Midline sagittal MRI slice exhibiting the subnuclear divisions of the lateral nuclear masses of the thalamus. The small cursor notes the superior aspect of the thalamus selected on the lateral sagittal slice in Fig. 10.3. The AC−PC distance and thalamic height are annotated on the bottom left. The surgeon selects a point with the cursor approximately 2.5 mm above AC−PC, in the posterior portion of VOP, 1 mm anterior to the junction of VOP and VIM on the midline image (large cursor).

usually performed on the same day as CT and MRI database acquisition. A coronal burr hole is made and a positive contrast ventriculogram is performed, with the patient in the stereotactic headholder on the stereotactic positioner and with the patient under local anesthesia. The z coordinate of the thalamic coordinate (VOP) is calculated from a point 3 mm above AC−PC, and the y coordinate is determined from a point 2 mm behind the midpoint of AC−PC. The laterality (x coordinate) of the target is confirmed by microelectrode recording.

The microelectrode recording trajectory is directed from the stereotactic frame and passes through ventralis caudalis externus (VCE) toward a point 1 mm anterior to PC, and initially

11.5 mm lateral to the lateral wall of the IIIrd ventricle on the AC−PC line. The final laterality of the target in VOP/VIM is determined from the somatotopy of the evoked responses, as described in other publications [6].

Discussion

Several authors have proposed proportional adjustments of stereotactic coordinates generated from anatomic atlas sections to account for individual spatial anatomic variability. Positive contrast ventriculography is used to determine actual anatomic measurements and these are then compared with measurements in the atlases as a scaling factor.

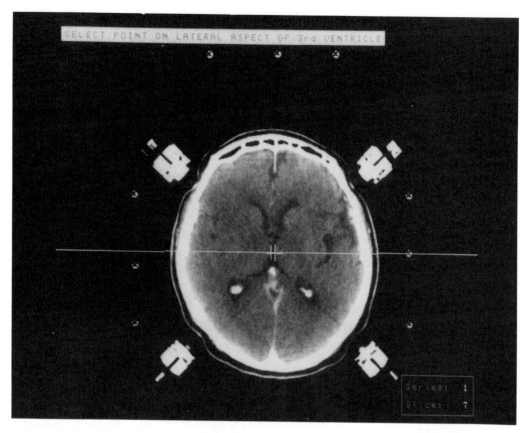

FIGURE 10.5 Correlated CT axial slice and point (smaller cursor) corresponding to the point selected on Fig. 10.4 with line drawn parallel to the midline. The surgeon selects a point on the lateral wall of the IIIrd ventricle (larger cursor).

Talairach proposed a proportional grid system derived from a line drawn between the anterior and posterior commissure (AC−PC line) and the height of the thalamus from this line [7]. The accuracy of the anterior and posterior dimensions was increased in the Schaltenbrand and Bailey atlas, and later in the Schaltenbrand and Wahren atlas, when the coronal zero plane was defined at the midpoint of AC−PC [5,8]. A statistical system, based on the midline and a line connecting the foramen of Munro and the pineal recess, was later proposed by Andrew and Watkins [9]. Each of these techniques increased the accuracy in the anterior−posterior and somewhat in the superior−inferior dimensions, especially when the anatomic target was near the midline. None of these techniques had an accurate means of adjusting mediolaterally.

The two techniques described in this chapter, the computer-resident atlas and multimodality correlation technique, are variations of previously reported techniques for calculating stereotactic coordinates of a point from CT and MRI. We have found that the targets generated from these techniques, and especially from the new multimodality technique, provide reasonable stereotactic coordinates when compared to actual targets determined from positive contrast ventriculography modified by microelectrode recording [4,10−12]. Both techniques are rapidly performed using the user-friendly stereotactic software. Nevertheless, stereotactic coordinates for neuroablative subcortical procedures should be determined from as many sources as possible, until one technique provides higher accuracy in every instance. The multimodality correlative technique holds much

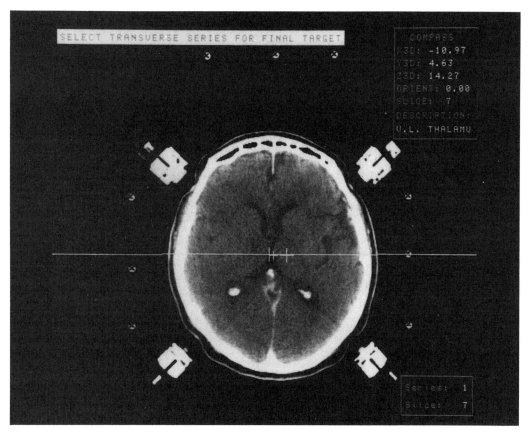

FIGURE 10.6 Large cursor indicates point on line 11.5 mm from point selected on the wall of the IIIrd ventricle (Fig. 10.5) and its stereotactic coordinates (top right).

promise in the years ahead to provide these results, as the spatial accuracy and resolution of these radiologic images increases, and their thickness decreases.

References

1 Brierley, J. & Beck, E. The significance in human stereotactic brain surgery of individual variation in the diencephalon and globus pallidus. *J. Neurol. Neurosurg. Psychiatr.* **22**: 287–98 (1959).

2 Van Buren, J. & Maccubbin, D. An outline atlas of human basal ganglia with estimation of anatomical variants. *J. Neurosurg.* **19**: 811–39 (1962).

3 Kelly, P.J., Derome, P. & Guiot, G. Thalamic spatial variability and the surgical results of lesions placed with neurophysiologic control. *Surg. Neurol.* **9**: 307–15 (1978).

4 Kall, B.A., Kelly, P.J., Goerss, S. & Frieder, G. Methodology and clinical experience with computed tomography and a computer-resident

stereotactic atlas. *Neurosurgery* **17**(3): 400–7 (1985).

5 Schaltenbrand, G. & Wahren, W. *Atlas for Stereotaxy of the Human Brain*, 2nd edn. Stuttgart: Thieme (1977).

6 Kelly, P.J. Microelectrode recording for the somatotopic placement of stereotactic thalamic lesions in the treatment of parkinsonian and cerebellar tremor. *Appl. Neurophys.* **43**: 262–6 (1980).

7 Talairach, J., David, M. & Tournoux, P. *Atlas d'Anatomie Stereotaxique*. Paris: Masson (1957).

8 Schaltenbrand, G. & Bailey, P. *Introduction to Stereotaxis with an Atlas of the Human Brain*, Vol. 1. New York: Grune and Stratton (1959).

9 Andrew, J. & Watkins, E.S. *A Stereotaxic Atlas of the Human Thalamus and Adjacent Structures*. Baltimore: Williams and Wilkins (1969).

10 Kelly, P.J., Kall, B. & Goerss, S. Functional stereotactic surgery utilizing CT data and computer-generated stereotactic atlas. *Acta Neurochir.* **33** (suppl.): 577–83 (1984).

11 Kelly, P.J. Applications and methodology for con-

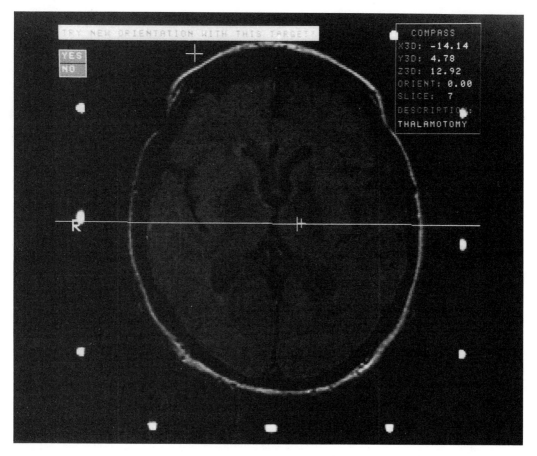

FIGURE 10.7 Transverse MRI slice correlated to point selected on Fig. 10.6. Large cursor indicates point of correlation. Smaller cursor further to right on the line indicates the final stereotactic coordinate selected by the surgeon as the proposed surgical target. The stereotactic coordinates for this target appear in the upper right quadrant.

temporary stereotactic surgery. *Neurol. Res.* **8**: 2–12 (1986).

12 Kelly, P.J., Ahlskog, J.E., Goerss, S.J., Daube, J.R., Duffy, J.R. & Kall, B.A. Computer-assisted stereo-tactic ventralis lateralis thalamotomy with micro-electrode recording control in patients with Parkinson's disease. *Mayo Clin. Proc.* **62**: 655–64 (1987).

Three-dimensional Maps by Interpolation from the Schaltenbrand and Bailey Atlas

Masafumi Yoshida

Introduction

During stereotactic functional neurosurgery, voluminous amounts of neurophysiologic data are obtained from subcortical structures of the human subjects, who undergo this procedure in a waking state under local anesthesia. This information is extremely valid for target localization and, at the same time, for understanding the underlying pathology and physiology of human subcortical structures.

Since these data usually come with three-dimensional (3-D) coordinates, they can be fed into a computer to create a huge 3-D data library, to be processed and displayed three-dimensionally for efficient use of this information for intraoperative guidance in target localization, and also for visualization of the functional organization of subcortical structures. In past decades, computer-assisted integration of functional and anatomic organization was attempted by plotting neurophysiologic data on an anatomic atlas, thus creating a functional atlas [1–4]. For this purpose, 3-D display using a 3-D atlas is useful.

In this chapter, a 3-D atlas [5], created by interpolation from the Schaltenbrand and Bailey atlas [6], on which functional data is plotted, will be presented along with a description of our comprehensive minicomputer data processing system for use in functional neurosurgery.

Basic concept

Stereotactic surgery is based on the fact that the 3-D relationship of intracranial structures is reasonably constant and, therefore, any anatomic structure can be located on a 3-D coordinates system within the limits of individual anatomic variation.

The armamentarium for stereotactic surgery consists of: (1) an anatomic atlas (or 3-D matrix system) which is based on the anatomy of the standard human brain (or 3-D voxels in computed tomography (CT) scan or magnetic resonance (MR) images of a particular patient) for the calculation of 3-D coordinates; (2) a purely mechanical device to fix the patient's head securely, and to accurately access any intended target on a 3-D coordinates system constructed on the headframe; and (3) an interface to link the two different 3-D coordinates systems, so that 3-D coordinates on one system can be interchangeably converted to those on the other system.

Stereotactic functional neurosurgery

In functional neurosurgery, an anatomy-based 3-D coordinates system is usually constructed on cerebral reference points in and around the IIIrd ventricle, which is in close proximity to the usual target area in functional neurosurgery. The most popular example of such a system is the Schaltenbrand and Bailey atlas [6], whose 3-D coordinates system is constructed on the anterior and posterior commissures (AC and PC), with the origin of the coordinates system at the midpoint of a line drawn between AC and PC (AC–PC line).

With the patient's head securely fixed to the stereotactic headframe, the anatomic 3-D coordinates system rests upon the headframe-based coordinates system. Therefore, localization of at least three cerebral reference points (or their equivalents) on the headframe-based coordinates system (either by ventriculogram or CT image data processing) will give conversion parameters for the two coordinates systems. Provided the patient's head is securely fixed to the headframe, and using the same conversion parameters, any point localized on the frame-based 3-D coordinates system can be converted to 3-D coordinates of the AC–PC system, or vice versa, during the entire procedure.

Digitization of intraoperative film for intraoperative data input

In the author's institution, intraoperative ventriculograms are used for visualization of cerebral reference points, for determination of coordinate conversion parameters, and for verification of electrode positions, and all necessary 3-D coordinates calculations are performed by digitized data of intraoperative X-ray films.

The purposes of digitization of intraoperative X-rays are: (1) calculation of the magnification factor of the X-ray film, and of the 3-D coordinates on the headframe axes at various digitized points; (2) calculation of coordinates conversion parameters between the two different 3-D coordinate systems; (3) calculation of trajectory coordinates by digitization of positions of electrodes introduced into the subcortical structures; and (4) acquisition of basic morphologic data for each patient, which appears on the intraoperative ventriculograms and which may be later used as filtering parameters.

Calculation of magnification rate and 3-D coordinates on frame axes

For precise calculation of 3-D coordinates on frame axes from digitized data of intraoperative

X-ray films, complicated software is required to correct the radial divergence of the X-ray beam and parallax. However, most of the commercially available stereotactic instruments are so designed that, without complicated calculations, reasonably accurate 3-D coordinates on the frame coordinates axis can be obtained from X-ray films.

In the stereotactic apparatus in use in the author's institution (Sugita's apparatus), the headframe is basically rectangular in shape, and each of the four side elements of the frame is equipped with a "pin-hole window" at the center of which the axes of the frame-based coordinates system are located. Therefore, before fixing the patient's head to the frame, the X-ray bulb is optically aligned so that an optical beam passes through each of the "pin hole windows" of opposite side elements. The precise alignment of the X-ray beam to the two axes of the frame-based coordinates system is confirmed by X-ray picture.

The headframe is also equipped with a pair of reference pins located precisely 5 cm from the center of the "pin-hole window" on each of the side elements (each pair of reference pins is 10 cm apart); these are for calculation of magnification factors. Therefore, X-ray film taken in this situation will show two sets of reference pins with two different magnification factors, the greater being the magnification factor for the side element close to the X-ray bulb, and the smaller being that for the side element distant from the bulb. The magnification factor for any point located on the X-ray film can be calculated as a factor of location of a particular point on the axis aligned to the X-ray beam between these two side elements, provided the X-ray magnification factor is relatively small (1.065 for lateral views and 1.11 for anterior–posterior (A/P) views, in the author's setting).

Thus, based on digitized data of X-ray films, the magnification factor of each of the digitized points can be calculated, and 3-D coordinates can be obtained from the frame-based coordinates system.

Calculation of 3-D coordinates conversion parameter

Calculation of the 3-D coordinates conversion parameters is possible if the following values on the frame coordinate axes are known: (1)

rotation angle of the head; (2) tilting angle of the head; and (3) 3-D coordinates of the mid-commissural point.

For determination of rotation and tilting angles of the head, recognition of the mid-sagittal plane, precisely aligned to the AC−PC axis, is necessary. Although this is difficult, because some sort of asymmetry of the cranium and intracranial structures is noted in virtually every patient, reasonably accurate rotation and tilting angles can be determined: the rotation angle by location of the zygomatic process of the frontal bone and the lateral margin of the skull in A/P view; and the tilting angle by the position of the sagittal suture and the center of the odontoid process in A/P view.

The midcommissural point is determined from the location of AC and PC in lateral view, and the lateral coordinate from the center of the IIIrd ventricle in A/P view.

Calculation of trajectory coordinates

The purposes of digitization of electrode positions visualized on X-ray are: (1) confirmation of proper electrode position; and (2) calculation of the 3-D coordinates along the trajectory, as correlated to depth of the advancing electrode tip, i.e. the distance between the tip of an electrode and the target point, which can be read as a calibrated number on the stereotactic device.

For the latter purpose, the penetrating electrode tip is digitized at two different points at least, with different depth readings. Once these data are obtained, 3-D coordinates of any data recording point along the trajectory can be calculated by linear interpolation or extrapolation, as a factor of the depth reading. As a result, given the trajectory identification number and the depth reading at the recording point, intraoperative physiologic data will be inputted automatically, together with 3-D coordinates of that point.

Acquisition of basic morphologic data for each patient

Basic morphologic data are acquired from intra-operative ventriculograms for each patient, and include IIIrd and lateral ventricles, the aqueduct of Sylvius with cerebral reference points,

and the inner and outer tables of the cranial vault with their cranial landmarks.

Creation of 0.5 mm-step maps by interpolation from the Schaltenbrand and Bailey atlas

The Schaltenbrand and Bailey atlas [6] has reasonable continuity for practical usage. However, a 3-D serial equidistance atlas, when displayed appropriately, is convenient and visually expressive for plotting out 3-D physiologic data, to create a functional atlas and for understanding of the 3-D anatomy [5,7].

The 3-D atlas introduced in this chapter is a 0.5 mm-step atlas, created by interpolation of the Schaltenbrand and Bailey atlas. With use of this atlas, any three-dimensionally located point can be displayed on a map within a perpendicular distance of 0.25 mm from the point.

Interpolation is performed using subnuclei of the same nomenclature which appear on both of the two adjacent parallel sections and, therefore, the Schaltenbrand−Bailey atlas has to be digitized by subnuclei prior to interpolation.

The algorithm for interpolation is: (1) recognition of the same structure in two adjacent parallel sections; (2) recognition of a portion of a boundary line which has anatomic or geographic characteristics commonly shared by the structures on both sections, i.e. recognition of corresponding portions of the boundary lines which are to be interpolated. Once one or several such portions, if not all, are recognized, the remaining portions can be correlated, and virtually all portions of the structure boundary can be interpolated. The criteria found most useful for identifying "common characteristics" were: (1) a portion of a boundary line which crosses same common neighboring structure; and (2) where no common bounding structure can be identified, a common configuration of line, such as a portion of acute angulation.

A fairly satisfactory new map was created by this method. (Figs 11.1 and 11.2). This was only a simulated, and not a truly 3-D atlas, since interpolation was performed with only two parallel adjacent sections. For example, when a new coronal map was to be created by interpolation, the interpolation was performed only between two adjacent coronal sections and no attention was paid to either the sagittal or hori-

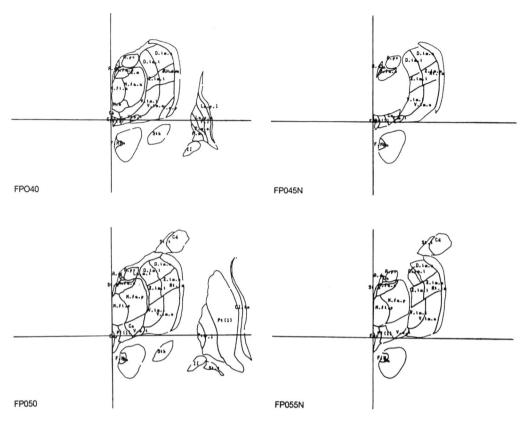

FIGURE 11.1 Interpolation in frontal (coronal) plane. From the Fp 4.0, Fp 5.0, and Fp 7.0 plates of the original atlas (left), new plates Fp 4.5N and Fp 5.5N were created by interpolation (the newly created plates have suffix letter 'N'). Note the "blank area" in Fp 4.5, where interpolation was impossible with the current algorithm because of the absence of the same subnuclei in both the sections being interpolated.

zontal sections covering the 3-D area being interpolated. Therefore, the interpolation was based on the assumption that, in the 3-D area being interpolated, the structure would follow an almost straight line through the two vertically placed anatomic sections, and would not be a complicated, e.g. zigzag-shaped, line.

Also, when a particular structure appears in only one of two adjacent sections, interpolation is impossible and, as a result, this particular area remains as a blank area in the newly created map (Fig. 11.1). Sometimes, this blank area is compensated when surrounding structures can be interpolated, and therefore the structure is "passively" interpolated. However, in such a situation the exact name that should be assigned to the "passively" interpolated structure cannot be determined with certainty when each of two

"blank" structures is present on two adjacent maps under a different name.

With 0.5 mm-step serial anatomic maps, a wide variety of forms of 3-D display are possible, but basically they are determined by: (1) a number of serially placed sections; (2) 3-D rotation angle of the section; and (3) the spatial relationships of each group of serially displayed sections. The display method varies in accordance with the purpose of display. For plotting out 3-D functional data on anatomic maps to make functional maps, the method the author found most useful was displaying a group of 2–3 sections with 3-D rotation, and placed sufficiently far apart to avoid overlapping of two adjacent groups (Fig. 11.3). In effect, this form of display simulates the effect of viewing the sliced brain three-dimensionally [7].

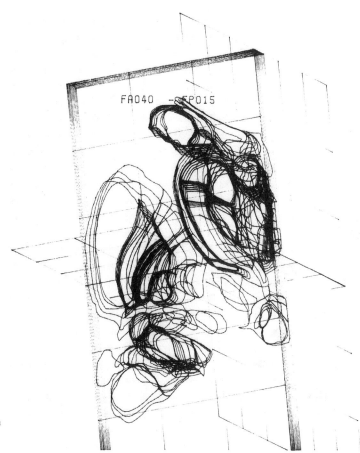

FIGURE 11.2 An example of serial display of a 0.5 mm-step atlas display in the frontal (coronal) plane with axis rotation, for 3-D demonstration of anatomy. Display range = Fa 4.0–Fp 1.5.

Source of intra- and perioperative information

The types of intraoperative neurophysiologic data fed into the computer for creation of functional maps depend on the purpose of study. Along with physiologic data, clinical parameters that might influence the organization of the 3-D functional map, and therefore could be potentially used as filtering parameters for specific selection of data for 3-D display, are also fed into the computer.

Intraoperative electrophysiologic data acquisition

Neurophysiologic data to be plotted onto an anatomic map for the creation of a functional map are always inputted with 3-D coordinates of either the stimulating point or the recording point corresponding to each functional datum.

Such electrophysiologic data include: (1) spontaneous field potentials (neural noise) obtained from semi-microelectrode [8–10]; (2) thalamocortical evoked potentials; (3) evoked potentials recorded from subcortical structures upon stimulation of the contralateral median nerve; and (4) sensory and motor responses upon stimulation of subcortical structures.

Apart from sensory and motor responses, which are coded and subject to keyboard input, these data are fed into the computer by analog-to-digital (AD) conversion, to be processed in suitable form and coded for display. Among these functional data, field potentials seem to primarily reflect anatomic (cytoarchitectural) organization [9], and with various digital processing methods may delineate the boundaries of parcellated subnuclei of the thalamus [11, 12]. Other electrophysiologic data are more oriented to functional representation.

Besides these functional data, the 3-D positions of therapeutic coagulating or stimulation electrodes are fed into the computer, together with coagulation or stimulation parameters.

Clinical parameters

Clinical parameters, which are used primarily for filtering neurophysiologic data, are: (1) basic clinical data; (2) pre- and postoperatively obtained symptom-related data; and (3) intraoperatively obtained anatomic data, especially in the vicinity of the target area of each patient.

Basic clinical data which potentially influence the organization of a neurophysiologic map include such basic features of the patient's profile as age, sex, diagnosis, age at onset, basic neurology, heredity, previous toxicity and central nervous system (CNS) infection, and basic psychometric tests.

Pre- and postoperative data are obtained outside the operating room, usually in the outpatients' clinic, and for this purpose a laptop type personal computer is used. The patients were periodically evaluated in the outpatients' department using a physical examination scale, a functional disability scale, a complication scale, and so on. These data are used for assessment of immediate clinical responses and long-term follow-up results after surgery. Although these data cannot be directly correlated to intraoperative physiologic data, by processing such data immediate and long-term effects of surgery can be correlated to the site of a therapeutic ablative lesion or deep brain stimulation (DBS) electrode, and further to the neurophysiologic data obtained in the vicinity of the strategic site. In this respect these data can also be plotted on 3-D maps in relation to strategic sites for coagulation and stimulation.

Intraoperative data are those visualized on intraoperative ventriculograms, and they are obtained as 3-D data by digitization of X-ray films, as described above. Structures or reference points on intraoperative ventriculograms which are to be digitized include: outlines of

the IIIrd and lateral ventricles with AC, PC_7 and foramen of Monro, the massa intermedia if present, and the cranial vault; other cranial landmarks such as the external auditory meatus, inferior orbital margin, tuberculum sellae, posterior margin of foramen magnum, basion, asterion, and bragma.

Data processing and display

In a functional atlas, 3-D maps serve as anatomic landmarks upon which 3-D functional data are displayed. Sections of the atlas and their rotation angle on an axis and position are freely selected. Category of data displayed and the filtering parameters and their range are also selected to create various types of functional atlas.

Since each 0.5 mm-step map consists of two-dimensional (2-D) coordinates, one can create 3-D coordinate data by the addition of 0.5 mm-step coordinates in the direction of a line perpendicular to the map (an exception to this is a horizontal map, which is not aligned to the horizontal plane of the AC−PC axis, so that additional coordinates conversion is required). For simultaneous display of an anatomic map and functional data, 3-D coordinates of both the 3-D map and the physiologic data should be processed with the same conversion parameters. Since data-processing parameters for each of the anatomic maps often vary, each of the three-dimensionally placed functional data has to be assigned to the topographically closest section with which the datum is to be displayed, i.e. data have to be selected so that their coordinates on the axis perpendicular to the displaying section are within ± 0.25 mm of each section number.

An example of 3-D functional maps

An example of a functional map created by the process described above is shown in Fig. 11.3. This functional map is based on intraoperatively obtained sensory and motor responses to stimulation of subcortical structures. These data were obtained from seven patients (four with parkinsonism, one with post-traumatic tremor, one with thalamic pain, and one with pseudo-thalamic pain), who underwent either nucleus

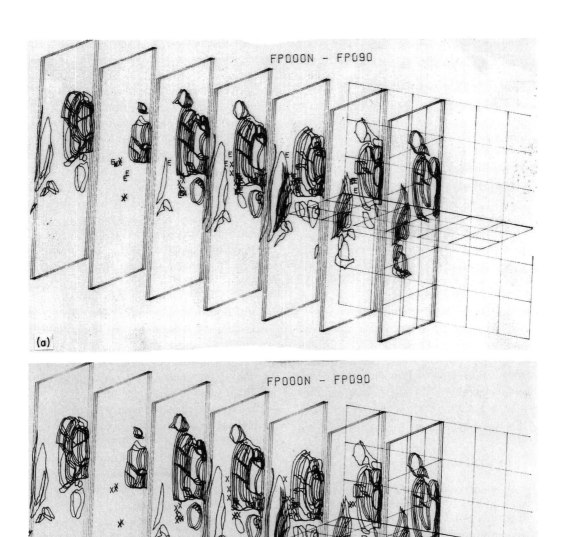

FIGURE 11.3 Examples of functional atlas based on (a) sensory and (b) motor response elicited on electrical stimulation of subcortical structures. Response modality is coded and plotted at stimulation sites. Note that the motor response is elicited on stimulation in the rather confined vicinity of VIM, whereas the sensory response is elicited on stimulation in a wide area. Display range = Fp 0.0N–Fp 9.0. (a) E = electrical; H = heat; S = stiff; T = tingling; W = warm; X = no response. (b) A = tremor arrest; E = tremor enhanced; R = irregular movement, S = tremor suppression; T = twitch; X = no response.

ventralis intermedius (VIM) thalamotomy or DBS electrode insertion to the nucleus ventralis posterolateralis (VPL)-internal capsule region. The stimulating electrode used is a coaxial stain- less steel or tungsten bipolar electrode, whose outer diameter is 0.8 mm, interpolar distance 0.5 mm, and tip diameter 50 μm. The stimu- lation parameter is 2 mA, 0.2–0.5 ms, square pulse wave with frequency range of 5–90 Hz. Data were stored as coded information representing the modalities and somatic distribution of the stimulation responses. Sensory and motor response modalities are plotted to create a functional map. In both displays, the stimulation site is indicated by an alphanumeric code corresponding to the response modality, as shown in Fig. 11.3a and b, in which the letter "X" represents a point where no response was elicited on electrical stimulation. Although geographic freedom of placement of the exploratory electrode is limited, and therefore the trajectory is more or less confined to the vicinity of the ventrolateral nuclear groups of the thalamus, it is apparent that sensory responses of various modalities, mostly electrical sensations, were elicited by stimulation of rather broad areas, whereas motor responses were primarily localized in the vicinity of VIM. The similar display based on the somatic distribution of stimulation response (not shown) indicated that the majority of these responses had their somatic distribution in either the face, the hand, or the upper limb.

Use of 3-D atlas in stereotactic surgery

The 3-D atlas presented here is a product of relatively simple mathematical interpolation, and is not a truly 3-D atlas as described above. Creation of a truly 3-D atlas requires detailed anatomic study; however, since the post-mortem brain is subject to anatomic deformity during preparation, creation of a truly 3-D atlas from post-mortem material might be difficult. In any event, the organization of anatomic structures as defined by information on microcytoarchitecture (line drawings from microscopic anatomic study, and anatomic nomenclature, of Hassler [13]) are most commonly referred to when anatomic locations are to be cited. Therefore, for study of deep subcortical structures, comprehensive data collection in the form of data on the AC–PC axis is felt to be essential. This will facilitate quick reference of stored data to a microsurgically cytoarchitecture-based anatomic atlas. For display of such data, the 3-D atlas in 0.5 mm sections created by interpolation of the Schaltenbrand and Bailey atlas is useful.

The usefulness of this sort of 3-D atlas is apparent when it is incorporated into a comprehensive computer data processing system for stereotactic functional neurosurgery. Here it is used to show anatomic landmarks for the display of various computer-stored data, because of its ability to produce various types of 3-D display, with a wide range of flexibility in both display modality and data filtration. Thus, the functional atlas created will give a clear view of the functional organization of the subcortical structures, based on a huge pool of 3-D oriented data which otherwise may be difficult to understand. With this comprehensive approach, it might be possible to solve some of questions inherent in stereotactic functional surgery, which the author considers the ultimate goal of this computerized stereotactic data processing system, such as (1) the anatomic variations of each of the subcortically located parcellated structures; (2) the basic physiologic profile of the subcortical structures; and (3) their alteration in pathologic states.

In the operating room, display of such a functional atlas, based on accumulated data and with appropriate data filtration, together with displays of trajectory location and physiologic data obtained along the trajectory of a particular patient, will be very helpful in optimal target selection [14,15].

On the other hand, the disadvantages and limitations of this approach in the clinical setting are: (1) the requirement for an invasive procedure; (2) the limitation of the clinical material to a particular patient group affected by a particular pathology; and (3) limitation of the anatomic area available for trajectory placement, and therefore for physiologic exploratory study.

To compensate for these disadvantages and limitations, the idea of a centralized databank system is worth considering. With a standardized data format and 3-D coordinates system, inter-institutional data comparison, and accumulation of a wider range of data about pathology and trajectory locations [16], could become possible.

Application of the system

Any information which involves 3-D coordinates, and which can be converted to AC–PC axis coordinates, can be integrated into this computer data-processing system to create a new data library.

Various such data, in the form of 3-D voxels, are now widely available. They include voxel data from CT, MRI, and positron emission tomography (PET). These data are non-invasively obtained, are particular to an individual patient, and cover all cranial and intracranial structures.

The accuracy of images depends on voxel size. In recent CT, the voxel size can be sufficiently small to localize fine structures, including AC and PC. Since 3-D coordinates of structures visualized by CT imaging are precise, by direct reading of the 3-D coordinates from CT images of at least three points, including AC and PC, conversion to the AC−PC axis is possible [15,17].

The MR image is superior in its resolution and can visualize more detail of anatomy, but its spatial or 3-D coordinates' accuracy may be less than that in CT. In PET, 3-D voxel data are of low resolution, and calculation of accurate 3-D coordinates of cerebral reference points is difficult. Sine voxel data of MRI and PET are obtained on essentially the same principles as those of CT, with use of a localizer (or mechanical interface) which can be, preferably non-invasively and securely, fixed to the patient's head, and can be precisely visualized in all CT, MRI, and PET images, 3-D coordinates of essential cerebral reference points can be localized on voxel data of MRI and PET by the position of a localizer on three types of images and coordinates of necessary reference points on the CT image as interface.

Once this has been done, 3-D voxel data of CT, MRI, and PET can be reformatted to be aligned to the AC−PC axis. Thus, as in the functional atlas described above, anatomic or functional maps based on the voxel data library can be displayed with the 3-D anatomic atlas or, conversely, voxel data of an individual patient can be reconstructed so that they are aligned to the AC−PC axis, and can be displayed together with the appropriate 3-D anatomic map [15,17].

In recent years, new subdivision of the thalamus based on histochemical study has been published [18]. In this context, it might be interesting to incorporate PET data to this system, since PET is a biochemically and metabolically oriented diagnostic modality. This approach means integration of: (1) intraoperatively obtained neurophysiologic data from a group of patients who have undergone stereotactic functional neurosurgery; (2) non-invasively and relatively easily available morphologic (CT and MRI) and biochemical (PET) data, both from control groups and from patients with a wide range of pathology; and (3) microscopic anatomy as defined by cytoarchitecture. This comprehensive approach is expected to contribute to the understanding of the anatomic, physiologic, and biochemical organization of deep subcortical structures and their modification by various pathologic conditions.

References

1 Tasker, R.R., Hawrylyshyn, P. & Organ, L.W. Computer mapping of brainstem sensory centers in man. *J. Neurosurg.* **44**: 458−64 (1976).

2 Hardy, T.L. Bertrand, G., & Thompson, C.J. The position and organization of motor fibers in the internal capsule found during stereotactic surgery. *Appl. Neurophysiol.* **42**: 160−70 (1979).

3 Hardy, T.L., Bertrand, G. & Thompson, C.J. Organization and topography of sensory responses in the internal capsule and nucleus ventralis caudalis found during stereotactic surgery. *Appl. Neurophysiol.* **42**: 335−51 (1979).

4 Tasker, R.R., Organ, L.W. & Hawrylyshyn, P. *The Thalamus and Midbrain of Man. A Physiological Atlas using Electrical Stimulation.* Springfield: C.C. Thomas (1982).

5 Yoshida, M. Creation of a three-dimensional atlas by interpolation from Schaltenbrand-Bailey's atlas. *Appl. Neurophysiol.* **50**: 45−8 (1987).

6 Schaltenbrand, G. & Bailey, P. (eds). *Introduction to Stereotaxis with an Atlas of Human Brain.* Stuttgart: Thieme (1959).

7 Yoshida, M. Mapping of semi-microelectrode stimulation response in and around the thalamus. *Stereotact. Funct. Neurosurg.* **52**: 171−5 (1989).

8 Bertrand, G., Jasper, H., Wong, A. & Mathews, G. Microelectrode recording during stereotaxic surgery. *Clin. Neurosurg.* **16**: 328−55 (1969).

9 Fukamachi, A., Ohye, C. & Narabayashi, H. Delineation of the thalamic nuclei with a microelectrode in stereotaxic surgery for parkinsonism and cerebral palsy. *J. Neurosurg.* **39**: 214−25 (1973).

10 Ohye, Ch., Saito, A., Fukamachi, A. & Narabayashi, H. An analysis of the spontaneous rhythmic and non-rhythmic discharges in the human thalamus. *J. Neurol. Sci.* **22**: 245−59 (1974).

11 Yoshida, M. Electrophysiological characterization of human subcortical structures by frequency spectrum analysis of neural noise (field potential) obtained during stereotactic surgery. *Appl. Neurophysiol.* **50**: 471−2 (1987).

12 Yoshida, M. Electrophysiological characterization of human subcortical structures by frequency spectrum analysis of neural noise (field potential) obtained during stereotactic surgery. Preliminary presentation of frequency power spectrum of various subcortical structures. *Stereotact. Funct. Neurosurg.* **52**: 157−63 (1989).

13 Hassler, R. Anatomy of the thalamus. In: Schaltenbrand, G. & Bailey, P. (eds) *Introduction to Stereotaxis with an Atlas of Human Brain*. Stuttgart: Thieme (1959).

14 Bertrand, G., Olivier, A. & Thompson, C.J. The computer brain atlas: its use in stereotaxic surgery. *Appl. Neurophysiol.* **36**: 312−3 (1974).

15 Hardy, T.L., Koch, J. & Lassiter, A. Computer graphics with computerized tomography for functional neurosurgery. *Appl. Neurophysiol.* **46**. 217−26 (1983).

16 Laitinen, L.V. Brain targets in surgery for Parkinson's disease. Results of a survey of neurosurgeons. *J. Neurosurg.* **62**: 349−51 (1985).

17 Kall, B.A., Kelly, P.J., Goerss, S. & Frieder, G. Methodology and clinical experience with computed tomography and a computer-resident stereotactic atlas. *Neurosurgery* **17**: 400−407 (1985).

18 Hirai, T. & Jones, E.G. A new parcellation of the human thalamus on the basis of histochemical staining. *Brain Res. Rev.* **15**: 1−34 (1989).

B

On-line Analysis and Functional Mapping

12

Computers in Functional Stereotactic Surgery

Ronald R. Tasker and Jonathan O. Dostrovsky

Introduction

Most functional stereotactic operations require the neurosurgeon to locate a given target within the central nervous system, guide a suitable probe towards it, confirm arrival within the target, and then to manipulate it as needed.

The likely location of the target is first determined by imaging with an appropriate stereotactic frame rigidly attached to the head. Although, historically, this was done with ventriculography or pneumoencephalography, current practice is to employ computed tomography (CT) or magnetic resonance imaging (MRI). Next a suitable probe is selected, depending on the type of target manipulation required: destructive, with radiofrequency current, extreme cold, particle beams, or focused electromagnetic radiation; or modulatory, with electrical stimulation or drug infusion. Corroboration of localization of the probe in the intended target is usually done physiologically, using macro- or microstimulation or else macro- or microelectrode recording of spontaneous and/or evoked neuronal activity. Although motor and sensory consequences of macrostimulation are usually the features studied, there is a growing tendency to use microelectrode recordings of single unit activity and microstimulation. Finally target manipulating is done.

These various activities require a graphic display of three-dimensional (3-D) localization of sites in the brain and of probe trajectories with reference to a standard brain atlas, the results of imaging, stereotactic frame coordinates, and physiologic data collected along probe trajectories. These displays should allow replotting of physiologic data with respect to anatomic data, to reflect individual variations and for storage for future reference, both of individual and pooled patient data. Such tasks, tedious to accomplish by hand, are admirably suited to the use of computers.

This chapter will focus on the study of physiologic data with respect to brain anatomy, a field to which my attention was drawn by my colleagues Leslie Organ and Peter Hawrylyshyn.

Historical

Peluso and Gybels [1,2] appear to have been the first to produce techniques to calculate the stereotactic positions of probes and side protruding electrodes during stereotactic operations with the use of tables derived from computers. Similar methods were developed for use with specific types of stereotactic frames [3–5]. However these programs produced a tabular, not a visual, output, and were used to read off probe position with respect to 3-D locations within the brain, relative to selected brain landmarks.

Computer capabilities were taken a step further by Bertrand *et al.* [6,7] who developed on-line graphic displays in various atlas planes of the course of a probe through brain structures. Probe site was extrapolated from the plates of the atlas by Schaltenbrand and Bailey [8], by superimposing the locations of the patient's anterior and posterior commissures upon those of the atlas diagrams. This was done by digitizing the atlas data, storing them in computer memory and then displaying them as needed in the operating room on a graphics terminal.

Mundinger *et al.* [9] developed an elaborate computer program which incorporates atlas data, cranial X-ray loci, and CT scan upon which electrode trajectories can be plotted in three dimensions.

Hardy *et al.* [10−15] expanded this concept one step further by producing a computer graphics display of physiologic data, collected with microelectrodes in the form of alphanumerics superimposed on the atlas diagrams described above. Both individual and pooled patient data could be so displayed. Hardy and co-workers extended this technique to include imaging data collected by CT and MRI [16−18], leading to the commercially available CASS system (Medical Instrumentation and Diagnostics Corporation, Albuquerque, NM), which can be adapted to any stereotactic frame capable of graphically displaying physiologic data on appropriately scaled atlas diagrams in various planes with superimposed CT, MRI and positron emission tomography (PET) images.

Our group at the Toronto General Hospital, led by Peter Hawrylyshyn, began, in 1974, the development of an interactive on-line graphics system to assist the neurosurgeon in carrying out functional stereotactic procedures [19−24]. The system software, written in FORTRAN, depended upon linkage to the nearby powerful, but massive, IBM 3033 computer, housed in the University of Toronto, with a Tektonix 4014 computer graphics terminal located in the operating room. A Gould 5000 electrostatic printer provided hard copies.

The sagittal diagrams from the Schaltenbrand−Bailey atlas [8] were digitized and stored on-line. As soon as the stereotactic 3-D coordinates of the anterior and posterior com-

missures (our landmarks for stereotactic surgery) were measured in a particular patient, using positive contrast ventriculography [24, pp. 5−12], they were fed into the computer, which then drew a full set of atlas sagittal diagrams, stretched or shrunk as needed until their intercommissural distance matched that of the particular patient being operated upon. It proved impossible to rescale dorsoventrally. The computer then superimposed upon these diagrams a 1 mm grid reading in the antero-posterior and dorsoventral scales of the Leksell stereotactic frame, according to its position on that particular patient's head. The whole was displayed both in hard copy and on the video screen on-line. Subroutines permitted rotation and translation of the display about selected points and selection of any portion of it within specified boundary limits.

On these diagrams the surgeon could select the desired stereotactic anatomic target and read off its 3-D frame coordinates. Of course, this selected anatomic target would be the actual site to be manipulated by the surgeon only if the patient's brain conformed exactly to the brain from the Schaltenbrand−Bailey atlas [8], from which the diagrams were prepared — an unlikely possibility. Even so, the match is good to within ± 1 mm in up to 45% of patients. But the 55% or so in which the fit was less good constitute the reason that physiologic localization is essential.

Our program was developed for data obtained by macrostimulation with a concentric bipolar electrode, having a 1.1 mm diameter, a 0.5 mm bare tip, and a 0.5 mm pole separation, and estimated to produce effective stimulation over a sphere 2 mm in radius when currents up to 1.0 mA were used [24, p. 31]. With the program displayed, correctly spatially oriented on the computerized sagittal maps, the physiologic data were collected as the stimulating electrode was advanced in 2 mm steps through the brain towards the target. Data analysis was facilitated by placing the access burr hole in the same sagittal plane as the intended target, so that physiologic data from the entire trajectory could be displayed in a single sagittal diagram.

The plotting of physiologic data was accomplished by first calling up, by number, one of six stylized diagrams (see Fig. 12.1), dis-

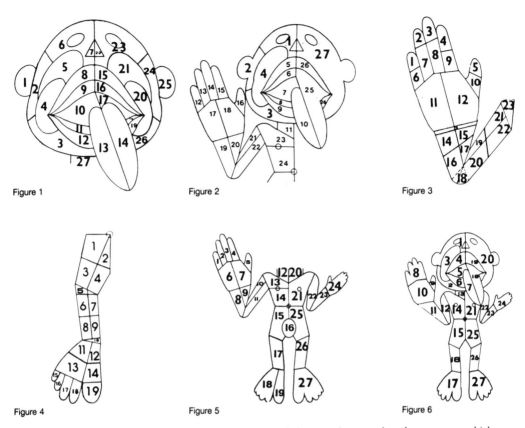

Figure 1   Figure 2   Figure 3

Figure 4   Figure 5   Figure 6

FIGURE 12.1 Set of six numbered figurine diagrams, divided in turn into numbered parts, upon which physiologic responses are indicated. From Tasker *et al.* [24].

playing all or part of the patient's body, each of which was subdivided into numbered parts. Next, one or more of these numbered parts was chosen and shaded in, to indicate those parts of the body affected by stimulation at each stimulation site. Different patterns of shading reflected differing thresholds. Finally, alphanumerics (see Table 12.1) were added to the figurine at each site to indicate the quality of response reported there: P for paresthetic, H for hot, TA for tremor arrest, MR for motor, a triangle for no response, and so on. As plotting was completed at each site the electrode was advanced to the next site, where the process was repeated, and so on until the trajectory was completed. Additional trajectories in the same or another sagittal plane were similarly studied, until enough data had accrued to permit unequivocal identification of the target, which the program then marked on the appropriate brain diagram (see Figs 12.2 and 12.3). Such com-

pleted maps were stored in the memory of the computer. For simplicity, mappings were identified as either contralateral or ipsilateral, regardless of which side of the patients' brain was explored. The computer diagram was completed by the addition of the patient's name, age, and diagnosis and the sagittal plane explored. If the physiologic data collected and plotted failed to conform to that expected from the various brain structures across which the computerized diagram suggested the trajectory passed, it was possible to translate, rotate or replot the physiologic data until an appropriate match was attained.

With this program each patient's data, stored in memory, could be retrieved in hard copy or on screen at any time. In addition, the stored records of all patients studied could be scanned for responses of a given type within given threshold limits, etc., and the resulting pooled selected data replotted on a set of sagittal

TABLE 12.1 Alphanumeric symbols used to further describe physiologic data. From Tasker *et al.* [24], by kind permission of Charles C. Thomas

Cold, cool	K	Vestibular	
		Clockwise	Vc
Warm	W	Anticlockwise	Va
		Left	Vl
Hot	H	Right	Vr
		Other	V?
Burning	B		
		Dizzy	Di
Vibration	Vi		
		Tremor	
Paresthesia,	P	Drive	Td
tingling,		Reduction	Tr
numbness		Arrest	Ta
Faint, woozy	F	Dystonia	
		Drive	Mid
Nausea	N	Arrest	Mia
Smell, olfactory	Sm	Motor	
		Response	Mr
Taste, gustatory	G	Twitch	Mt
Auditory		Emotional	Et
Ipsi	Ai		
Contra	Ac	Vocal, speech	Vo
Other	Au		
		Pain	Do
Visual			
Ipsi	Oi	Pial response	★★
Contra	Oc		
Other	Ot	Other, miscellaneous	??

diagrams, all scaled to a standard intercommissural distance, as seen in Fig. 12.4. It was also possible to reformat the physiologic data from sagittal diagrams onto coronal displays. Alternatively, all types of response seen in a particular anatomic region could be plotted, and statistical analyses performed to determine the percentage of responses of different types seen at different sites in the brain.

This program was used to review our experience collected with macrostimulation in *The Thalamus and Midbrain of Man. A Physiological Atlas of the Human Brain* [24].

Current developments

Developments in two areas have revolutionized the role of computers in functional stereotactic surgery — imaging and computer technology. The superb imaging of an individual patient's brain possible with CT or MRI has added a new dimension to the background across which the course of a probe can be followed through the brain, and upon which physiologic data can be displayed. On the other hand, advances in computer graphics technology have facilitated exploitation of improved imaging, as described elsewhere in this book, with feats that once required the use of a massive mainframe now performed using a small desktop personal computer (PC).

For example, Giorgi *et al.* [25] and Lipinski and Struppler [26] described a program run on a Tesakeg P114 graphic processor capable of displaying atlas diagrams upon which radiologic, including CT, and pooled physiologic

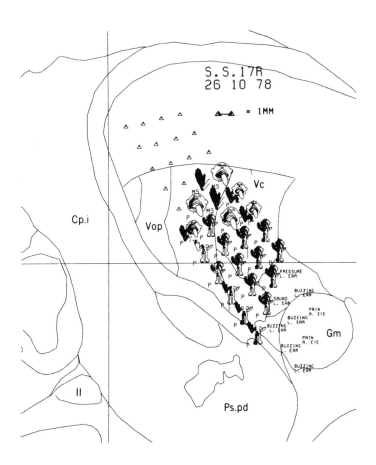

FIGURE 12.2 Completed computer-plotted diagram for patient SS in the 17 mm right sagittal plane, demonstrating sites where paresthetic (P), and auditory responses were elicited by macrostimulation, and where such stimulation elicited a sense of muscle movement (MS), all on the contralateral (left) side of the body. Experience of pain in right (ipsilateral) eye is caused by pressure of tip of the electrode against the surface of midbrain. Cp.i = internal capsule; II = optic nerve; Ps.pd = cerebral peduncle; Vop = ventral oral posterior nucleus; Vc = ventral caudal nucleus; Gm = medial geniculate nucleus.

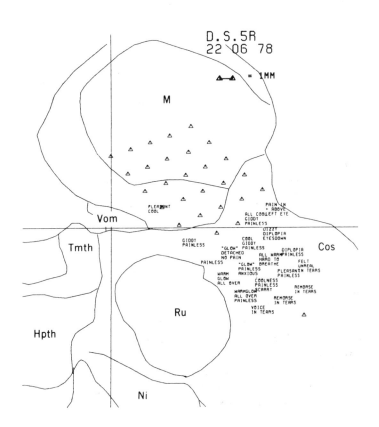

FIGURE 12.3 Similar diagram for patient DS in the 5 mm right sagittal plane, illustrating the use of alphanumerics to plot unusual physiologic data. M = dorsomedian nucleus; Vom = ventral oral medial nucleus; Ru = red nucleus; Tmth = mamillothalamic tract; Hpth = hypothalamus; Ni = substantia nigra. From Tasker et al. [24].

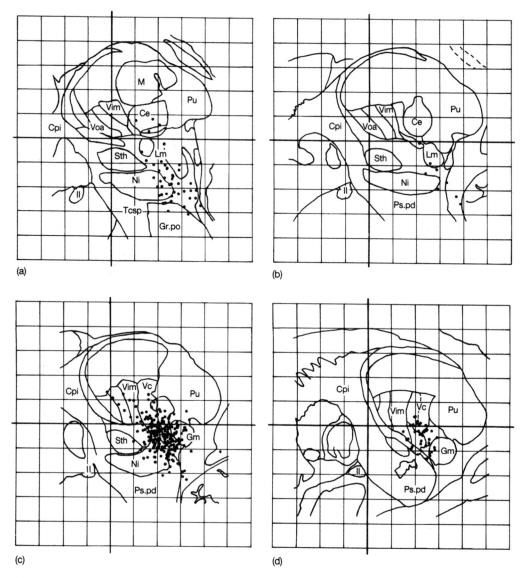

(a) (b) (c) (d)

FIGURE 12.4 Computer-generated display of sites at which paresthetic responses were elicited by macrostimulation below 0.2 mA in all patients studied (24), in the (a) 9, (b) 11, (e) 13.5 and (d) 16.5 mm lateral sagittal planes. Voa = anterior ventral oral nucleus; Vim = ventral intermediate nucleus; Sth = subthalamic nucleus; Ce = centre median; Pu = pulvinar; Lm = medial lemniscus; Tcsp = corticospinal tract; Gr.po = pontine gray; other abbreviations as in Fig. 12.3. From Tasker *et al.* [24].

data can be displayed and color-coded with a digital PDP11/23 or DEC LSI 11/73 computer. Nagaseki *et al.* [27] have produced a program written in BASIC, using a PC NECPC9801 which displays, in 3-D, semi-microelectrode trajectories, neuronal noise levels, and lesion sites and shapes on a set of coronal sections. Goodman *et al.* [28] have incorporated a stereotactic atlas with variability studies into a micro-

computer. Yoshida [29,30] has transferred a stereotactic atlas to a 3-D computer program upon which physiologic data can be appropriately displayed.

Favre [31] has prepared a digitized version of an atlas, capable of being stretched or shrunk to suit individual brain dimensions, upon which electrode trajectories and physiologic events can be superimposed. Rayport and Davis [32] describe a technique for applying a stereotactic reference system to MR images, using a Vectra RS/20 computer with the Autocad system.

We, on the other hand, have concentrated on producing graphics displays of physiologic data, using PCs instead of more complex equipment. This was readily accomplished in the following way. The original program referred to above, written in FORTRAN for the IBM 3303, was rewritten in C for use on a PC. For the past 5 years we have been using this program to plot digitized sagittal brain diagrams, based on those from the Schaltenbrand–Bailey atlas [8], stretched or shrunk as need be to fit the patients' intercommissural distance, upon which are superimposed a 1 mm grid representing the coordinates of the Leksell frame as it is applied to the head of the patient in question. The resulting maps are plotted out on an HP Laserjet printer (Fig. 12.5). The surgeon scans

the appropriate sagittal map, selecting the anatomic target of interest, and reads the frame coordinates off the map, ready to be set on the Leksell frame. Trajectories can be planned to include or avoid structures along the way by reading off the angles of approach, applying them to the frame, and making the twist drill hole at the appropriate site. Such trajectories, and any physiologic information collected en route, are usually sketched in by hand in the course of the surgery upon enlarged copies of appropriate portions of the map.

On the other hand, we have also made use of commercially available software for IBM-compatible PCs to aid in data analysis. Using Autocad 9 (Autodesk Inc., Sansalito, CA), a predigitized outline of the body or of one of its component parts (similar to the diagrams described for the IBM 3303 mainframe) is inserted along a schematic representation of the elec-

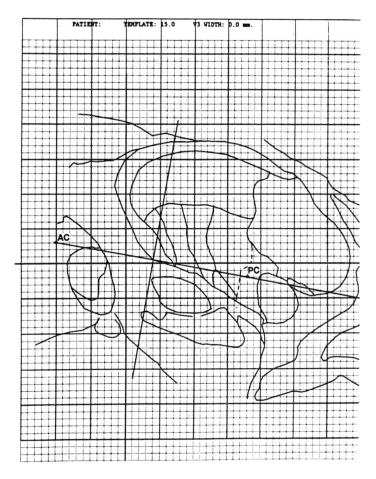

FIGURE 12.5 Computer plot of a sagittal map (15.0 mm lateral to midline) of human thalamus, superimposed on the stereotactic coordinates of the Lexell frame. To produce this map the coordinates of the anterior commissure (AC) were chosen to be 3.0 mm above the frame horizontal zero plane and 10.0 mm anterior to the frame's zero vertical plane, and those of the posterior commissure (PC) 2.0 mm below and 18.0 mm posterior to frame zero. The plot was generated on a Hewlett-Packard Laserjet printer.

trode trajectory at the appropriate depth relative to target. Upon this, receptive fields or sites to which the effects of stimulation are referred (projected fields) can be shaded in by hand (Fig. 12.6), along with descriptive data to indicate quality of response, threshold, neuronal type, etc. But this can also be accomplished with the software program, if desired, in a similar fashion to that for our previously described program with the IBM 3303 mainframe.

Finally, database programs such as Reflex (Borland) can be used to help tabulate and retrieve data pooled from large numbers of patients (Fig. 12.7).

Conclusions

The rapidly expanding fields of brain imaging and computer technology have brought within reach of most functional neurosurgeons the

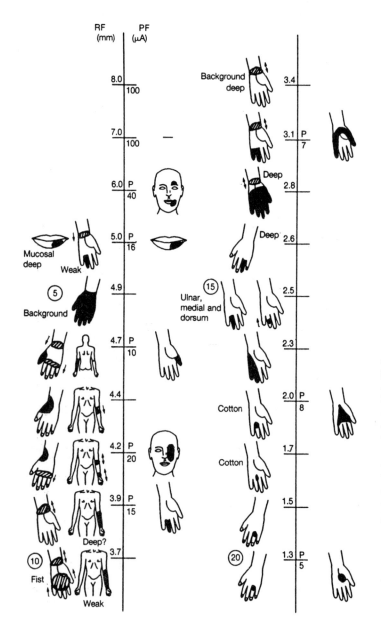

FIGURE 12.6 Plot generated by the program Autocad on a Hewlett-Packard Laserjet printer of a segment of an electrode trajectory (from 8.0 mm to 1.3 mm above target) through thalamus of patient RM. The figurines on either side of the vertical line were drawn from a set of standard figurines of different body parts that were prepared for this purpose. The actual receptive fields and projected fields (regions of body where patient perceives sensation evoked by microstimulation) are drawn by hand on the body parts. RF = receptive field; PF = projected field.

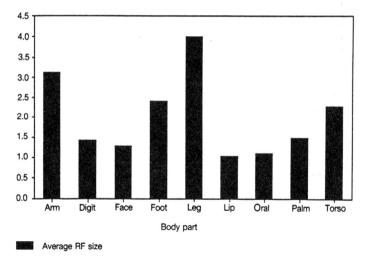

FIGURE 12.7 Bar-graph plot from the program Reflex showing average receptive field (RF) size of neurons in the somatosensory thalamus (on a scale of 1−4) as a function of the receptive field location on the body. The program extracted these data from a large database containing various different parameters for each patient.

possibility of making individual brain maps upon which to display surgery, including physiologic data, and of coordinating it with the results of various types of imaging.

References

1 Peluso, F. & Gybels, J. Calculation of position of electrode point during penetration in the human brain. *Confin. Neurol.* **32**: 213−8 (1970).

2 Peluso, F. & Gybels, J. Computer calculation of position of the side-protruding electrode tip during penetration in the human brain. *Confin. Neurol.* **34**: 94−9 (1972).

3 Birg, W. & Mundinger, F. Computer calculations of target parameters for a stereotactic apparatus. *Acta Neurochir.* **29**: 123−9 (1973).

4 Colloff, E., Gleason, C.A., Alberts, W.W. & Wright, E.W. Computer-aided localization techniques for stereotactic surgery. *Confin. Neurol.* **35**: 65−80 (1973).

5 Dervin, E., Heywood, O.B., Crossley, T.R. & Dawson, B.H. The use of a small digital computer for stereotactic surgery. *Acta Neurochir.* (suppl.) **21**: 245−52 (1974).

6 Bertrand, G., Olivier, A. & Thompson, C.J. Computer display of stereotactic brain maps and probe tracts. *Acta Neurochir.* (suppl.) **21**: 235−43 (1974).

7 Bertrand, G., Olivier, A. & Thompson, C.J. The computer brain atlas: its use in stereotactic surgery. *Confin. Neurol.* **36**: 312−3 (1975).

8 Schaltenbrand, G. & Bailey, P. *Introduction to Stereotaxis with an Atlas of the Human Brain.* Stuttgart: Thieme (1959).

9 Mundinger, F., Birg, W. & Klar, M. Computer-assisted stereotactic brain operations by means including computerized axial tomography. *Appl.*

Neurophysiol. **41**: 169−82 (1977).

10 Hardy, T.L., Bertrand, G. & Thompson, C.J. Thalamic recording during stereotactic surgery. II. Location of quick-adapting, touch-evoked (novelty) cellular responses found during diencephalic recording. *Appl. Neurophysiol.* **42**: 198−202 (1979).

11 Hardy, T.L., Bertrand, G. & Thompson, C.J. Organization and topography of sensory responses in the internal capsule and nucleus ventralis caudalis found during stereotactic surgery. *Appl. Neurophysiol.* **42**: 335−51 (1979).

12 Hardy, T.L., Bertrand, G. & Thompson, C.J. Position and organization of thalamic cellular activity during diencephalic recording. I. pressure-evoked activity. *Appl. Neurophysiol.* **43**: 18−27 (1980).

13 Hardy, T.L., Bertrand, G. & Thompson, C.J. Position and organization of thalamic cellular activity during diencephalic recording. II. Joint and muscle evoked activity. *Appl. Neurophysiol.* **43**: 28−36 (1980).

14 Hardy, T.L., Bertrand, G. & Thompson, C.J. Topography of 'bilateral-movement-evoked' thalamic cellular activity found during diencephalic recording. *Appl. Neurophysiol.* **43**: 67−74 (1980).

15 Hardy, T.L., Bertrand, G. & Thompson, C.J. Touch-evoked thalamic cellular activity. The variable position of the anterior border of somesthetic S1 thalamus and somatotopography. *Appl. Neurophysiol.* **44**: 302−13 (1981).

16 Hardy, T.L. & Koch, J. Computer-assisted stereotactic surgery. *Appl. Neurophysiol.* **45**: 396−8 (1982).

17 Hardy, T.L., Koch, L. & Lassiter, A. Computer graphics with computerized tomography for functional neurosurgery. *Appl. Neurophysiol.* **46**: 217−26 (1983).

18 Hardy, T.L. A method for MRI and CT mapping of diencephalic somatotopography. *Stereotact. Funct. Neurosurg.* **52**: 242−9 (1989).

19 Hawrylyshyn, P., Rowe, I.H., Tasker, R.R. & Organ, L.W. A computer system for stereotactic neurosurgery. *Comput. Biol. Med.* **6**: 87−97 (1976).

20 Tasker, R.R., Rowe, I.H., Hawrylyshyn, P. & Organ, L.W. Computer mapping of brainstem sensory centres in man. *J. Neurosurg.* **44**: 458−64 (1976).

21 Hawrylyshyn, P.A., Tasker, R.R. & Organ, L.W. CASS: computer-assisted stereotactic surgery. *Proc. Sigraph.* **77**(July) (1977).

22 Tasker, R.R., Hawrylyshyn, P., Rowe, I.H. & Organ, L.W. Computerized graphic display of results of subcortical stimulation during stereotactic surgery. *Acta Neurochir.* (suppl.) **24**: 85−98 (1977).

23 Tasker, R.R., Hawrylyshyn, P. & Organ, L.W. Computerized graphic display of physiological data collected during human stereotactic surgery. *Appl. Neurophysiol.* **41**: 183−7 (1978).

24 Tasker, R.R., Organ, L.W. & Hawrylyshyn, P. *The Thalamus and Midbrain of Man. A Physiological Atlas using Electrical Stimulation.* A monograph in the Bannerstone division of American Lectures in Neurosurgery, Wilkins, R.H. (ed.) pp. 36−45. Springfield: Thomas (1982).

25 Georgi, C., Cerchiari, U., Broggi, G., Birk, P., Struppler, A. Digital image processing to handle neuroanatomical information and neurophysiological data. *Appl. Neurophysiol.* **48**: 30−33 (1985).

26 Lipinsky, H.G. & Struppler, A. New trends in computer graphics and computer vision to assist functional neurosurgery. *Stereotact. Funct. Neurosurg.* **52**: 234−41 (1989).

27 Nagaseki, Y., Horikoshi, T., Fukamachi, A. & Ohye, C. A three-dimensional display of stereotactic ventralis intermedius thalamotomy reproduced with a personal computer. *Appl. Neurophysiol.* **49**: 293−4 (1986).

28 Goodman, J.H., Watkins, E.S., Davis, J.R. & Mullin, B.B. Microcomputer stereotactic atlas. *Appl. Neurophysiol.* **50**: 49−52 (1987).

29 Yoshida, M. Creation of a three-dimensional atlas by interpolation from Schaltenbrand-Bailey's atlas. *Appl. Neurophysiol.* **50**: 45−8 (1987).

30 Yoshida, M. Mapping of semimicroelectrode stimulation response in and around the thalamus. *Stereotact. Funct. Neurosurg.* **52**: 171−5 (1989).

31 Favre, J. Digitized stereotactic atlas for personal computer. *Stereotact. Funct. Neurosurg.* **54 & 55**: 240 (1990).

32 Rayport, M. & Davis, J.R. Computerized coplanar stereotactic imaging of normal cerebral structures and lesions in the brain. Presented at Xth meeting of the World Society for Stereotactic and Functional Neurosurgery, Maebashi, October 1989.

13

Computer Processing and Anatomic Correlation of Somatosensory Evoked Potentials in the Ventrolateral (VL) Thalamus

Albrecht Struppler and Hans-Gerd Lipinski

Introduction

There are some clinical and neurophysiologic findings which lead us to assume that special types of hypertonia or pathologic tremor are facilitated by sensory motor afferents originating in the skeletal muscle. Microtechniques such as electrophysiologic stimulation and recordings allow us to identify the function of these neuronal systems. With recent computer techniques, such as computed tomography (CT) and magnetic resonance imaging (MRI) we are able to identify the morphology of brain structures. Our goal was to correlate functional characteristics, e.g. somatosensory evoked potentials, with brain structures by computer assisted techniques. In this chapter we describe a transformation mode which allows correlation of intrathalamic stimulation sites with Schaltenbrand and Wahren's atlas [1].

Computer arrangement

Computer processing for anatomic correlation in functional neurosurgery requires sufficient computer hardware. Besides high-speed A/D-converting of neuronal signals, digital image processing as well as computer graphics should be available. Such a configuration allows combination of neural signals, digital images of the brain, and stereotactic atlas, necessary to match neuronal activity and reference anatomy.

Figure 13.1 shows a possible computer arrangement for functional neurosurgery. The probe, moved to the target by a hydraulic motorized microstepper, is controlled by the computer via a D/A-converter channel. The position of the probe along the trajectory is simultaneously recorded by an electromechanical converter connected to an A/D-converter channel. Further A/D-channels are used to convert the neuronal signal recorded by microelectrodes. Intrathalamic or somatosensory evoked stimulations are performed by the computer using further D/A-converter channels. Both A/D- and D/A-converters are connected to the computer, upmounted with an image processing board. Such a board is needed to analyze digital images (e.g. CT images) for the target calculations. Man–machine communication takes place by keyboard, optical mouse, and display. Digital images and computer graphics are presented on a separate color monitor. Data, including digital images, atlas data and signal data, are stored in a large memory (e.g. optical laser disk).

Minicomputers, like DEC's LSI 11, fulfill the prerequisite to perform both signal processing and image analysis if the LSI is upmounted with appropriate boards. The adequate operating system is the RT11 system; the programs can be written in FORTRAN and MACRO ASSEMBLER, respectively. We installed SIGNUM's IS 100 image processing module, and a 16-channel A/D-converter combined with a four-channel

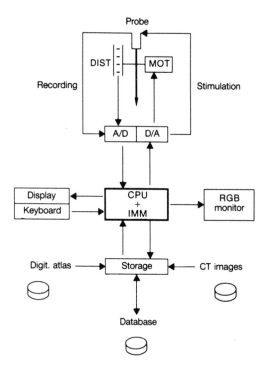

FIGURE 13.1 Computer hardware arrangement for correlating sites of intracerebral electrophysiologic registration and anatomic structures.

D/A-converter on an LSI 11/73 computer [2]. The A/D-converter allows one to digitize neural noise at a sample rate of 500 kcps (kHz). The image processing system generates images of $4 \times 512 \times 512$ picture elements (pixels) of 8-bit gray tone values each (1 Mbyte image storage capacity). The digitized images and atlas planes can be visualized on a color monitor. An additional A/D-converter allows one to digitize the video signal of a CCD camera. This enables us to analyze conventional X-ray ventriculograms by the computer (e.g. measurements of ventricle widths and distances between the anterior and posterior commissures).

During recent years personal computer hardware has become available. On the basis of a MS-DOS machine like IBM's AT computer, it is also possible to arrange a low-cost hardware configuration for the anatomic correlation procedure. Utilizing a standard frame grabber (e.g. ITI's PC-vision frame grabber) for image processing, and high-speed A/D-converters for

digitizing neuronal signal, we also have sufficient PC hardware for the computation. The very powerful programming language C and the ASSEMBLER language, which are available for MS-DOS machines, allow for very efficient programming of localization routines and A/D- and D/A-converting.

The localization procedure

The borders of the commissures and the foramen of Monro served as references for the target coordinates. These references can be obtained from diverse images (X-ray ventriculograms, sagittal CT reconstructions, and MR images). The most important stereotaxic atlases are also based on two of these three reference points. Schaltenbrand and Wahren's atlas [2] is based on the anterior commissure (AC) and posterior commissure (PC); Andrew and Watkins' atlas [3] is based on the foramen of Monro (FM) and PC. For the individual patient's brain, a Cartesian coordinate system similar to that of Schaltenbrand and Wahren can simply be defined. Its origin is at half the distance between AC and PC within the midventricular plane. The x axis is oriented in the anterior–posterior direction (frontal is positive), and called the "S" axis; the y axis is oriented laterally (left is positive), and called the "L" axis; and the z axis is oriented perpendicularly (cranial is positive) and called the "H" axis (Fig. 13.2). This coordinate system allows comparison of individual brains with the atlas of Schaltenbrand and Wahren.

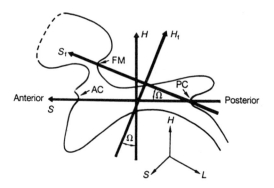

FIGURE 13.2 Definition of Schaltenbrand and Wahren's and Andrew and Watkins' Cartesian atlas coordinate systems.

$$\begin{bmatrix} S^c{}_f \\ L^c{}_f \\ H^c{}_f \end{bmatrix} = \begin{bmatrix} \cos\Omega & 0 & \sin\Omega & \frac{1}{2}(c.\cos\Omega - f) \\ 0 & 1 & 0 & 0 \\ -\sin\Omega & 0 & \cos\Omega & -\frac{1}{2}.c.\sin\Omega \end{bmatrix} \begin{bmatrix} S^c \\ L^c \\ H^c \\ 1 \end{bmatrix} \qquad \text{(F1)}$$

If Andrew and Watkins' atlas is used, the coordinate system has to be modified. In this case the S axis penetrates the foramen of Monro instead of the AC. Hence, this coordinate system is rotated within the midventricular plane relative to the PC at the angle Ω. Let H be replaced by H_f, S be replaced by S_f and L be replaced by L_f (Fig. 13.2). The origin of Andrew and Watkins' coordinate system is at half the distance between FM and PC, within the midventricular plane. Let c be the distance between PC and AC, and f the distance between the FM and PC. Any point $Q \equiv (S^c, L^c, H^c)^T$ within the AC–PC coordinate system can be transferred to the FM–PC coordinate system as $Q^t \equiv (S^c{}_f, L^c{}_f, H^c{}_f)^T$ by the transformation (see F1 above).

We used the Todd–Wells frame for the stereotaxic operations. The target coordinates in reference to the frame were conventionally evaluated by the sites of the AC and PC, and by the maximal lateral extension of the IIIrd ventricle. Based on the target coordinates, the trajectory of the movable electrode was defined in reference to the starting coordinates of the electrode, which was mounted on the frame. The frame coordinate system is a spherical system. The origin of the frame system is located at the defined target point, which has the coordinates $P_0 \equiv (S_0, L_0, 0)^T$, where S_0 is the distance between the origin and half of the AC–PC distance in the anterior–posterior direction. L_0 is the lateral component of the target coordinates relative to the midventricular plane. Let $P_1 = (S_1, L_1, H_1)^T$ be a reference point within the frame system, and let α be the tilt angle of the trajectory in the frontal plane, and

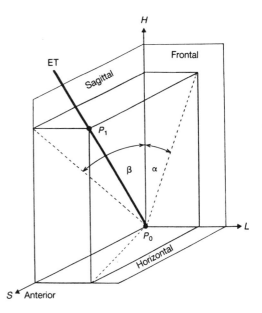

FIGURE 13.3 Correlation of a spherical frame coordinate system and a Cartesian atlas coordinate system (ET = electrode trajectory).

β the tilt angle of the trajectory in the sagittal plane (Fig. 13.3). A point $P = (\alpha, \beta, d)$ within the spherical coordinates of the frame can simply be transferred to the Schaltenbrand and Wahren AC–PC system by the transformation F2 (see below).

Spontaneous neural noise was registered by tungsten microelectrodes (tip diameter ≈ 50 μm, impedance < 100 kΩ), driven forward to the target to control the trajectory by electrophysiologic detection of the thalamus border. The thalamus border was reached when

$$\begin{bmatrix} S_1 \\ L_1 \\ H_1 \end{bmatrix} = \frac{d}{\sqrt{\Gamma}} . \begin{bmatrix} \tan\beta \\ \tan\alpha \\ 1 \end{bmatrix} + \begin{bmatrix} S_0 \\ L_0 \\ 0 \end{bmatrix} \qquad \text{(F2)}$$

where d is the euclidian distance between P_0 and P_1 and $\Gamma = 1 + \tan^2\alpha + \tan^2\beta$.

a spontaneous change in neuron noise level was registered, indicating that the electrode had reached the nucleus reticularis thalami, or had exited the thalamus at the region of the radiatio praelemniscalis or the zona incerta, respectively [1,4,5].

In order to match the electrophysiologically explored thalamus borders with atlas borders, sites of noise changing and digitized atlas planes were displayed on the monitor. Before display, individual intracerebral coordinates were weighted proportionally by the quotient of the AC−PC distances of the atlas and the patient in all three dimensions (the so-called AC−PC transformation) as described elsewhere [2,6−8]. Following the AC−PC transformation, the sites of noise changing were found to deviate markedly from atlas borders (see Fig. 13.5a) [5]. This was mainly due to the fact that the lateral coordinate of the target area in reference to the atlas could not be calculated precisely on the basis of the AC−PC distance ratio. Conventionally generated positive X-ray ventriculograms (anterior−posterior (A/P) direction) do not present a practicable value of the target laterality, for the A/P ventriculogram presents a projection of the IIIrd ventricle, hence only maximal lateral ventricle widths occur. From CT images, however, the laterality of the target area was derived in an applicable manner. Thalamus outlines could be calculated by different tools of image processing procedures, using a technique based on the fact that the thalamic nuclei and capsula interna fibers differ in their Hounsfield units and hence in their gray tone values.

Digital computer tomograms which contained the thalamus region were selected from the original stack of CT scans. In each of these images the thalamus area served as a region of interest marked by an image window. Within this image window the gray tone values were low-pass filtered by a digital median filter to reduce image noise. The sites of AC and PC were obtained from parasagittal reconstructions of the CT scans. Following rotation and linear shifting, images were created from that set of CT images which were orientated: (1) perpendicular to the midventricular plane; and (2) parallel to the AC−PC plane. These computations were done by linear gray tone interpolation. From this set of images, the image which was 4 mm above the AC−PC plane was selected. Within this image the thalamus was segmented by binary coding following "optimal" gray tone thresholding [9]. Picture elements (pixels) which had a gray tone value equal to that of the thalamic nuclei region were coded as "1"; otherwise, the pixels were coded as "0." Unfortunately, gray tone thresholding resulted in background noise. Small areas which were part of the thalamus were coded as "0," such as the capsula interna fibers, while some small areas within the capsula interna were coded as "1," such as the thalamic nuclei. In contrast to the whole thalamic area, these "wrongly coded" areas were rather small and could easily be detected and eliminated by different tools of mathematic morphology, such as erosion and dilatation [10]. Finally, the thalamic outlines and outlines of other diencephalic structures were derived from the Laplace filtered binary image (Fig. 13.4).

From these outlines the lateral extension of the thalamus was computed at two-thirds of the AC−PC. The quotient of this value and the corresponding atlas value were then used for weighting the coordinates in the lateral and vertical directions. The lateral component was weighted by the ratio of the thalamus laterality, whereas the vertical component was weighted by the mean of the AC−PC distance ratio and thalamus laterality ratio. No anatomic reference was found to standardize the vertical coordinate. Therefore, the mean value of the thalamus laterality ratio and the AC−PC distance ratio were used for the transformation of the "H" coordinate. Hence, any point which has the coordinates (S_p, L_p, H_p) within the patient's brain can be transferred to the atlas coordinates (S_A, L_A, H_A) according to the simple formula F3 (opposite). In cases where the thalamus laterality ratio was equal to the AC−PC distance ratio, formula F3 reduces to an AC−PC transformation. Sites of noise changing, determined using the compound transformation, were again compared to the atlas thalamus borders. Figure 13.5b shows the result of that computation for Schaltenbrand and Wahren's sagittal atlas plane 12.0. In contrast to the AC−PC transformation, the CT-based transformation generated a better fit between electrophysiologically registered

$$\begin{bmatrix} S_A \\ L_A \\ H_A \end{bmatrix} = \begin{bmatrix} q_C & 0 & 0 \\ 0 & q_L & 0 \\ 0 & 0 & q_H \end{bmatrix} \bullet \begin{bmatrix} S_p \\ L_p \\ H_p \end{bmatrix} \tag{F3}$$

where q_c is the quotient of AC−PC distance in the atlas and in the patient: q_L is the quotient of the thalamus lateral extension in the atlas and in the patient; and $q_H = \frac{1}{2}(q_L + q_C)$.

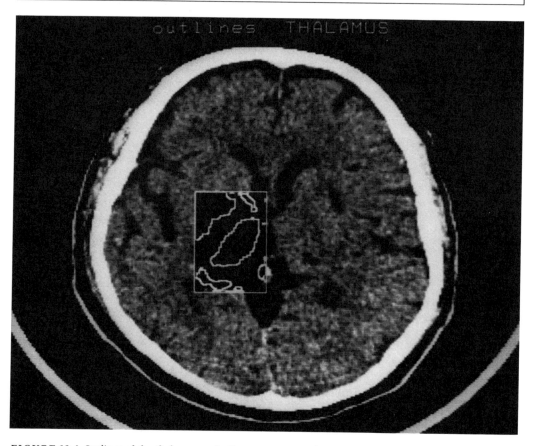

FIGURE 13.4 Outlines of the thalamus and adjacent structures derived from a Laplace filtered binary image of the thalamus area in a CT image 4 mm above the AC−PC plane.

FIGURE 13.5 Sites of noise changing measured by a microelectrode when the electrode penetrated the thalamus, compared to Schaltenbrand and Wahren's sagittal atlas plane 12.0 (a) using conventional AC−PC transformation; (b) sites of noise changing were transferred to the atlas plane by a CT-based transformation.

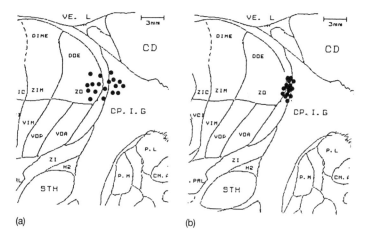

(a)   (b)

thalamus borders within the patient's brain and corresponding atlas borders.

A graphic multidisplay (Fig. 13.6) was created which shows the actual site of the electrode and the trajectory in relation to the atlas plane, as well as important data of the trajectory permanently available during the stereotaxic intervention [2]. On the basis of this display, anatomic correlation of somatosensory evoked potentials could be monitored on-line during the stereotactic operation.

Correlation of somatosensory evoked potentials and stereotaxic atlas

Monopolar recording of somatosensory evoked far field potentials (SEPs) was performed by tungsten electrodes which had an impedance of

less than 100 kΩ [11,12]. To localize neuronal activity, difference potentials were recorded with a multielectrode. The potentials were recorded between first and second poles and third and fourth poles of a four-pole multielectrode. For single unit recording, a tungsten semi-microelectrode was used, which had an impedance of about 1 MΩ. To avoid damage to the tip, the electrode was directed to target without directly penetrating the brain tissue situated above. This was accomplished using a protective inner guide tube which exactly fitted the outer one. An outer guiding tube is used for the recording electrodes. Electrical stimulation within the target area was routinely performed. For the most effective localization, minimal stimulus amplitude was used. The correlation of all physiologic data with the respective

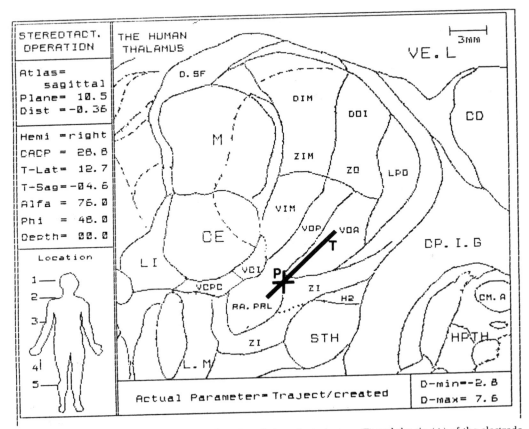

FIGURE 13.6 Computer graphic multidisplay. Correlation of a trajectory (T) and the tip (+) of the electrode at the position P and Schaltenbrand and Wahren's sagittal atlas plane 10.5. The patient was operated on for the right hemisphere, the AC–PC distance was 28.8 mm, the target laterality relative to the midventricular plane was 12.7 mm, the target was 4.6 mm behind the half of AC and PC. The tilt angles of the electrode in the spherical frame coordinate system were $\alpha = 76°$ and $\Phi = 90° - \beta = 48°$. The tip of the electrode matches the target coordinates (depth = 0.0).

affected anatomic structures was performed by a computer system, as described above.

The SEP was recorded monopolarly within subthalamus, thalamic border region, and inside the ventrolateral thalamus (Fig. 13.7, positions 1–3). In general, the potentials were quite reproducible. The latencies following stimulation of both the ulnar and median nerve at the brachial sulcus varied between 8 and 9 ms (Fig. 13.7, patients A–D). At position 1, amplitudes varied between 50 and 60 μV; at position 2, between 30 and 40 μV; and at position 3 between 20 and 30 μV. The latencies were about 14 ms when the median nerve was stimulated at the wrist (Fig. 13.7, patients E, F).

The difference potentials were recorded by a multipole electrode from the same area as the SEPs, and were related to the atlas. The median nerve was stimulated at the wrist. The potentials were recorded between first and second poles and the third and the fourth poles of the multipole electrode. A phase reversal between curve 3 and curve 4 located at the thalamic–subthalamic border is shown in Fig. 13.8. Monopolar stimulation within the target area caused slow tonic contractions of peripheral muscles and subsequent modification of the tremor in 28 patients. Stimulation effects elicited with minimal stimulus amplitudes occurred from stimulation sites predominantly located in the prelemniscal area (Fig. 13.9).

Summary

Since electrophysiologic techniques (recording and stimulation) have become applicable

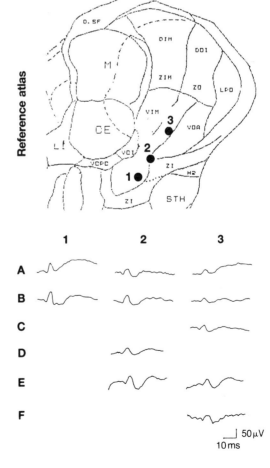

FIGURE 13.7 Correlation of recording sites of somatosensory evoked potentials in the subthalamus (1), in the thalamic border region (2), and within the thalamus (VL) (3), related to Schaltenbrand and Wahren's sagittal atlas plane 10.5. Patients A–D: both the ulnar and median nerve were stimulated at the brachial sulcus. Patients E and F: the median nerve was stimulated at the wrist.

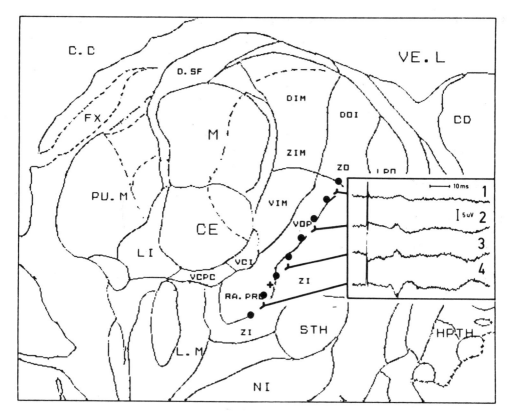

FIGURE 13.8 Evoked potentials following contralateral median nerve stimulation recorded within the thalamic area by a multipole electrode. Phase reversal occurs between trace 3 and trace 4 which was related to the thalamic–subthalamic border (+). Active areas of the multielectrode (●) were related to Schaltenbrand and Wahren's sagittal atlas plane 10.5.

methods for controlling the target coordinates within the individual brain [13–18], and CT and MR images are handled in functional stereotaxy, computers have been successfully used in different ways to aid target point evaluation [1,4,5,7,14,19,20,22–24].

A stereotaxic atlas commonly served as a reference to relate intrathalamic stimulation and registration sites to anatomic structures. Based on computerized graphical methods, those sites could be transferred to the atlas in an applicable manner.

Coordinates from the individual brain are commonly transferred to the atlas proportional to the quotients of the AC–PC distances of the individual brains and the atlas. This conventional method is rather ineffective, since the variability of the lateral component does not simply depend on the AC–PC extension. A mean thalamus lateral width was derived from

the binary image of the thalamic area in CT images. This value could be efficiently used to standardize the individual brain in the lateral and the vertical directions, respectively. The AC–PC distance was used to standardize in the anterior–posterior direction. This provided a satisfactory transformation from the individual brain to the atlas. Using this method, sites of intrathalamic registrations of somatosensory evoked far field potentials were transferred to the atlas of Schaltenbrand and Wahren, which allows a good correlation between anatomic structure and neuronal function.

References

1 Schaltenbrand, G. & Wahren, W. *Atlas for Stereotaxy of the Human Brain*. Stuttgart: Thieme (1977).
2 Lipinski, H.G., Birk, P. & Struppler, A. Computerized stereotaxic neurosurgery. In: Lemke,

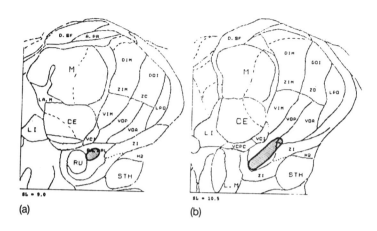

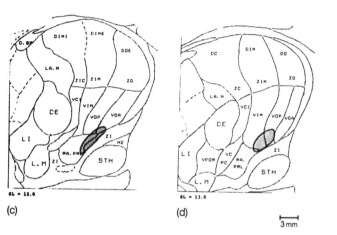

FIGURE 13.9 Distribution of stimulation sites correlated to Schaltenbrand and Wahren's sagittal atlas planes (a) 9.0; (b) 10.5; (c) 12.0; and (d) 13.0; where motor effects were elicited at the body with minimal stimulus amplitude mainly in lower nucleus ventralis intermedius (VIM) and ventralis oralis posterior (VOP) region and prelemniscal area.

H.U., (ed.) *Computer-aided Radiology* (*CAR 1987*), pp. 348–52. Berlin: Springer (1987).

3 Andrew, J. & Watkins, E.S. *A Stereotaxic Atlas of the Human Thalamus and Adjacent Structures.* Baltimore: Williams & Wilkins (1969).

4 Lipinski, H.G. & Struppler, A. New trends in computer graphics and computer vision to assist functional neurosurgery. *Stereotact. Funct. Neurosurg.* **52**: 234–41 (1989).

5 Lipinski, H.G. & Struppler, A. A computer-based stereotaxic localization method utilizing brain atlas and CT images. *Comput. Biomed. Res.* (submitted).

6 Banks, G., Vries, J.K. & McLinden, S. Radiologic automated diagnosis (RAD). *Comput. Meth. Progr. Biomed.* **25**: 157–68 (1987).

7 Tasker, R.R., Hawrylyshyn, P. & Organ, L.W. Computerized graphic display of physiological data collected during human stereotactic surgery. *Appl. Neurophysiol.* **41**: 183–7 (1978).

8 Velasco, F., Molina Negro, P., Bertrand, C. & Hardy, J. Further definition of the subthalamic area for the arrest of tremor. *J. Neurosurg.* **36**: 184–91 (1972).

9 Gonzales, R.C. & Wintz, P. *Digital Image Processing.* London: Addison Wesley (1977).

10 Serra, J. *Mathematical Morphology.* London: Academic Press (1982).

11 Birk, P., Riescher, H., Struppler, A. & Keidel, M. Somatosensory evoked potentials in the ventrolateral thalamus. *Appl. Neurophysiol.* **49**: 327–35 (1986).

12 Birk, P. & Struppler, A. Functional anatomy of the target area for the treatment of pathological tremor: an electrophysiological approach. *Stereotact. Funct. Neurosurg.* **52**: 164–70 (1989).

13 Albe-Fessard, D., Arfel, G, Guit, G., *et al.* Activités électriques charactéristiques de quelques structures cérébrales chez l'homme. *Ann. Chir.* **17**: 1185–214 (1963).

14 Giorgi, C., Cerciari, U., Broggi, G., Birk, P. & Struppler, A. Digital image processing to handle neuroanatomical information and neurophysiological data. *Appl. Neurophysiol.* **48**: 30–3 (1985).

15 Luecking, C.H., Struppler, A., Erbel, F. & Reiss, W. Spontaneous and evoked potentials in the human thalamus and subthalamus. *Electroenceph. Clin. Neurophysiol.* **31**: 351–60 (1971).

16 Momma, H., Sabin, H.I. & Branston, N.M. Clinical evidence supporting origin of the P15 wave of the somatosensory evoked potentials to median nerve stimulation. *Electroenceph. Clin. Neurophysiol.* **67**: 134–9 (1987).

17 Narabayashi, H. & Ohye, C. Parkinsonian tremor and nucleus ventralis intermedius of the human thalamus. *Prog. Clin. Neurophysiol.* **5**: 165–72. (1978).

18 Struppler, A. Stereoencephalotomy and control of skeletal muscle tone. *Stereotact. Funct. Neurosurg.* **52**: 205–18 (1989).

19 Birg, W. & Mundinger, F. Computer calculations of target parameters for a stereotactic apparatus. *Acta Neurochir.* **29**: 123–9 (1973).

20 Birg, W. & Mundinger, F. Direct target point determination for stereotactic brain operations from CT data and the calculation of setting parameters for polar-coordinate stereotactic devices. *Appl. Neurophysiol.* **45**: 387–95 (1982).

21 Kelly, P.J., Kall, B. & Goerss, S. Functional stereotactic surgery utilizing CT data and computer generated stereotactic atlas. *Acta Neurochir.* (suppl.) **33**: 577–83 (1984).

22 Mundinger, F., Birg, W. & Klar, M. Computer assisted stereotactic brain operations by means of including computerized axial tomography. *Appl. Neurophysiol.* **41**: 169–82 (1978).

23 Ohye, C., Kawashima, Y., Hirato, M., Wada, H. & Nakajima, H. Stereotactic CT scan applied to stereotactic thalamotomy and biopsy. *Acta Neurochir.* **71**: 55–68 (1984).

24 Peluso, F. & Gybels, J. Calculation of position of electrode point during penetration in human brain. *Confin. Neurol.* **32**: 213–8 (1970).

Electrophysiologic Data Reduction

14

Computer Evaluation and Display of Seizure Activity Recorded from Chronically Implanted Depth Electrodes

Heinz G. Wieser

Introduction

In epileptology, and in particular in the course of presurgical evaluation of candidates for epilepsy surgery, computers have gained increasing importance. This is partly the consequence of having to analyze the overwhelming amount of data which is produced during long-term monitoring of a patient's habitual seizures. Data acquisition, storage and processing of electroencephalography (EEG) and simultaneous behavioral observations during *seizure monitoring* is hardly manageable without the aid of computers. Today there is general agreement that, for the precise definition of the primary epileptogenic area (the structures responsible for initiating recurrent seizures), ictal information is of utmost importance, if not indispensable. On the other hand, *interictal epileptic graphoelements and abnormal background EEG* cannot be neglected, so that interictal data must also be carefully analyzed. A third, perhaps even more beneficial, reason is the need for more comprehensive *computer-assisted analyses* of raw multichannel EEG data. Another aspect making computers indispensable is *statistical processing* of clinical and research data [1,2].

In this chapter these four aspects are illustrated. First, some examples are given of how computers can be used to facilitate the physician's daily burden of seizure monitoring. This concentrates on on-line seizure detection, quantitative automatic regional spike analysis, and on-line analysis of background EEG, as routinely performed today by most centers offering surgical treatment of epilepsy. Second, an example is given of a so-called "phase and coherence" analysis of epileptic activity with the aim of determining the site or side of its origin. This type of analysis is increasingly used to detect so-called secondary bilateral synchronous (or better synmorphous) EEG phenomena. Patients with such EEG characteristics constitute an important population which, when suffering from frequent seizures with violent falls, might favorably respond to callosotomy. Finally, with respect to the facilities offered by computers for statistical analysis of data from many patients, reference is made to two studies. The first is an electroclinical spatiotemporal analysis of spontaneous complex partial seizures [3]. The other, more recent, study deals with the clinical effects of intracerebral stimulation (Schmid & Wieser, in preparation).

Seizure monitoring

Since the electroclinical analysis of the patient's habitual seizures is usually *the* significant step in the presurgical evaluation of a candidate for surgical therapy, special techniques of data acquisition, i.e. recording and transmission, become an essential prerequisite in order to fulfill the high demands in terms of both time-span (long-term recording) and space (bedroom or even domiciliary recordings). The need for simultaneous recording of behavior and electrical brain activity, the latter often simultaneously from intracranial and scalp electrodes, together with polygraphy, produces voluminous data which are difficult to assimilate and interpret. Therefore, computer-aided meaningful data reduction is necessary at an early stage, and usually an essential part of an integrated telemetry–computer system.

Integrated telemetry–computer system

Transmission of EEG signals from the subject to the recording apparatus, or from recording facilities to other places, can be done by a signal lead (cable telemetry) or by radiotelemetry. EEG recording/storage on videotapes might make use of an audio channel of the tape that also contains the behavioral information, or might — after reformatting — be recorded on the same video image as that recording behavior.

Figures 14.1 and 14.2 illustrate the main principles of a radiotelemetric video/EEG monitoring system, currently used at our institution.

The simultaneously recorded bioelectric signals and behavior is, at this stage, available on cheap VHS video tapes in split-screen fashion and the bioelectric signals are available as on-line or off-line paper printout, in either continuous, random, or selective fashion.

The bioelectric signals are fed in parallel into a PC equipped with software to accomplish on-line event detection and/or quantitative background EEG analysis.

Automatic seizure detection programs (we use that of Stellate Systems) complement the signaling of seizure occurrence by a button press by the patient or another observer (nurse, visitor). Seizure events are stored and available for further off-line analysis (see Fig. 14.7). Spike detection can be quantitatively displayed over time by location (see Fig. 14.6), and data can be documented in a meaningful fashion for inclusion into a patient's file and medical reports.

Automatic seizure detection

With the advent of the computer era, several methods have been developed for automatic seizure detection. Early attempts concentrated on spike-wave recognition or the detection of generalized seizures. Gotman [4] developed a computer method based on measurements of characteristics "paroxysmal" compared to background, "rhythmic" and "sustained" in duration. Basically, in these algorithms, the EEG is first decomposed into half-waves, and then, for every 2-second epoch, the average amplitude of the half-waves relative to the background (indicating whether an epoch was paroxysmal), the average duration of the half-waves (indicating frequency), and the coefficient of variation of half-wave duration (indicating rhythmicity) are measured. According to currently used criteria, a detection takes place when the relative amplitude reaches 3, the frequency is between 3 and 20 Hz, and the coefficient of variation is below 60%. Another especially valuable criterion has been added for detection of seizures with low amplitude but high frequency: relative amplitude at least 1, the frequency at least 60% that of background, and the coefficient of variation is below 60%.

Our procedure has been to identify depth-EEG recorded seizures by measuring "functional" versus anatomic distances, and to visualize the results directly on a television screen [5]. For this purpose, the correlation matrix for all intracerebral EEG signals is calculated and the first three coordinates of the (usually 32) eigenvectors is mapped into an idealized unit sphere, representing the skull with the brain. In case of identical intracerebral signals, the vectors, indicated by differently colored lines in the television display, would all point to a common location. If only one location, i.e. one vector, moves off, the activity of this location is unrelated to all others and is therefore a candidate for defining a seizure-initiating area (Fig. 14.3). Progressive coupling of other vectors, i.e. brain areas, with such an aberrant activity vector could then be interpreted as a progressive ictal synchronization. Such an analysis is possible in real-time. By defining vector aberration behavior, this analysis can be used for seizure detection as well as for the

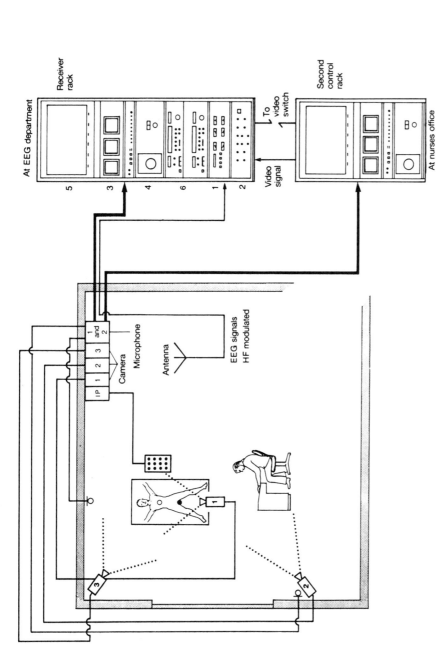

FIGURE 14.1 Block diagram of a multichannel radiotelemetric video/EEG system. With the patient in his or her room or in the hall, the bioelectric signals (scalp and/or intracranial EEG, including two-channel DC-EEG, or other polygraphic signals such as electrocardiogram, respiration, electro-oculogram, or electromyogram) are transmitted (PMC-Telemetry, BIOMES 80 GLONNER) on a 433 MHz receiver. The patient's behavior is monitored simultaneously by several cameras (1–3: AQUA-TV CCD SM 72A). In this diagram, camera 1 monitors the bed, camera 2 the site of sitting, and camera 3 the whole room. Behavioral monitoring in the dark at night is achieved by using infrared lighting. Two microphones allow for acoustic monitoring. The "receiver rack" is located at the EEG department and consists of: 1, the VHF receiver with battery load control of the transmitter as well as control of its input; 2, the videometry processor (GLONNER DR 16); 3, three control monitors from the three cameras, with switch; 4, loudspeaker; 5, the line monitor; and 6, two video recorders (VHS system) in serial connection, with an automatic switch from recorder 1 to recorder 2 as soon as the first videocassette is completed. The 16 bioelectric signals are amplified, and can be displayed on paper and further processed, either continuously on-line, or selectively off-line after visual inspection on the screen. A second control rack is located at the nurses' office on the ward, and once again consists of the line monitor, the three control TV monitors with camera-selector switch, loudspeaker, as well as the battery load of the transmitter and its input. From Wieser & Moser [12].

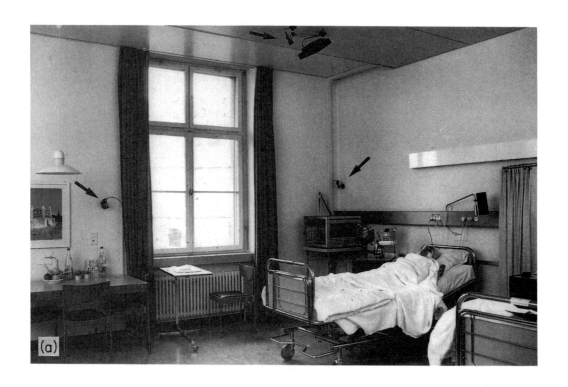

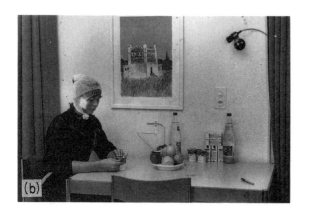

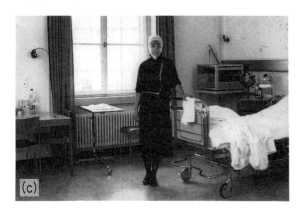

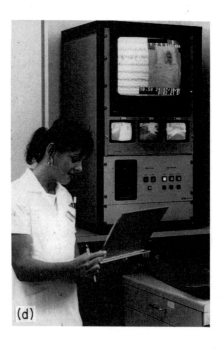

FIGURE 14.2 *Continued opposite.*

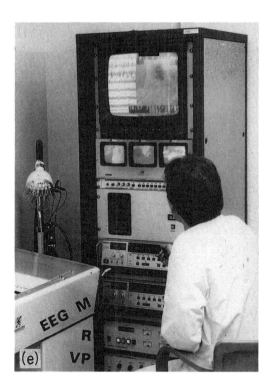

FIGURE 14.2 Photographs of the TV/ radiotelemetric EEG monitoring system, as described in Fig. 14.1 (a) The patient's room, with the three cameras (arrows 1−3) and the infrared emitter; (b) behavioral and bioelectric monitoring at the site of sitting (camera 2); (c) behavioral and bioelectric monitoring with the patient moving unrestricted in the room; (d) control rack in nurses' office; (e) control rack at the EEG department with the elements described in the legend of Fig. 14.1, with an EEG machine, used for conventional EEG paper printout. From Wieser & Moser [12].

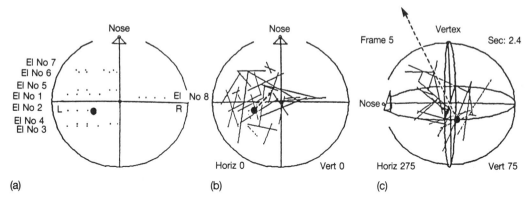

FIGURE 14.3 Example from a movie, illustrating the measurement of functional versus anatomic distances. In (a), dots indicate anatomic locations, as given by the depth electrodes of the patient. ● = left hippocampus. (b) Essential coherent activity of most locations during the preictal period results in a vector configuration without any gross aberrant single vector; (c) the strong individual activity of the left hippocampus (vector marked by dotted line) indicates the seizure origin at this location. Note that display of the electrode assemblies is originally identified by color on the TV screen. From Wieser [5].

analysis of seizure propagation phenomena. Because of the increasing availability of other seizure detection methods, our approach has not been fully evaluated in terms of clinical usefulness for routine seizure monitoring.

As a very simple on-line detection method, we also use on-line compressed spectral array (CSA), as provided, for example, by Spectralab[R] (Fig. 14.4). CSA usually allows for easy and convenient recognition of ictal discharges, and in addition supplies further information on the background activity in terms of vigilance-dependent fluctuation and pathologic alteration. Besides the quantification of abnormal

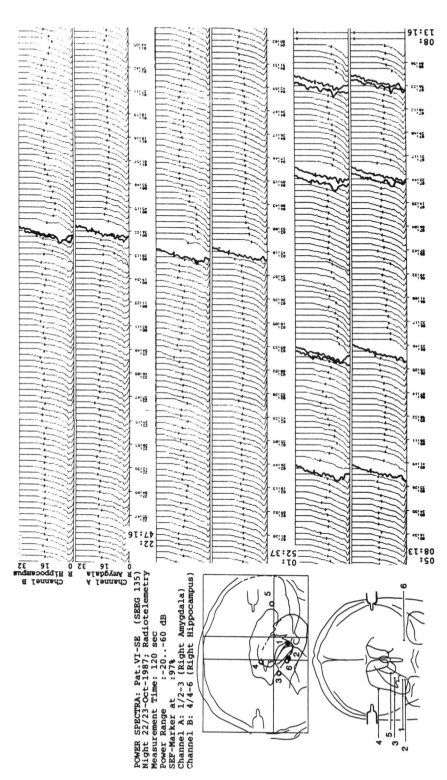

POWER SPECTRA: Pat.VI-SE (SEEG 135)
Night 22/23-Oct-1987; Radiotelemetry
Measurement Time: 120 sec
Power Range   :-20..-60 dB
SEF-Marker at :97%
Channel A: 1/2-3 (Right Amygdala)
Channel B: 4/4-6 (Right Hippocampus)

FIGURE 14.4 On-line compressed spectral analysis (CSA) from stereotactic depth recordings of the right amygdala and the right hippocampus during more than 9 hours, with clear indication of six complex partial seizures with increasing frequency towards early morning.

EEG spectra (e.g. increased pathologic frequency content), the behavior of the spectra in terms of their independence from different vigilance states ("rigidity") has turned out to be a very valuable indicator of the "primary epileptogenic zone" [6].

Automatic spike detection; combined display of spikes and EEG background descriptors

Automatic spike detection

Today, sophisticated automatic spike recognition programs are available which use either mimetic or parametric models. Because of the difficulties in accurately identifying which characteristics define a spike, none of them has proved completely satisfactory. Despite these shortcomings, automatic spike detection is very useful, provided the detected event can be visually controlled by an experienced electroencephalographer.

The Montreal approach makes use of decomposed half-waves after digital filtering. The duration and the amplitude of each half-wave are measured, the latter relative to the average amplitude in the preceding 5 s. If two adjacent half-waves fall within a set of thresholds for relative amplitude and duration, the sharpness of the apex relative to the background is then also measured. Thresholds are such that the wave of a relatively small amplitude has to be very sharp to be detected, whereas a large relative amplitude does not require as sharp an apex for detection. Other centers, for example University of California, Los Angeles (UCLA), use the "second derivative technique" to detect spikes. Such a system (for example UCLA's COUNTR, realized with an ASSEMBLER language computer program) computes the amount of sharpness and the degree of variation in sharpness in the background EEG, by computing mean and standard deviation of the analog second derivative of the low-pass prefiltered signal. Usually, sharp transients are detected as those which are a set number of standard deviations above the mean (threshold level). Periodically renewed estimates of the mean and standard deviations of the background EEG are derived from these time points, which are defined as the so-called checking level [7].

Combined display of spikes and EEG background descriptors

A very convenient way to display both paroxysmal events and background EEG is to combine spike detection algorithms with EEG-chronotrend curves. Chronotrend curves are based on the extraction of certain EEG parameters, such as "vigilance-descriptors" [8]. Figure 14.5 illustrates the most commonly used ones: spectral edge frequency, peak frequency, and ratios of certain frequency bands. Plotting such descriptors over time results in chronotrend curves to which the detected spikes can be added in a quantitative and time-locked fashion (Fig. 14.6). Since these spikes, which exhibit an "autonomy" from different states of vigilance, mark the "primary epileptogenic area" much better than those which show a vigilance-dependent occurrence, this kind of display is of particular value.

Computer-aided analysis of ictal activity

An important issue in the context of presurgical evaluation of candidates for epilepsy surgery is the reliability of the recorded seizures, i.e. the extent to which recorded seizures are typical for the patient's habitual attack pattern(s). Electroclinical coincidence, correspondence of the reported/observed aura-phenomena with the distribution of the initially observed seizure discharge at scalp and/or depth EEG, formal characteristics of the epileptic discharge at seizure onset (pattern), etc., must be given careful consideration. Electrically, the distribution of the "abnormal seizure discharge" at seizure onset is important with regard to definition of the primary epileptogenic zone which, if surgery is considered, has to be resected in order to achieve the best possible seizure control.

Although there are many problems inherent to the term "onset," clinically it may be characterized as the stage at which we first detect a significant and specific change of the electrical activity recorded by a given and limited set of electrodes placed at and within certain structures. The types of electrodes, and the resolution in terms of electrode spacing, remain crucial. Seizure onset is commonly described as being "focal," "regional," or "generalized." "Focal"

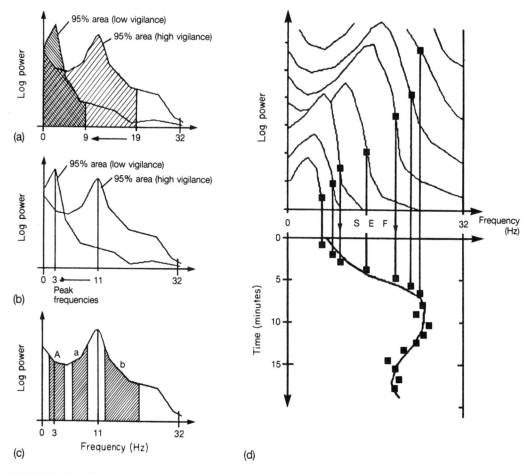

FIGURE 14.5 Illustration of frequently used EEG-vigilance parameters (a)–(c) and relationship of spectra with spectral edge frequency (SEF) marks and the corresponding chronotrend-curve (d). (a) Power spectra during waking state with high vigilance and during slow-wave sleep (low vigilance). Hatched areas denote 95% of the total area between 0 and 32 Hz. The *SEF 95%* is that particular frequency at which 95% of the power is reached (in the example, 9 and 19 Hz). The *median frequency* is a special case of SEF, i.e. SEF 50%; (b) in spectra with a clear peak the *peak frequency* can be advantageously used; (c) a very sensitive and flexible vigilance descriptor is the *ratio of the power in various frequency bands*. In this example, the ratio R is given by $R = (a + b)/A$. (A, a, b are the hatched powers in the respective frequency bands.) From Wieser [8].

seizure onset is often electrically characterized by a high frequency–low amplitude discharge at onset, with a progressive slowing of discharge frequency, paralleled by a progressively increasing amplitude (at least in intracranial recordings). With the spread of the seizure, the activity of more distant electrodes undergoes characteristic changes, displaying either the same pattern as seen at the onset sites, or specific alterations. This spread can occur progressively with a certain "propagation time," but sometimes — following a relatively stable discharge pattern (in terms of location and formal

characteristics) — sudden metamorphoses ("paroxysmale Umschaltungen" according to Petsche *et al.* [9]) can be observed.

There are good reasons to adhere to the operational concepts of the "initial locus" as opposed to that of the so-called "pacemaker focus", which might not be identical. In fact, experimental data suggest that, during the seizure, secondarily involved brain sites might become the "driving" source(s). Clinically, such notions led us to offer so-called "palliative" amygdalohippocampectomy to patients with a secondary pacemaker focus in the hippocampal

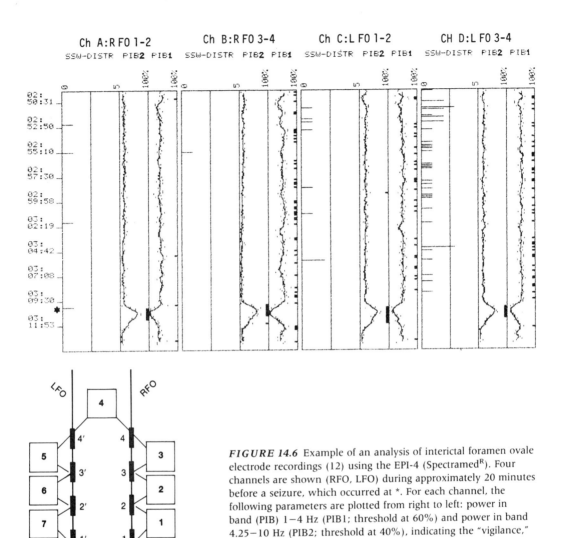

FIGURE 14.6 Example of an analysis of interictal foramen ovale electrode recordings (12) using the EPI-4 (Spectramed[R]). Four channels are shown (RFO, LFO) during approximately 20 minutes before a seizure, which occurred at *. For each channel, the following parameters are plotted from right to left: power in band (PIB) 1–4 Hz (PIB1; threshold at 60%) and power in band 4.25–10 Hz (PIB2; threshold at 40%), indicating the "vigilance," and the spike rate (SSW-DISTR; full scale equals 5 spikes). (The example comes from a study concerned with the question of whether there are characteristic preictal EEG changes, in particular a decrease of interictal spikes; see also Wieser [16].)

formation and the seizure onset located in Wernicke's area. Since the pioneering work of Brazier [10], the concept of causality or "driving" in electrophysiologic signal analysis has been substantially elaborated using modern computer technology. The basic assumptions in this respect are that similarities of signal characteristics are indicative of transmission in the neural connections between locations, and that the direction of transmission can be inferred from phase lags at those frequencies at which they are significantly similar. The method of coherence and phase of Gotman [11], see also

[15], allows the quantitative estimation of differences on the order of 5–50 ms, consistently present between two channels during a section of an epileptic discharge. Although the interpretation of such time delays must be done carefully with regard to possible origins and significance, such analyses offer valuable information.

Figure 14.7 gives an example. It illustrates the ictal EEG during an automatically detected epileptic discharge, its computer display, and its off-line analysis using the programs Rhythm[R] and Monitor[R] (Stellate System). The example is

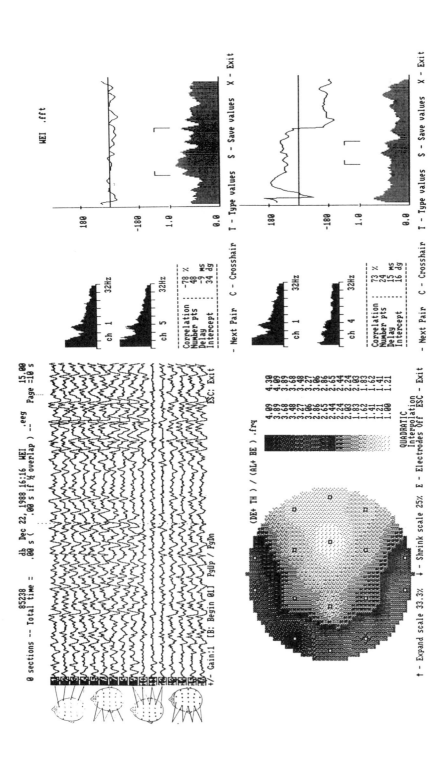

FIGURE 14.7 Example of an EEG analysis of slow sharp wave—slow wave discharges (*"petit mal variant discharge"*) in a patient with a Lennox—Gastaut syndrome. Left: raw EEG as detected, stored and displayed by the computer (top), and EEG power map (bottom), showing a left frontotemporal maximum of slow waves (display of the ratio of the classically defined frequency bands (delta + theta)/(alpha + beta)). Right: coherence and phase analysis between 2 pairs of EEG signals. Dotted vertical lines indicate the analyzed segment. At top. right frontal (channel 1) versus left frontal (channel 5) derivations; at bottom, right frontal (channel 1) versus right occipital (channel 4) are compared. Black figures are the power spectra (middle of the figure), hatched figures (right) the coherence between the indicated pairs of channels. Above the coherence the phase is plotted. The calculated delays indicate that the discharges originate at left frontal (channel 5). "driving" the right frontal EEG signal (channel 1) with a delay of 9 ms. The comparison between channel 1 (right frontal) and channel 4 (right occipital) indicates that the frontal signal "drives" the occipital (delay 15 ms). (Gotman's software; Monitor[R] and Rhythm[R] — Stellate Systems; see Gotman [11].)

taken from a candidate for anterior callosotomy because of medically refractory seizures with frequent violent falls.

Statistical analysis of clinical and research data collected from a group of patients

Electroclinical spatio-temporal seizure analysis

In an attempt to study the characteristics of psychomotor seizures (complex partial seizures), recorded in 29 selected patients referred for surgical treatment, we have encoded 80 observed clinical signs and symptoms and 80 ictally active brain locations which we recorded during stereo-electroencephalographic evaluation. Two hundred and thirteen spontaneous seizures, resulting in 563 10-second seizure intervals, were selected for this study [3]. The seizure symptoms were encoded when first observed. The ictally discharging brain sites were encoded, according to their electrical discharge patterns, within 5 degrees at the end of a 10-second interval, ranging from autochthonous high-frequency low-amplitude discharges (degree 1) to "epileptic modification of background EEG rhythms" (degree 5). Each seizure was followed in 10-second epochs until it reached its full expression, which sometimes coincided with its termination. In this manner, 80×80 matrices (symptoms × ictal brain locations) were obtained for each 10-second epoch, with preservation of their time sequence. Thus, the further analysis could make use of any particular epoch during the seizure course, i.e. the ones at seizure onset or at termination, etc., or analyze them according to chronology. In applying cluster analyses, multidimensional scaling methods, and principal component analyses, the relationship between signs and symptoms and location of ictal discharges could be evaluated over time. The results of this study, published in a monograph [3], led us to classify psychomotor seizures in five subtypes, viz. mesiobasal limbic, temporal polar, frontobasal–cingulate, temporal lateral neocortical posterior, and opercular–insular. The mesiobasal limbic subtype is the most important, both in terms of frequency and surgical consequences. The findings were the basis for the introduction of the so-called selective amygdalohippocampectomy for treatment of patients suffering from medically intractable seizures of this type [13]. To date, 267 patients have been operated on with this operative procedure at our institution, with rather favorable results [6,14].

Figure 14.8 gives an example of this kind of computer-aided analysis. It illustrates the principal component analysis with the four strongest factors, out of the 48 factors described. As can be seen from (a), the sorted eigenvalues do not show any steep bend, leaving the dimensionality of the described epileptic seizure process unclear; (b) depicts the four strongest factors with eigenvalues from 7 to 4. Factor 1 contains no ictal symptoms, but is composed of ictally active brain sites which delineate the core structures of the limbic system of one hemisphere. Only after subtracting factor 1 and repeating the procedure, the second factor combines ictal active brain sites and clinical symptoms. As has been shown by other means, this factor indicates a late seizure stage. Factor 4 is the most distinct and delineates the opercular–insular subtype of psychomotor seizures.

Such "synthetic" variables (here factors) might produce straightforward results which are clinically meaningful and easy to interpret. However, they also allow for new hypotheses and therefore may lead to new insights. An example to illustrate this can be given in the form of an interpretation of factor 1:

1 The observed clinical signs and symptoms are less reliable in defining the psychomotor seizure than the ictal discharge recorded from the limbic system.
2 Therefore, the psychomotor seizure can be best defined as being a limbic seizure. Attempts to define it by a list of "characteristic" seizure symptoms are less successful.
3 As a consequence we have to accept that for exact characterization of this seizure, depth recording remains essential, at least if selective resective surgical procedures are intended.

Statistical analysis of clinical signs and symptoms evoked by electrical brain stimulation

Together with Schmid (Schmid and Wieser, in preparation) we have analyzed 2670 electrical

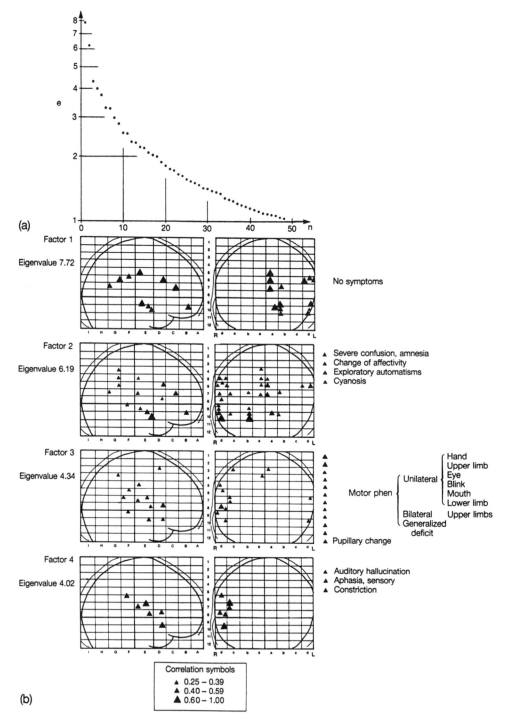

(a)

(b)

Correlation symbols
▲ 0.25 – 0.39
▲ 0.40 – 0.59
▲ 0.60 – 1.00

FIGURE 14.8 Principal component analysis of stereo-electroencephalographically recorded brain sites (80 locations) and 80 ictal symptoms in 563 10-second intervals of 213 psychomotor seizures. (a) Sorted trace of decomposed correlation matrix, dimension 160, rank 134. First 48 factors explain 73% of total variance. First 17 factors contain most activity. (b) Graphical display of the 4 strongest "factors" (principal components), sorted according to their eigenvalue. Only one lateral view is shown, which superimposes left and right hemisphere locations. Information about lateralization is as follows: factor 1 has a stronger adherence to the left hemisphere than to the right hemisphere, whereas factor 4 has a stronger adherence to the right hemisphere than to the left hemisphere. Both factors are "unilateral" ones, whereas factors 2 and 3 are "bilateral," i.e. the ictal discharge involves both hemispheres. From Wieser [3].

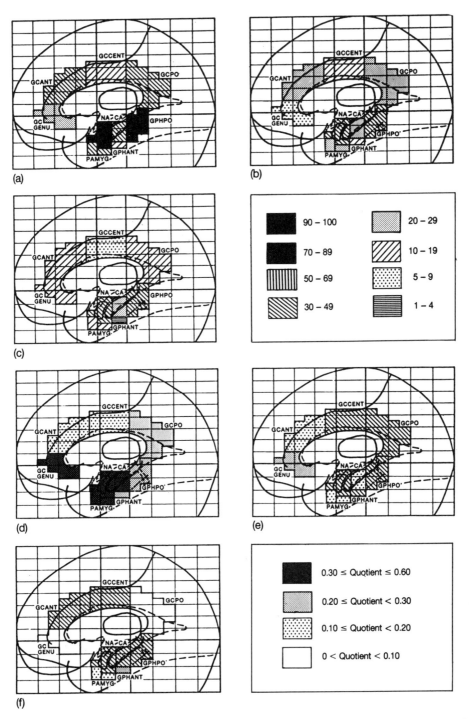

FIGURE 14.9 (a)−(c) Topographical distribution of 386 electrical stimulations in the limbic system, evoking a clinical symptom but no afterdischarge. Frequency distribution (absolute values) for both hemispheres together (a), as well as for the right (b) and the left hemisphere (c). (d)−(f) Relative frequency of certain symptom classes evoked by stimulation. The code denotes the "ratio" of total number of stimulations per area, divided by stimulations which evoked a clinical symptom, falling into the indicated categories: "visceromotor" (d); viscerosensory" (e); and "emotions" (f).

brain stimulations performed so far at our institution during presurgical evaluation of patients who underwent so-called "chronic" depth recording (i.e. prolonged stereo-EEG exploration [15]). By comparison to the analysis of spontaneous seizures, the main advantage of this stimulation study is that the localizational uncertainties are smaller as the site of stimulation is precisely known. Except for the stimulated site, which was not monitored during stimulation and for a short period after the end of stimulation, our laboratory conditions allowed us to record from all other explored brain sites during stimulation. Therefore, clinical signs and symptoms evoked by electrical stimulation of various brain sites could be divided into those *without* any detectable afterdischarge, those accompanied *with local* afterdischarge, and those *with regional* afterdischarges. It is evident that evoked symptoms without afterdischarges constitute the "purest," i.e. most appropriate, category for the study of the functional anatomy of epileptic brains. Figure 14.9 illustrates this kind of study. In this example, only limbic stimulation sites were analyzed which, when stimulated, led to clinical symptoms without any detectable afterdischarge. The results indicate that within the limbic system there exists a clear-cut functional specialization of anatomically different brain structures.

References

1 Mazzola, G., Wieser, H.G., Brunner, V. & Muzzulini, D. A symmetry-oriented mathematical model of classical counterpoint and related neurophysiological investigations by depth EEG. *Comput. Math. Applic.* **17**(4–6): 539–94 (1989).

2 Meles, H.P. & Wieser, H.G. Computer-generated dynamic presentation of functional versus anatomical distances in the human brain. *Appl. Neurophysiol.* **45**: 404–5 (1982).

3 Wieser, H.G. *Electroclinical Features of the Psychomotor Seizure.* Stuttgart-London: G. Fischer–Butterworth (1983).

4 Gotman, J. Automatic recognition of epileptic seizures in the EEG. *Electroencephalogr. Clin. Neurophysiol.* **54**: 530–40 (1982).

5 Wieser, H.G. Automatic analysis of electrocerebral activity. *Acta Neurochir.* **33**(suppl.): 17–33 (1984).

6 Wieser, H.G. Selective amygdalo-hippocampectomy for temporal lobe epilepsy. *Epilepsia* **29**(suppl.): 100–113 (1988).

7 Wieser, H.G. Data analysis. In: Engel J. Jr (ed.), *Surgical Treatment of the Epilepsies*, pp. 335–60. New York: Raven Press (1987).

8 Wieser, H.G. Verhalten epileptischer Herde im Schlaf; Befunde bei intrakraniellen Ableitungen. In: Meier-Ewert, K. & Schulz, H. (eds), *Schlaf und Schlafstörungen*, pp. 58–69. Berlin: Springer (1990).

9 Petsche, H., Rappelsberger, P., Lapins, R. & Vollmer, R. Rhythmicity in seizure patterns: topographical aspects. In: Speckmann, E.-J. & Caspers, H. (eds), *Origin of Cerebral Field Potentials*, pp. 60–79. Stuttgart: Thieme (1979).

10 Brazier, M.A.B. Spread of seizure discharges in epilepsy: anatomical and electrophysiological considerations. *Exp. Neurol.* **36**: 263–72 (1972).

11 Gotman, J. Measurement of small time differences between EEG channels: method and application to epileptic seizure propagation. *Electroenceph. Clin. Neurophysiol.* **56**: 501–14 (1983).

12 Wieser, H.G. & Moser, S. Improved multipolar foramen ovale electrode monitoring. *J. Epilepsy* **1**: 13–22 (1988).

13 Wieser, H.G. & Yasargil, M.G. Selective amygdalohippocampectomy as a surgical treatment of mesiobasal limbic epilepsy. *Surg. Neurol.* **17**: 445–7 (1984).

14 Wieser, H.G., Siegel, A.M. & Yasargil, M.G. The Zurich amygdalo-hippocampectomy series: a short up-date. *Acta Neurochir.* **50**(suppl.) 122–7 (1990).

15 Wieser, H.G. & Elger, C.E. (eds) *Presurgical Evaluation of Epileptics.* Berlin: Springer (1987).

16 Wieser, H.G. Preictal EEG findings. *Epilepsia* **30**: 664 (1989).

part IV

Stereotactic Surgical Planning and Simulation

A

Computer Systems

A Personal Computer-based Workstation for the Planning of Stereotactic Neurosurgical Procedures

Terry M. Peters, G. Bruce Pike, and John A. Clark

Introduction

Stereotactic surgery procedures are used to approach deep-seated brain lesions with a probe by way of a small twist-drill hole in the skull, or by an external narrow beam of high energy ionizing radiation [1−3]. They are also employed to place electrodes deep within the brain for EEG recording or stimulation. Before any of these procedures can be attempted, the precise locations of the "target" points (with respect to some fixed reference) within the brain must be accurately determined.

In order to accomplish this task, a reference structure (stereotactic headframe) of some kind is rigidly fastened to the patient's head during the imaging and surgical procedures. Marker structures associated with the frame allow the localization of targets within the brain to be determined from tomographic or projection images [4,5]. Engraved scales on the frame structure allow the target to be localized prior to being approached by frame-mounted instruments or isocentric photon beams.

Imaging modalities used for stereotactic neurosurgery planning include X-ray computed tomography (CT), digital subtraction angiography (DSA), and magnetic resonance imaging (MRI). With such a variety of image data from different sources, we need to easily relate structures and targets that are identified on images from each of the different modalities. This can only be achieved by establishing a consistent imaging environment within a computer program that allows the free interchange of parameters between images from different sources.

The software package described here achieves these goals and has been written specifically for use with, and is available commercially for the Olivier−Bertrand−Tipal (OBT) [6] and Leksell [7] stereotactic frames, each of which is compatible with MR, CT, and DSA imaging systems.

We present clinical examples of the use of this system in typical stereotactic neurosurgery procedures, and discuss the results of inter-modality tests to establish the accuracy of the technique.

Materials and methods

The headframe

The stereotactic headframe (Fig. 15.1) is fitted to a patient's head prior to an imaging study, and remains rigidly fixed to the patient in this manner throughout the imaging examinations and surgery. In exceptional circumstances it may be removed and replaced in the same position at a later date through the use of locking chucks attached to the fixation pins. During the imaging session, the frame supports the appropriate fiducial marker plates [4] which are described below. At the time of surgery, the frame is used to support the surgical instruments

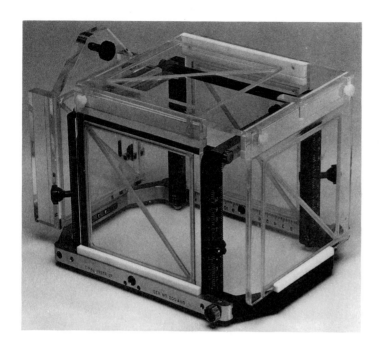

FIGURE 15.1 OBT stereotactic frame with MRI marker plate set in place.

as well as to maintain the reference coordinate system employed during the imaging procedure.

In order that the frames have a minimum impact on the quality of the resulting images, they are constructed from an aluminum alloy, or aluminum and plastic materials, in such a manner as to provide maximum strength while minimally impacting on the quality of the images (i.e. avoiding the introduction of image artifacts). The frame referred to in the remainder of this paper is the OBT unit (Tipal Instruments Inc., Montreal, Canada) [5], although the image analysis system is applicable to both this frame and the similar Leksell apparatus (Elekta Instruments AB, Stockholm, Sweden) [6].

The OBT frame consists of a lower ring on which four support posts are mounted, along with a series of bars at the top to complete the structure. This assembly is sufficiently light for it to be accommodated by the patient without discomfort, while being strong enough to support a variety of surgical instruments. The sides of the frame are engraved with millimeter scales that allow accurate positioning of the instruments during surgery.

Fiducial markers

CT and MRI In order that the coordinates of structures in an image may be calculated, the scaling and positions of two-dimensional (2-D) tomographic slices within the three-dimensional (3-D) frame must be determined accurately. To achieve this goal, the frame is surrounded with a series of plastic plates in which are embedded markers in the shape of a Z or N pattern. Any cross-sectional slice through the brain and the frame (including the marker plates), displays three sets of three points surrounding the image. Analysis of the positions of these points in the images, combined with the knowledge of their frame coordinates, enables the location and scale of the slice within the 3-D frame of reference to be precisely determined. The 3-D coordinates of any point within the frame volume may be calculated by analyzing the images in this manner.

If it can be guaranteed that the scanning axis of the machine is parallel to the sides of the frame, only one such set of marker plates is sufficient to localize the position of the slice. However, this may be difficult to achieve in practice, for example when the scanning gantry is tilted or when movement of the patient occurs during the scanning procedure. The inclusion of the two additional sets of markers in each slice enables its exact position and angulation to be determined unambiguously.

The markers must be made from substances which exhibit a strong signal from the modality being used. For this reason, aluminum or copper, each of which has a relatively high radiopacity, is used for CT, and a copper sulfate solution (high nuclear magnetic resonance signal) enclosed in channels in the plastic plates is used for the markers in MRI examinations.

Since CT images are generally transverse, the minimum of three marker plates is required to identify coordinates from a set of images. MRI, on the other hand, allows images to be acquired in sagittal and coronal planes as well as transverse, and so five sets of plates must be provided in this case, to allow for the intersection of the images with three of the marker-sets for each orientation.

A stereotactic CT scan, in which the fiducial markers are clearly evident at the top and sides, is shown in Fig. 15.2. Sagittal and coronal images that are recorded directly by the MRI

system may be analyzed (subject to the limitations discussed below) in the same manner as transverse images. Orthogonal CT views, derived from the transverse data by standard reformatting techniques, may also be generated and analyzed by the software. At any time in the analysis, a scale corresponding to that engraved on the frame may be overlaid on the images.

DSA Since the DSA technique yields projections of the brain (Fig. 15.3), rather than cross-sections, a different approach to that described above is used to analyze the images. In this case, rather than the Z markers appropriate for CT and MRI, the fiducial markers consist of small metal pellets embedded in the front, back, and side plates. Although these points are placed at the corners of identical squares on opposite

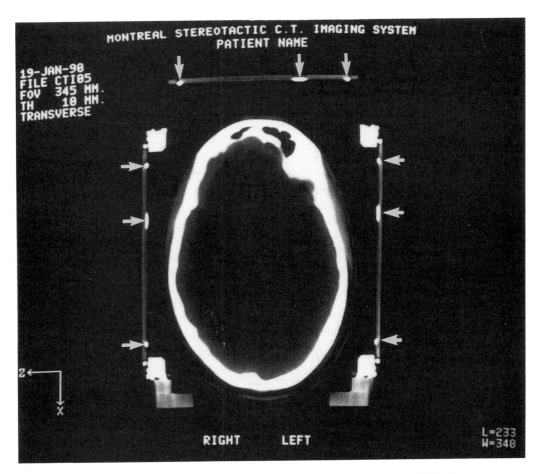

FIGURE 15.2 Stereotactic CT scan showing fiducial markers surrounding image, overlaid with computer-generated scale.

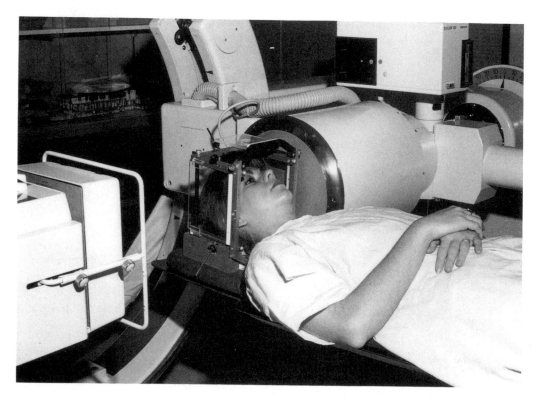

FIGURE 15.3 Patient with frame during DSA examination.

sides of the frame, they appear in the image (because of differential magnification) to be on squares of different sizes (Fig. 15.4). The positions of these points nevertheless precisely define the X-ray beam geometry of the imaging system. By analyzing images of the same structure in both anterior–posterior and lateral projections, the 3-D frame coordinates of structures may be identified from the subtracted angiograms (see Appendix).

Computer system

Other computer systems exist to handle multi-modality image data for stereotactic surgery planning [7], but most require extensive and expensive hardware facilities. While our system does not have the capability to display 3-D rendered images, for example, it nevertheless allows the surgeon to work within a 3-D environment. The computer hardware is based on a standard IBM PC-AT or compatible system, running MS-DOS and equipped with a math coprocessor. The only additional hardware

required is an inexpensive $512 \times 512 \times 8$ bit imaging board and monitor, and an industrial standard nine-track 1600 bits-per-inch magnetic tape unit. Tapes generated by a number of popular diagnostic imaging modalities may be read by the system, and images are stored on an 80 Mbyte hard disk.

The user interface is via a mouse which selects menu entries, and also controls image window and level (contrast), as well as the cursor movement on the screen. The image monitor is a color (RGB) system allowing for display of either black and white or pseudocolor images. In addition there is an optional video hard-copy unit for permanent recording of images and analyses generated during the planning session. The entire hardware configuration is shown in Fig. 15.5.

Image analysis

General features Having scanned the patient with one or more imaging modalities, the images may be analyzed by the software pack-

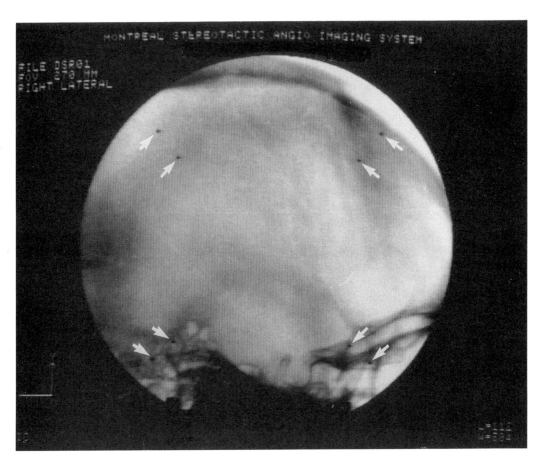

FIGURE 15.4 Lateral unsubtracted digital angiogram image. Note the two sets of four markers which the software uses to determine the geometry of the imaging beam.

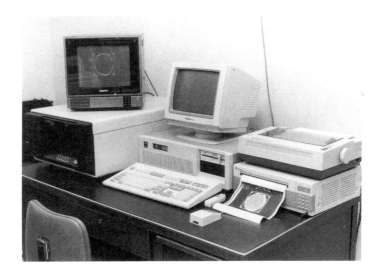

FIGURE 15.5 The hardware configuration used for the stereotactic planning system.

age, which has been specifically developed for stereotactic surgery planning. The unique feature of this package is that it enables images read from several different modalities to be analyzed in a common consistent environment. This means that target points identified in an image of one scanning modality (e.g. MRI) may readily be transferred to the images of another (e.g. DSA).

The first time each image is accessed, the fiducial markers associated with that image are identified automatically (in the case of CT or MRI) or with user guidance (for DSA), and the appropriate scaling and positional factors for that slice (or projection) are computed and saved for later use.

In the case of the tomographic imaging modalities, targets may be located on the basis of the originally scanned slices, or on sagittal and coronal slices reconstructed from the original data-set. Target identification in CT or MRI is by a simple linear transformation, based on the known positions of the markers and their resulting positions in the images. For DSA, however, the target must be identified in two orthogonal projections to determine the "third coordinate" of the point. Here the operator locates the target in one of the image pairs, estimating the value of the third coordinate. He or she then views the orthogonal image, and refines the value of the estimated coordinate. In this manner he may quickly "zero in" on the actual 3-D coordinate of the structure of interest.

Coordinates of target points may be determined on the basis of CT or MRI scans, but the path of approach to these targets is generally planned in conjunction with the DSA images, in order to avoid passing through major blood vessels on the way.

Specific program facilities Having read the appropriate data into the computer and identified the fiducial markers in each of the images, the operator is presented with the master menu for the analysis system appropriate to the images being considered. The example for CT analysis is presented in Table 15.1.

The menu for MRI is virtually identical with that in Table 15.1, and for DSA, items 1 to 4 relate to the display of an anterior–posterior (A/P) or lateral projections, otherwise all other entries are common for all modalities.

Radiosurgery dose planning

In addition to the straightforward stereotactic localization procedures described above, an enhancement to this package enables it to also be used to calculate the isodose distributions resulting from accelerator-based stereotactic radiosurgery. Such approaches utilize a highly collimated beam of high energy (≈ 10 MeV) X-rays, in order to concentrate the delivered dose to a volume of only several milliliters encapsulating a lesion or the nidus of a vascular malformation. Such a tightly controlled dose distribution may be achieved using one of a variety of techniques, including multiple arcing beams [8] or dynamic radiosurgery [9]. Most of these approaches yield dose distributions that are similar to those attainable with the Gamma Knife [10].

In order to plan a radiosurgical procedure, the operator selects the target points as if he were about to perform a conventional stereotactic procedure, then selects the machine parameters (beam diameter, photon energy), and the arcing parameters (number of arcs of the accelerator gantry, positions of the patient table, or, in the case of dynamic radiosurgery, the

---

TABLE 15.1 Master menu for CT analysis

Master menu	Meaning
1 Display a transverse section	Display of section that operator selects from the menu of slices from the current study that has been stored on disk
2 Alternate view at cursor (Only defined for DSA)	Selection is only defined for the DSA analysis module, and allows the operator to toggle between anterior–posterior and lateral views.

3 Reconstruct a coronal section	Reconstruct section from the stack of transverse images at the position currently indicated by the cursor, or with a selected slice coordinate
4 Reconstruct a sagittal section	As above, for sagittal sections
5 Overlay the coordinate scale	The coordinate scale, corresponding to that engraved on the frame, and appropriate to the slice currently being viewed, is overlaid on the screen
6 Clean-up display	All non-archived markings, such as vectors, text, or scales already displayed on the screen are erased
7 Calculate distances	Distances between any two points within the 3-D volume may be calculated, along with the shortest distance between any point and any probe placed within the volume
8 Calculate angles	Angles between any two vectors defined in the image may be determined
9 Determine coordinates	Frame coordinates of any point identified by the cursor may be determined in real time
10 Locate a point with coordinates	The point corresponding to the entered frame coordinates is automatically located and marked on the slice that contains it
11 Mark a point on the display	A target point designated by the cursor position is labeled and saved in the database for future reference. Such a labeled point will be subsequently displayed in any recalled or reconstructed section that contains the point
12 Delete a marked point	Delete marked point from screen and database
13 Mark a trajectory on the display	Mark a proposed trajectory, from any point within the volume to a previously marked target point. The positioning of such a target may be accomplished interactively, using the mouse. Trajectories marked in this manner remain part of the analysis database for the study, and as such will be displayed each time a section that contains all or part of such a trajectory is displayed. The azimuthal and declination angles of the probe track, relative to the frame arc system, are calculated and displayed along with the target point
14 Contour a region	Regions within the image may be contoured manually or automatically, using an operator-selected intensity threshold
15 Draw annotation lines	Annotation lines for display purposes may be superimposed on the images
16 Write annotation text	Arbitrary text may be added to the images
17 Save the current analysis	The database associated with the current analysis may be saved for future use, either within the same study or with a different modality study of the same patient
18 Retrieve coordinates	A previously saved database may be recalled. If the current modality matches that of the saved data, all of the probes and points marked by the previous analysis are restored, and the operator is returned to the same point in the analysis reached just prior to the saving operation. If the modality is different, the targets and probes marked for the previous modality are transferred to the new images.
19 Print current analysis	A permanent record of all the target points and probe trajectories established during a planning session is printed
20 EXIT	Exit to the study selection menu

start and end of the continuous rotations of both the gantry and the table). He also initiates an automatic contouring procedure that defines the cranial surface required by the dose-planning algorithm. Dose planning is achieved using a standard Milan and Bently [11] algorithm modified for 3-D calculations [9]. The set of isodose curves resulting from the chosen scanning geometry may be computed on any of the tomographic planes in the image data sets (Fig. 15.6), or superimposed upon the subtraction angiograms demonstrating the lesion.

Results

Clinical applications

During the last 4 years, several hundred patients at the Montreal Neurological Institute have undergone stereotactic surgical procedures based on planning performed on the computer system described here. These operations include the implantation of depth electrodes [12], tumor biopsy, cyst aspiration, thalamic stimulation, and radiosurgical treatment of arteriovenous malformations [13] and stereotactic radiotherapy of astrocytomas [14]. Most of the procedures are performed with images from two modalities (DSA, and either CT or MRI), while some use information from all three sources.

The images presented in Fig. 15.7 demonstrate the integrated nature of this software package. The patient whose images are shown here was scanned with CT, DSA, and MRI, for the purposes of planning a depth electrode implantation procedure. Rather than display all ten of the placements on these images, only two are shown for clarity.

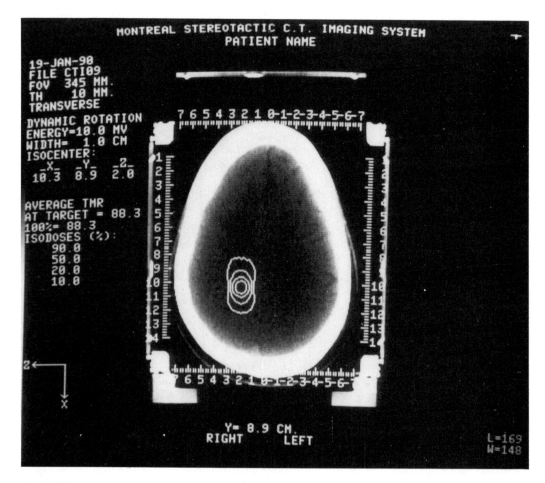

FIGURE 15.6 A typical set of isodose curves calculated by the radiosurgery dose-calculation option of the system, as they are displayed superimposed on a CT scan.

In these examples, the original targets and angles of approach are determined on the basis of the CT data-set on both transverse and coronal images (Fig. 15.7a,b). Note the coordinates of the targets and the angulations of the probes displayed on the upper right.

When a displayed slice intersects a probe, that segment of the probe within the slice is displayed. Fig. 15.7c shows one of these targets having been transferred to the set of transverse MR images, while Fig. 15.7d shows the probe destined for the target labeled "A" passing through a coronal slice just posterior to the target. Finally, Fig. 15.7e and f demonstrate the appearance of the probes, as seen on the DSA A/P and lateral images of the patient. The magnification of the displayed scale is appropriate for structures at a selected depth (e.g. Z = 3.4 cm displayed below the scale on Fig. 15.7f) within the image.

Accuracy

We have demonstrated a localization accuracy of ± 1 mm when the images are geometrically accurate. This goal has been achieved in our institute with CT, DSA, and transverse MR images. We have discovered, however, that the geometrical reliability in sagittal and coronal MR images is poor. Part of this problem can be attributed to the alloy components of the metal parts of the frame, but even using a completely plastic prototype frame we found inconsistencies of up to several millimeters for sagittal images when the MRI readout gradient was in the axial direction. This is indicative of problems in the homogeneity of the main field or the gradients, and may be eddy-current related. We emphasize that such problems will vary from magnet to magnet, and that it is extremely important when using MRI for stereotaxis that the limitations of the imaging systems be fully appreciated. If the distortions can be sufficiently well characterized, then it is possible that the image could be corrected prior to analysis [15]. Likewise, the geometrical accuracy of some DSA imaging chains (the image intensifier and the TV camera) often suffers from some pin-cushion distortion which must be considered. While the system installed at this institute suffers this problem to an insignificant degree, the distortion on some units may exceed several millimeters at the periphery of the image [16].

Table 15.2 details the results of the accuracy measurements made using MRI, CT, and DSA, along with a physical measurement to localize the positions of 16 randomly placed pellets within the frame. It also gives the mean error and the standard deviation of this error when the image coordinates were compared with the

TABLE 15.2 Errors in coordinate measurements of test pellets in the stereotactic phantom

Imaging technology	Error in each coordinate (mean ± SD)			
	Δx (mm)	Δy (mm)	Δz (mm)	Dist
CT transverse	−0.4 ± 0.5	−0.2 ± 1.1	0.4 ± 0.6	0.6 ± 1.3
DSA	−0.4 ± 0.8	−0.7 ± 1.1	0.3 ± 0.1	0.8 ± 1.6
MRI transverse AP readout	−0.7 ± 1.1	−0.1 ± 2.7	0.1 ± 1.0	0.6 ± 2.7
MRI transverse LR readout	−0.8 ± 0.9	−0.8 ± 1.6	0.3 ± 0.8	1.1 ± 1.9
MRI sagittal CC readout	−2.4 ± 1.3	−0.1 ± 0.8	1.7 ± 1.4	2.5 ± 1.7
MRI coronal CC readout	0.5 ± 1.7	−0.5 ± 0.6	0.6 ± 1.2	0.9 ± 2.1
MRI sagittal AP readout	−0.4 ± 0.8	3.4 ± 1.3	2.3 ± 2.5	4.0 ± 2.8
MRI coronal LR readout	−0.35 ± 1.4	0.7 ± 0.7	0.1 ± 0.8	0.8 ± 1.7

Sixteen point objects were distributed uniformly throughout the volume defined by the frame. AP, LR, and CC refer respectively to the anterior−posterior, left−right, and craniocaudal directions of the readout gradient used for the MR images. The first three entries in each row give the actual measured error in each coordinate, while the last combines these to give a linear distance error (Dist). The *x*, *y*, and *z* coordinates represent the AP, CC, and LR patient directions respectively. Note also that the SD of the error is always greatest in the slice-thickness direction for each imaging modality, as would be expected.

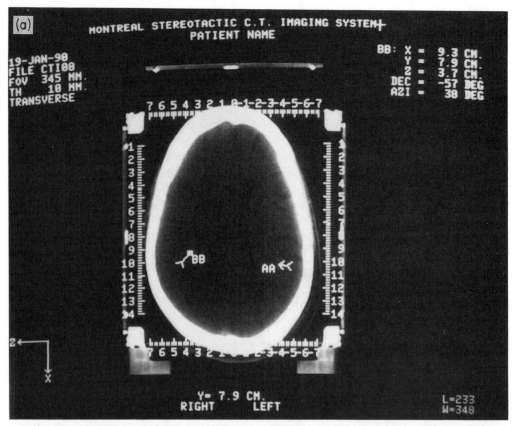

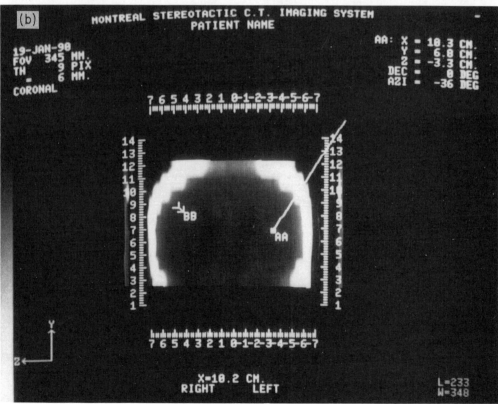

FIGURE 15.7 Target localization using multiple modalities. (a), (b) Transverse and coronal CT images defining targets and trajectories of probes.

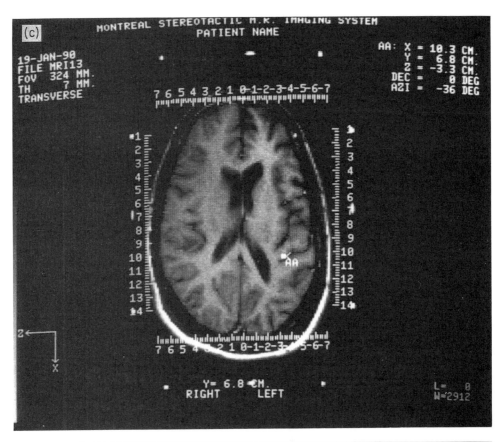

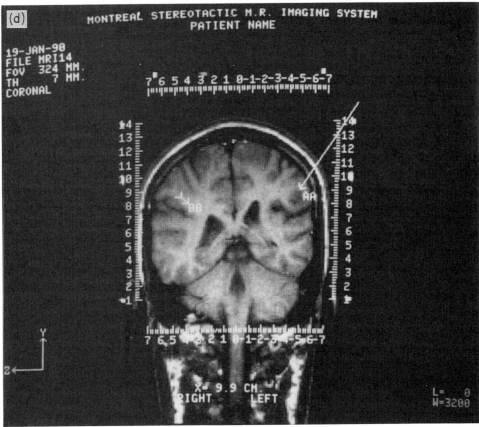

FIGURE 15.7 *continued* (c), (d) The same targets and probes seen on MR images. Note that in images (a)−(d) only the targets that fall within the slice are displayed.

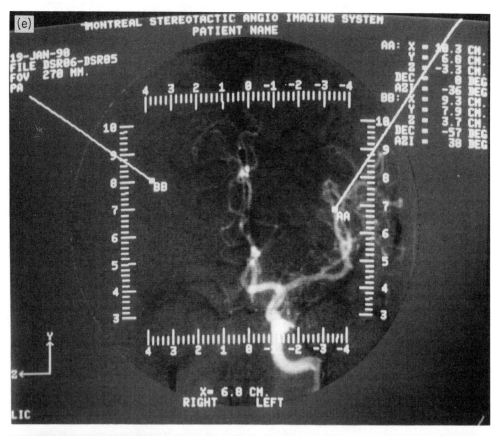

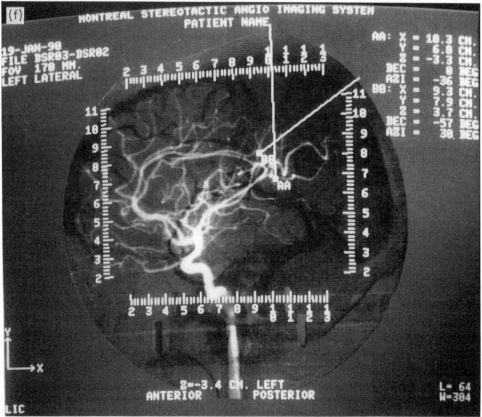

FIGURE 15.7 *continued* (e), (f) The targets and probes as seen in DSA anterior–posterior and lateral images.

coordinates that were physically measured within the frame. Since the frame is graduated in 2-mm steps, we estimate that the errors in the physical measurements are at least as great as the errors introduced by the digitization of the image data. The pixel size for the MR images is 1.27 mm, for the CT images 0.5 mm, and for the DSA images 0.3 mm. The slice thickness was 3 mm for CT and 5 mm for MR. We note that the geometric non-uniformities caused by the inhomogeneity in the main field may be partially overcome by increasing the bandwidth of the received signal (by increasing the strength of the readout gradient). This parameter may be adjusted in some systems by selecting a minimum "water−fat shift" in the image. (This parameter specifies the distance in the image between water and fat molecules that occupy the same spatial location.)

A further area where the accuracy of the coordinate calculation may be compromised is when the displayed image is reformatted from a series of original transverse images. If all of these images are exactly parallel and perpendicular to the axis of the frame, then a simple "restacking" and "reslicing" of the image volume will result in sagittal or coronal images which are consistent with the original data-set. If, however, some relative angulation is introduced between slices in the data-set (e.g. by patient movement), then such a calculated orthogonal image will not accurately reflect the geometry of the stereotactic volume, and coordinate calculations may be incorrect. For this reason, when we display the reformatted planes, the image lines from each slice are "painted" on the screen, each with its appropriate angulation as determined by the fiducial markers from each transverse image. The operator thus observes initially a sparse set of lines on the screen, one from each plane in the multislice data-set. The empty spaces are then immediately "filled in" by interpolation to form the full reformatted image. This procedure eliminates the situation of multiply defined points, and the associated error in the coordinate calculations caused by adjacent slices that may slightly overlap.

Conclusions

We have presented an inexpensive but effective PC-AT based workstation for the display and analysis of multimodality images for stereotactic surgery planning. The application of the system in routine operation, as well as the extension of the original ideas to include the planning of stereotactic radiosurgery, have also been discussed. The advantages of such a system, compared to manual planning from film or via the scanner console, are that: (1) all of the images from the various modalities are collected together on the same computer system; (2) they may be analyzed in a common environment; (3) the software is designed specifically for stereotactic image analysis; (4) no prior assumption is made regarding the orientation of the slices or DSA projections with respect to the frame; and (5) targets and probes defined on the basis of one modality are simply and automatically transferred and viewed in conjunction with images from another modality.

We note that while with care we may approach the desired goal of accuracy of ± 1 mm in each coordinate with all modalities, it may not be possible to achieve this level of accuracy with some scanning orientations with MRI without further geometric distortion correction.

Appendix

For every DSA image a minimum of six fiducial markers must be identified in order to subsequently identify the coordinates of structures from the images. Since the position of each identified marker is known precisely in frame coordinates, a series of simultaneous linear equations may be solved, using least-squares minimization techniques, to yield the 12 elements of a 4×3 homogeneous transformation matrix [17]. This matrix provides the transformation between a 3-D frame coordinate point and its displayed position:

$$[x \; y \; z \; 1] \times \begin{bmatrix} t_{11}t_{12}t_{13} \\ t_{21}t_{22}t_{23} \\ t_{31}t_{32}t_{33} \\ t_{41}t_{42}t_{43} \end{bmatrix} = \omega \; [u \; v \; 1]$$

where: x, y, z are the frame coordinates of the point; t_{ij} are the elements of the homogeneous matrix; ω is a constant; u, v are screen coordinates of the displayed (projected) point. Note that the perspective scaling is included implicitly within the x, y, z, ω homogeneous formulation.

These equations may be solved to obtain two equations relating the point's x, y, z coordinates and the displayed (screen) position u, v. Thus, if the frame coordinates x, y, z of a point are known, then its displayed position u, v can be found. If u and v are known on two single views, then an overdetermined set of equations results, allowing us to compute the frame coordinates using a least-squares technique.

From a stereoscopic pair of images, these equations may be solved in real time, allowing a cursor to be moved around in 3-D space with its frame coordinates instantly displayed (see Chapter 19).

References

1 Brown, R.A. A computerized tomography–computer graphics approach to stereotaxic localization. *J. Neurosurg.* **50**: 715−20 (1979).
2 Bergström, M. & Grietz, T. Stereotactic computed tomography. *Am. J. Roentg.* **127**: 167−70 (1976).
3 Kelly, P. Future possibilities in stereotactic surgery: where are we going? *Appl. Neurophysiol.* **50**: 1−8 (1987).
4 Peters, T.M., Clark, J.A., Olivier, A., *et al.* Integrated stereotaxic imaging with CT, MR imaging and digital subtraction angiography. *Radiology* **161**: 821−6 (1986).
5 Lundsford, L.D., Martinez, A.J. & Latchaw, R.E. Stereotaxic surgery with a magnetic resonance and computerized tomography-compatible system. *J. Neurosurg.* **64**: 872−8 (1986).
6 Leksell, L., Lindquist, C., Adler, J. *et al.* A new fixation device for the Leksell stereotactic system. *J. Neurosurg.* **66**: 626−9 (1987).
7 Kall, B. The impact of computer and imaging technology in stereotactic surgery. *Appl. Neurophysiol.* **50**: 9−22 (1987).
8 Hartmann, G.H., Schlegel, W., Sturm, V. *et al.* Cerebral radiation surgery using moving field irradiation at a linear accelerator facility. *Int. J. Radiation. Oncol. Biol. Phys.* **11**: 1185−92 (1985).
9 Pike, B., Podgorsak, E.B., Peters, T.M. & Pla, C. Dose distributions in dynamic stereotactic radiosurgery. *Med. Phys.* **14**: 780−9 (1987).
10 Leksell, D.G. Stereotactic radiosurgery, present status and future trends. *Neurol. Res.* **9**: 60−8 (1987).
11 Milan, J. & Bently, R.E. The storage and manipulation of radiation dose data in a small digital computer. *Br. J. Radiol.* **47**: 115 (1974).
12 Olivier, A. & de Lotbinière, A. Stereotactic techniques in epilepsy. *Neurosurgery: State-of-the-Art-Reviews* **2**: 257−85 (1987).
13 Souhami, L., Olivier, A., Podgorsak, E. *et al.* Dynamic stereotactic radiosurgery: treatment results on 33 patients with AVM. In: Heikkinen, E. & Kiviniitty, K. (eds) *Proceedings of the International Workshop on Proton and Narrow-beam Photon Therapy, Oulu, Finland*, pp. 72−6 (1989).
14 Souhami, L., Olivier, A., Podgorsak, E., *et al.* Fractionated dynamic stereotactic radiotherapy. In: Heikkinen, E. & Kiviniitty, K. (eds) *Proceedings of the International Workshop on Proton and Narrow-beam Photon Therapy, Oulu, Finland*, pp. 106−10 (1989).
15 Schad, L., Lott, S., Schmitt, F., *et al.* Correction of spatial distortion in MR imaging: a prerequisite for accurate stereotaxy. *J. Comput. Assist. Tomogr.* **11**(3): 499−505 (1987).
16 Casperson, L.W., Spiegler, P. & Grollman, J.H. Characterization of aberrations in image-intensified fluoroscopy. *Med. Phys.* **3**: 103−6 (1976).
17 Sutherland, I.E. Three-dimensional data input by tablet. *Proceedings of the Institute of Electronic and Electrical Engineers* **62**: 453−71 (1974).

16

Comprehensive Multimodality Surgical Planning and Interactive Neurosurgery

Bruce A. Kall

Introduction

The COMPASS™ stereotactic system has evolved over a period of more than 10 years into a fully functional, interactive, multimodality hardware and software surgical planning and therapeutic system. The system consists of off-the-shelf computer and imaging equipment, together with custom instrumentation and stereotactic software.

The COMPASS™ system offers the surgeon a broad range of planning and surgical options. This system is used for biopsies, cyst aspirations, IIIrd ventriculostomies, and deep-brain electrode placements, as well as functional procedures for movement disorders and chronic pain. The system has also been used for interstitial irradiation and radiosurgery. The COMPASS™ system specifically enables the volumetric removal of deep-seated, central or poorly located lesions whose removal would not be possible conventionally. Patients that would not be operated on with other techniques can safely undergo these computer-assisted stereotactic procedures.

This interactive system allows the surgeon to three-dimensionally model the various procedures in an efficient and rapid fashion before the patient enters the operating room. This saves valuable physician and operating room time. Target points may be calculated, three-dimensional (3-D) volumes reconstructed and

rendered, and surgical avascular trajectories determined. These targets, volumes, and trajectories may also be stereotactically correlated between the various diagnostic modalities. Furthermore, isodose volumes from interstitial irradiation and Gamma Knife-produced sources may be correlated and reviewed on stereotactically collected radiographic examinations and 3-D reconstructed lesion volumes. A computer-resident stereotactic atlas may also be overlayed onto diagnostic scans to annotate small subnuclei not visible with current imaging techniques.

The surgeon has full access to the computer and imaging system via a mouse and display monitors in the operating room to modify any of the preplanned parameters. Intraoperatively, the system controls a stepper motor-controlled, stereotactic, arc-centered, stereotactic slide, is used to monitor the position of probes with an interactive image intensifier-based X-ray interface, and provides the surgeon with valuable information within an intramicroscope display system during volumetric resections. This system has been employed in over 2000 stereotactic procedures over a 10-year period and will be described in this chapter.

Background

The COMPASS™ Stereotactic System (Stereotactic Medical Systems Inc., New Hartford, NY) evolved from an adaptation to a Todd-Wells stereotactic positioner (Trent Wells Inc., Southgate, CA) [1–2]. These adaptations and other developments described in this chapter evolved into the COMPASS™ Stereotactic System.

The development of the system began in early 1980 at the Erie County Medical Center in Buffalo, New York. Patrick Kelly, MD, in private practice, employed Stephan Goerss, and in late 1980 Bruce Kall, to begin applying their expertise in neurosurgery, machining, and computer science to modify the commercially available Todd–Wells device to make it computed tomography (CT) compatible. They furthermore integrated the use of a stereotactically directed CO_2 laser, computerized the calculation of stereotactic targets, and simultaneously developed the concept of *volumetric stereotaxis*. This team moved to the Sisters of Charity Hospital in Buffalo in late 1981, and the development of the system has continued from 1984 to the present at Mayo Clinic in Rochester, MN.

COMPASS™ instrumentation

The COMPASS™ system [3] is an arc-centered (or arc-quadrant) system. This type of hardware device defines a large sphere whereby all instruments approach the focus from any tangent of the sphere. Any target is moved (or translated) into the focus of the sphere. A probe is then inserted to the fixed distance from the tangent of the arc to accurately access the intracranial target. Arc-centered systems allow efficient access to any intracranial point.

The COMPASS™ hardware is discussed in detail in Chapter 6 of this volume. Briefly, the hardware consists of imaging compatible headframes, fiducial reference systems for each modality, a computer-interactive arc-quadrant stereotactic positioner, stereotactic retractors, an intramicroscope display device, fixed tube teleradiography and an interactive image intensifier-based X-ray acquisition unit.

Imaging compatible headframes

The system uses aluminum and nylon–carbon fiber composite round stereotactic headframes.

These are interchangeable by a reapplication methodology described below. The aluminum headring is utilized for CT, magnetic resonance imaging (MRI), and digital subtraction angiography (DSA) acquisition, as well as for interactive surgery. The nylon–carbon fiber headframe is used with some MRI scanners to reduce geometric distortions and to fit within the MRI headcoil.

Either headframe can be applied to the patient in the normal (headring by the patient's mouth) or inverted position (headring by the top of the head). The inverted headring position enables posterior fossa and brainstem access.

Fiducial reference systems

There is one fiducial reference device for each type of diagnostic scanner. These reference systems attach to the headring during the diagnostic study and leave markers on each collected image, allowing the computer to mathematically translate points and volumes from each image into the stereotactic coordinate system of the arc-quadrant device. A generalization of these techniques enables multimodality target and volume correlation.

Computer-interactive arc-quadrant stereotactic positioner

The computer-interactive arc-quadrant stereotactic positioner accepts the stereotactic headframe and positions it with four degrees of freedom (x, left to right; y, anterior–posterior; z, superior–inferior; and r, 360° circular rotation of the headframe in the positioner's receiving yoke). Each axis has vernier scales as well as optical encoders that transmit pulses to an x, y, z digital display device, outside of the operative field in a control panel. Stepper motors, attached to each axis, may be controlled manually by push buttons on a control panel or interactively by computer via a RS-232 interface. This allows easy and efficient access to multiple target points during craniotomies, deep brain electrode placements, and interstitial irradiation. Alternatively, and for backup, each axis may be moved with hand cranks.

The stereotactic sphere is defined by a 160

mm arc with two degrees of freedom. The *collar* angle rotates about the horizontal (left—right axis of the positioner). The collar moves an arc, which then allows the rotation of a probe holder, denoted as the *arc* angle. The arc angle rotates about the collar-modified vertical axis. The probe holder directs instruments perpendicular from a tangent of the arc to the focus. These six degrees of freedom (*x, y, z, r, collar, arc*), combined with the normal/inverted headframe option, allow precise access to any intracranial target or volume.

The positioner attaches to the side rails of a standard operating table, or may alternatively be used with a floor stand that fixes by vacuum to the floor. The floor stand is required for functional procedures and cases where the headframe is used in the inverted fashion.

Stereotactic retractor

A stereotactically directed, cylindrical retractor [4] is used for resecting deep-seated lesions. Cylinders of 2 and 3 cm diameters are available. The retractor attaches to the arc-quadrant with a special probe holder, and is thereby directed toward the focal point of the stereotactic positioner. Inscription marks on the outside of the retractor enable depth calculations in relationship to the target point. These retractors provide exposure to a lesion and act as a reference for superimposition of volumetric tumor information in the intramicroscope display device.

Intramicroscope display system

This device [5] superimposes computer-generated slices of a three-dimensionally reconstructed tumor, correlated in location and scale to the current surgical trajectory and depth, in a "heads-up" display attached to the surgical microscope. This device also displays the position of the surgical retractor for alignment. These intramicroscopically displayed images provide a template for the surgeon to follow in resecting a lesion. The surgeon interacts with this device to access the software system by menus appearing within the microscope display.

Fixed tube teleradiography/interactive image-intensifier-based X-ray acquisition

The COMPASS™ system uses fixed-tube teleradiography for stereotactic ventriculograms and to provide valuable feedback to the surgeon for measurements and confirmation of probe locations. Lateral and anterior-posterior (A/P) reticules (bomb-sites) attach to the system and provide focal references on each X-ray image. Lateral and A/P film cassette holders are provided for X-ray film acquisition. The X-ray film processors, however, are usually remotely located and may introduce long operative delays waiting for films.

A trolley that indexes into the stereotactic frame positions image intensifiers along the lateral and A/P planes of the stereotactic positioner. A video monitor attached to each intensifier provides a video signal that is fed back into the operative computer's video acquisition hardware. A special triggering device attaches to the X-ray generator to provide a signal to the computer to begin an acquisition. Intraoperative image intensifier-based X-ray images may be instantly collected and displayed directly on the operating room graphics monitors, saving valuable operating room time. These digital X-ray images may be windowed and leveled by the physician to bring out minute details that would not be possible by conventional film. Furthermore, image intensifier-based acquisitions involve less X-ray exposure to the patient than film imaging.

COMPASS™ computer and software

Computer system

The computer and imaging workstation currently consists of a scalable Sun Microsystems (Mountain View, CA) 4/300 Series workstation, connected to a Vicom Systems (Fremont, CA) VME image processing system. The Sun single-board 4/300 reduced instruction set computer (RISC) executes 16 million instructions per second (MIPS), contains 32 Mbytes of on-board memory, built-in small computer system interface (SCSI), ethernet controller, and high resolution 1152×900 monochrome display, more than one Gbyte of on-line disk storage, as well as ¼ inch and ½ inch magnetic tape drives.

The Vicom VME digital image processor is controlled by the Sun microcomputer, and uses a recursive pipeline processing structure in which memory, dedicated processors, and the Sun microcomputer are interconnected. The Vicom contains pipeline, spatial (array), point, ensemble, cursor, and video acquisition processors, as well as a display generator and three independent 16-bit display buffers, that may drive three separate monochrome monitors or be combined to display one 24-bit true color image. The Vicom contains its own image memory and also shares the address space of the Sun computer. A variety of built-in software features allow the Vicom to rapidly manipulate digital images for acquisition, storage, processing, and display.

A custom multiscreen display console was developed that contains three independent monochrome monitors and one color monitor, a mouse and controller as well as a terminal. Each monitor is capable of displaying and manipulating one 512×512 image at 12 bits of resolution with 4 bits remaining for graphic overlays. The multiscreen display was developed so that side-by-side multimodality correlation and comparisons would be possible at the full resolution of the original radiologic images, rather than trying to combine them on one screen. Furthermore, separation of the different modalities onto individual screens enables full window and level control of each image over the full range of its original intensity values. This is important in the treatment planning and interactive surgery process.

Software

The COMPASS™ stereotactic software has been developed and refined over a period of 10 years, and as such has been developed in FORTRAN, PASCAL and C. The first machines we used only supported graphics library interfaces using FORTRAN. Later generation devices offered PASCAL interfaces and present-day systems utilize C. The Sun system affords the possibility of combining source code from many languages that can be linked into a common program.

This provides several significant advantages. All volumetric software remains in FORTRAN because it just runs faster in our tests than the same program in C. Furthermore, this avoids having to rewrite previously written and extensively tested software. This would be very time consuming and could possibly introduce new errors and bugs.

The graphical user interface (GUI) employed throughout the COMPASS™ software system employs *stand-up* graphical menus and an interactive cursor that is manipulated by a mouse with three buttons (both the menus and cursor move automatically between the multiple screens as necessary). The entire interactive software package is utilized by the surgeon and is simple to use and intuitively based. The mouse has three buttons and each button has a standard function depending on the mode the software is currently in. It is important to maintain standard mouse functions to avoid user confusion.

The stereotactic software is used by picking items from a selection of items displayed on the multiscreen display, known as a menu. There are various levels of menus, which may be thought of as being organized into an *upside-down tree*. As one selects a menu item, another menu will appear that is a subsidiary of the item previously selected. Eventually one arrives at a menu item, analogous to the leaf of a tree, that performs a certain function. For example, to select a biopsy target on a CT image one would traverse the following menu path:

plan → *biopsy* → *target point* → *new target* → *CT*

where *plan* was a root menu selection, *biopsy* was a second level selection, *target point* the third, and *new target* was selected from the fourth level.

A variety of graphical prompts with various selections then easily walk the user through the variety of possibilities for each "leaf" function (i.e. which modality, which series within a modality, which slice, etc.). Confirmation of most functions also occurs at various locations (e.g. is the target point selected correct?).

Numbers and text can also be inputted from the graphics screen by numeric menus and an on-screen typewriter, freeing the surgeon from use of the keyboard (although it too may be used simultaneously with the numeric menu and on-screen typewriter). This keyboard-less methodology is especially important if any of the planned parameters need to be modified from the operating room once the surgeon is scrubbed in. The surgeon may simply run the menu software using the ceiling mounted monitors, entering numbers or text on the screen with a mouse or joystick contained in a sterile wrapper.

Images are selected from on-screen subimage panels. Each subimage panel contains 16 sub-sampled images from an original data-set. If there are more than 16 images, more than one subimage panel is available and the user moves between them by a *prior/next* menu selection. The user moves the cursor over any subsampled image on the subimage panel, and the original full-resolution image is displayed on an alternative screen as appropriate. This further avoids the use of the keyboard to select image numbers or to provide *prior* and *next* keyboard buttons.

System software capabilities

The COMPASS™ system may store as many patients as the disk capacity of the system will hold. Patients normally have 20–45 Mbytes of diagnostic imaging data as well as several Mbytes of information generated by the system for volumes and 3-D renderings. The information is automatically and invisibly organized by the stereotactic software under a patient identification (PID) number assigned by the institution. All diagnostic data are organized under the PID arrangement (as if in the same folder in a file cabinet), even though they may be inputted into the system from a variety of scanners with several different examination numbers.

The software automatically maintains a variety of files on an individual patient, in addition to the information described above. Each type of file contains redundant PID information so as to always ensure that the correct information is utilized for the correct patient.

There is a *description file* for each scan series containing information about every image in the data-set. This information, in addition to demographics and identification, includes the scanning parameters, as well as space for storage of stereotactic transformation statistics and the locations of the fiducial markings on each and every slice. Fiducial marker information for each image needs to be located only once, and is then automatically retrieved upon each successive use.

Every patient also has a *record file* that contains a variety of information: each patient may have up to 12 individual targets, known as *saved targets*. This allows the surgeon to preplan a variety of targeting options. Each *saved target* has an associated alphanumeric description stored with it, to enable easy classification. Only one of these *saved targets* may be "active" at one time. "Active" in this sense means that if the software was placed into its surgical mode, the currently active target would be confirmed to be placed in the focus of the stereotactic frame.

Each *saved target* may also have up to three individual trajectories recorded along with it, enabling the surgeon to preplan a variety of approaches and then select the desired option from the operating room. Furthermore, the location of collected biopsy specimens for each stored trajectory may be saved for later correlation with the histologic diagnosis. There can only be one "active" trajectory at a time.

Saved targets and *saved trajectories* may be retrieved at any time. For instance, a resident may plan the case and the surgeon may confirm the procedure by "playing back" the stored plan. This recording mechanism also allows the surgeon to plan the case on one day and then retrieve it for surgery another day without having to replan it.

Computer-assisted stereotactic surgery

Stereotactic surgery is performed in three steps: (1) diagnostic data collection; (2) treatment planning; and (3) interactive surgery.

Diagnostic data collection

Patients have one of the imaging-compatible stereotactic headframes applied under local anesthesia, using a carbon-fiber pin/locking collet fixation system. Briefly, a headframe is rigidly applied to the patient's skull through four $\frac{7}{64}$ inch twist-drill holes into the skull with locking collets, sleeves, and carbon fiber pins. Carbon fiber vertical supports offset the headring away from the intended surgical target.

Micrometer attachments are used to provide depth settings for each of the four carbon fiber pins, so as to enable accurate removal and replacement of the headring if data acquisition and surgery are not performed on the same day. This allows efficient use of physician time and operating room facilities. Furthermore, the headframe may be removed, for example, after a stereotactic biopsy, and reapplied up to several months later for a computer-assisted craniotomy without necessarily having to rescan the patient. Each headframe may be applied to the patient in the normal or inverted position.

Following the application, the patient is transported to the radiology department for CT, MRI, and DSA scanning. Although there is no required order, patients usually have DSA, followed by CT, and in some cases then undergo MRI.

CT SCANNING

An adaptation plate is attached to the scanning table and the headframe is securely attached. A CT localization system [1] is attached to the headholder during the diagnostic study. This system consists of three sets of two vertical and one oblique carbon fiber bars, arranged around the headframe both laterally and anteriorly. This deposits a set of nine reference marks on each axial image, by which the computer transforms any point or volume from each image into the stereotactic coordinate system. A set of contrast-enhanced CT images is then collected, with a 0.673 mm pixel size. Approximately 15–35 512 × 512 CT images are collected for each patient.

DSA SCANNING

An arteriographic reference system attaches to the headframe during digital subtraction angiography. This system is composed of four acrylic plates, each containing nine radiopaque markers, which are located laterally as well as anteriorly and posteriorly. An adaptation plate secures the patient's headframe to the scanning table, and also enables precise collection of 6° oblique stereoscopic pairs by rotating the headframe in its yoke. (This obviates the need for trying to rotate the C-arm of the angiographic unit 6°, which is not only cumbersome, but is also not usually mechanically accurate.) Standard orthogonal and oblique arterial and venous images are obtained in both lateral and A/P projections. Twelve 512 × 512 images make up a data-set for each vessel of interest when combined with the mask (unsubtracted) image. Up to 36 images may be collected for an individual patient in a three-vessel study.

MRI

Patients often undergo MRI following the CT and DSA scans. An MRI-compatible multiplanar localization system attaches to the headframe; it deposits references on images collected in the transverse, sagittal and coronal planes, allowing stereotactic transformations by the computer. The patient is located in the head coil of the unit in a snug fit, obviating the need for an adaptation plate. A variety of pulse sequences, acquisition modes, and thicknesses are possible for MRI, depending on the type of surgical procedure. Between 20 and 120 256 × 256 MRI images may be collected on a particular patient, using a 0.938 mm pixel size.

IMAGE TRANSFER

Each of the images from each modality is recorded onto a magnetic tape using the scanner's software. These tapes are then transported to the operative computer system and transferred into a format appropriate to the stereotactic software.

Treatment planning

Treatment planning is performed immediately after data acquisition if the surgical procedure is to follow, or may be performed at the surgeon's convenience when surgery is performed on another surgical day. This balances the needs of patients requiring immediate attention against optimal use of the surgeon's and operating room schedules.

Computer-assisted stereotactic procedures are categorized into point-in-space and volumetric procedures.

POINT-IN-SPACE PROCEDURES

Point-in-space procedures require access to a single point or multiple points within the brain, together with the determination of an avascular trajectory. These procedures include biopsy [6−14], IIIrd ventriculostomy [15], thalamotomy [16−19], Ommaya reservoir placement, and cyst aspirations. (*Note*: cyst aspirations may be considered a volumetric procedure if the surgeon desires a calculation of the cyst volume before the procedure.)

The stereotactic coordinates of the desired intracranial target point are easily and quickly determined with the COMPASS™ system, using CT, MRI, or DSA images.

CT and MRI

A target point from CT and MRI is similarly determined. The reference fiducials appearing on each slice allow the computer to determine the angulation of the slice (α = left−right; β = anterior−posterior; and γ = superior−inferior) and its height above a known location (e.g. transverse = distance above the headframe). These reference statistics allow any point on any slice to be transposed into the 3-D coordinates system of the stereotactic positioner.

The surgeon moves the cursor over the intended target and then presses a button on the mouse. The computer calculates an intermediate x, y, z coordinate and adjusts it for the slice's angulation. The user then selects the orientation of the headframe on the 3-D slide, and the software rotates the coordinates appropriately, resulting in the final stereotactic coordinate. The program prompts the user to enter an appropriate alphanumeric description to associate with this target, stores it in the record file, and displays all of this information on the imaging screen.

DSA

A vascular target point from DSA may be selected from orthogonal lateral and A/P pairs,

or alternatively using a 3-D cursor manipulated on stereoscopic pairs. This is useful for surgical procedures to treat arteriovenous malformations (AVMs).

Orthogonal determination The user selects the vessel of interest and a target location is initially selected on the lateral image. The software relates this point to the known mathematical relationships of the fiducial reference system and calculates an x, z coordinate pair (Fig. 16.1a). The computer displays the associated A/P image and interpolates a line at the calculated z coordinate, extending along the x axis (Fig. 16.1b). The user picks the target location on this line which the computer associates with a y, z coordinate. The true stereotactic x, y, z coordinate may be determined from these two coordinate pairs. The lateral image is again displayed, this time annotated with a Z line interpolated along the y coordinate. If the points selected on the lateral and A/P image match, this line should traverse the original point selected on the lateral image (Fig. 16.1c). These steps may be repeated if necessary to correlate these two points. In most cases this is not required.

Oblique target determination A corresponding region is selected and lateral and A/P stereoscopic pairs are displayed on two adjacent screens. The mouse's vertical and horizontal movements then move a 3-D line, projected on each of the stereoscopic pairs by mimicking the collar and arc rotations on the stereotactic frame. The surgeon manipulates this until a common point is selected. The 3-D stereotactic coordinates of this point are then calculated by a geometric coordinate transformation.

Each of the above-mentioned CT, MRI, and DSA targeting techniques results in an x, y, z stereotactic coordinate, the rotation of the headframe on the 3-D slide, and an alpha-numeric description of the target. These targeting functions may also be utilized to select and save an entry location, or a point within the substance of the brain, through which a probe should traverse (see "Trajectory determination: Two-point method," below).

Multimodality target correlation It is useful to cor-

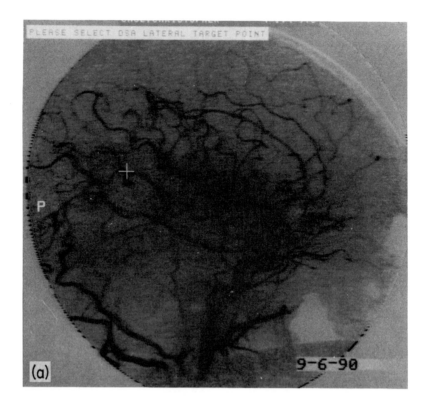

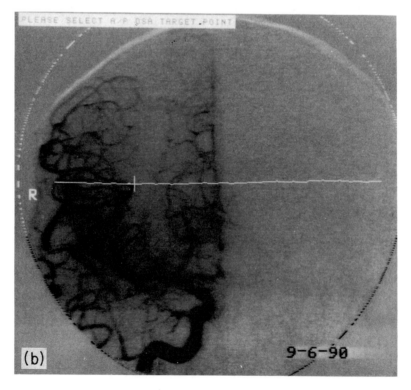

FIGURE 16.1 continued opposite.

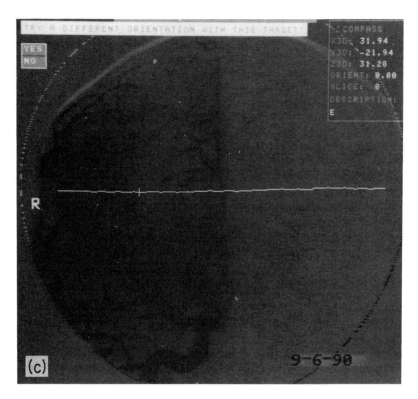

FIGURE 16.1 (a) To determine a stereotactic target point from orthogonal DSA images, the surgeon initially selects the target location on a lateral image. (b) The *z* coordinate determined from the target selected in Fig. 16.1a is used to interpolate a line along the *x* axis on an A/P image. The surgeon then selects the corresponding target location on this line with the cursor. (c) After the selection of the target point on Fig. 16.1b, the lateral image is annotated with an interpolated Z line along the *y* coordinate determined on Fig. 16.4b. This line will pass through the original target selected in Fig. 16.4a if the two selected targets match. The final stereotactic *x, y, z* coordinates are calculated from the lateral and A/P selected points.

relate a selected target point from one modality to its stereotactically correlated location on another modality and/or plane of section [9,13–14].

1 *CT to MRI correlation.* A target point, for example, is selected on an axial MRI slice. The software, by an exhaustive (but immediate) search, locates the closest CT slice and pixel within that image that minimizes the 3-D distance to the selected target (taking into account differing planes of section, thicknesses, and slice angulations). This image is then displayed on an adjacent screen, and annotated with its stereotactic coordinates and the 3-D distance between the digitized and correlated target location.

2 *CT/MRI to DSA correlation.* Any CT or MRI target may be correlated onto its closest location on lateral and A/P angiograms. The program computes the closest pixel within the angiogram image that corresponds stereotactically with the CT or MRI target by its relationship to the fiducial markings. This step is automatically performed under angiographic trajectory determination, described below.

Trajectory determination

In most cases, the surgeon desires to determinate an avascular trajectory to approach the target. There are three alternatives for selecting a trajectory: manually, calculation between two targets, and from angiography. Once the trajectory is calculated, it may then be reviewed on the CT and MRI planar images.

Manual determination The surgeon may desire to enter the patient through a specific location on the skull. He would place the patient on the 3-D positioner at the calculated target's coordinates, and would then extend a probe from the arc to the intended entry location. The surgeon would then read off the collar and arc settings, and input them into the software via numeric menus.

Two-point method A trajectory may be calculated in terms of collar and arc settings that would introduce a probe between any two previously saved targets. These are usually the target placed at the focus of the frame and an entry location. The computer first checks whether the two saved targets have the same patient orientation, and then calculates the collar and arc settings, as well as the 3-D distance between the two points. (This type of calculation is also useful, for example, during a cyst aspiration to measure the distance between the skull and the cyst wall.)

Alternatively, a IIIrd ventriculostomy for obstructive hydrocephalus [15] would necessitate determination of the trajectory between a target located in the midline between the dorsum sellae and the basilar artery and a traversal point on the foramen of Munro. The software determines the stereotactic coordinates for each point, as well as the collar and arc angles to traverse these points and the 3-D distance between them.

Angiographic determination Digital subtraction angiograms are most useful in determining an avascular surgical trajectory in addition to targeting calculations. Several available annotation options are available before the trajectory is actually selected: (1) identification of surface anatomy; (2) annotation of target and entry

points; and (3) display of volumetric lesion data.

The surface anatomy of the fissures and sulci may be identified by the surgeon before the trajectory is calculated. The surgeon selects a region of interest and the computer then displays the appropriate sections of stereoscopic arterial and venous images on adjacent screens. The surgeon identifies vessels that extend below the cortical surface in the sulci, and those that are on the surface of the brain. Deep segments of veins and arteries are traced by the surgeon by manipulating the cursor on the orthogonal views of the stereoscopic pairs. The software relates these "line segments" to the mask (unsubtracted image).

Slices of a CT and/or MRI-defined volume (described below) may be viewed on lateral and A/P angiographic views (Fig. 16.2a and b). This may be projected onto the angiogram images at any specified level on any specified image, arterial, venous, or mask, with or without sulcal annotation.

The selected target and entry point (if selected) from CT and/or MRI are projected onto mask, arterial, and venous images displayed on the three screens. Lateral and A/P views may be alternated as necessary.

The surgical trajectory may then be calculated on orthogonal images or alternatively on stereoscopic pairs.

1 *Orthogonal-calculated trajectories.* Collar and arc settings on the stereotactic frame are alternatively determined from lateral and A/P images. The computer calculates the appropriate angle between the location of the target point and a cursor interactively manipulated by the surgeon. The surgeon alternates between successive lateral and A/P pairs until an avascular approach is determined. This trajectory may be saved in the record file and later reviewed.

2 *Stereoscopic-calculated trajectories.* A surgical trajectory may also be calculated on stereoscopic pairs using a combination of the stereoscopic angiographic target technique and the two-

---

FIGURE 16.2 (*opposite*) Lateral (a) and A/P (b) DSA images, annotated with the CT or MRI derived target (small cursor at the center of the screen) and proposed entry point (end of projected line). A slice from a CT- and/or MRI-derived lesion volume at any level is then projected onto the DSA images.

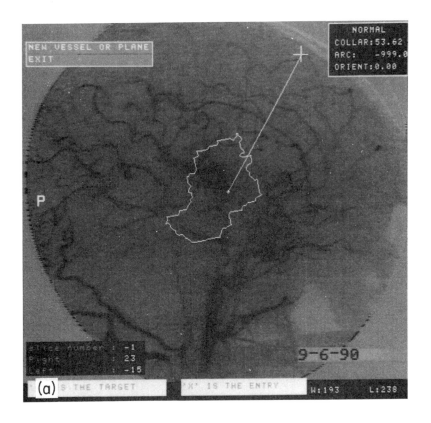

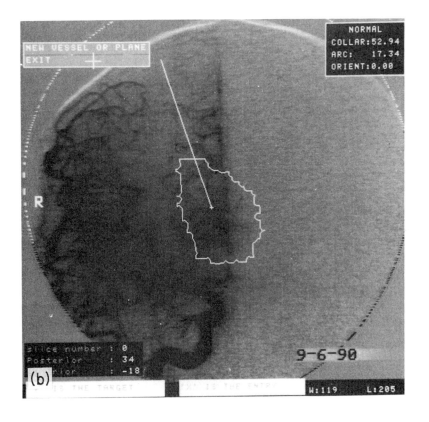

point target calculation algorithm. Lateral and A/P stereoscopic pairs are displayed on adjacent screens. The target location (and entry) is annotated on each image. The computer inter- actively calculates collar and arc settings as the surgeon simultaneously manipulates a 3-D cursor for each image. The computer instantly calculates a 3-D stereotactic coordinate for each pixel movement, and then pipelines the target and cursor x, y, z stereotactic coordinates through the two-point trajectory calculation to interactively determine collar and arc settings.

Trajectory review

Once the surgeon determines a tentative trajec- tory using one or more of the techniques described above, he or she may then pre- operatively review a simulated probe path on the CT and/or MRI images. This trajectory may be co-planar or oblique to the original images. Both of these techniques are also useful post- operatively to compare the histologic diagnosis to the tissue's originating location. This aids in the determination of the true boundaries of a lesion, as well as determination of appropriate treatment [13−14].

Co-planar   trajectories Co-planar   trajectories result when the surgical trajectory would intro- duce a probe parallel to an originally collected slice as adjusted by its angular deviations. In these cases, a set of serial biopsy locations may be annotated on a single image (Fig. 16.3a,b). The software annotates each biopsy location with its distance relative to the target location with proximal distances noted as positive and distal distance being negative.

Oblique trajectories Optimal surgical trajectories are often not co-planar to the imaging slices. Oblique trajectories may be annotated on a series of slices with a cursor indicating the

probe's position as it would pierce each slice. The distance from the target to the annotated point is also displayed. These are useful for stereotactic biopsy and interstitial irradiation planning.

Thalamotomy

An intracranial target point for a stereotactic thalamotomy may also be determined with the COMPASS™ system. This technique is discussed in detail in [16−19] and in Chapter 10 of this book.

VOLUMETRIC STEREOTAXIS − VOLUME RECONSTRUCTIONS

Three-dimensional volumes may be recon- structed from a series of contour outlines on a variety of diagnostic images for stereotactic craniotomy [18,20−33], or for planning inter- stitial irradiation [18,34−36], and more recently for radiosurgery. These techniques are useful for any stereotactic procedure, as the volume may be traced from any 3-D structure apparent on CT and/or MR images (e.g. ventricles). Primarily, lesion volumes are reconstructed for stereotactic craniotomies, interstitial irradiation and radiosurgery.

A variety of differing volumes may be inte- grated. For instance, the contrast-enhancing and hypodense region may be circumscribed on CT, while the T1- and T2-weighted contour may be outlined on transverse, sagittal and/or coronal MR images. The surgeon selects a modality and series to trace a volume. A range of contiguous slices exhibiting the lesion is then selected. The entire set of images is then read into the image memory from disk and a cine loop is initiated to allow the surgeon to view the changing nature of the volume.

The surgeon outlines the lesion on each CT and/or MRI slice, using the mouse and cursor

---

FIGURE 16.3 (*opposite*) (a) Surgical trajectory annotated on a CT image. This patient would be positioned in the prone position and would have had serial biopsies collected from −23 to +7 mm relative to the target point in this proposed trajectory. (Negative distances are proximal to the target, while positive distances are distal.) (b) The software automatically correlates the target and serial probe path on an MR image and is annotated accordingly. The 3-D distance is the distance between the target location on CT and the correlated target (biopsy location zero) on the MRI image.

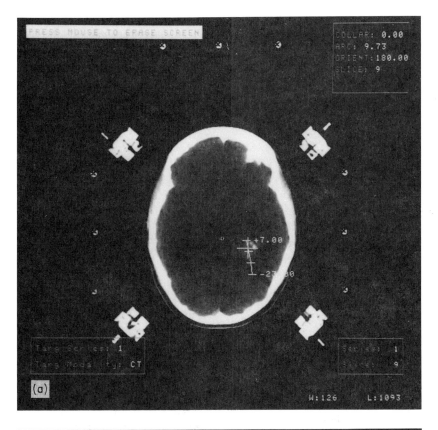

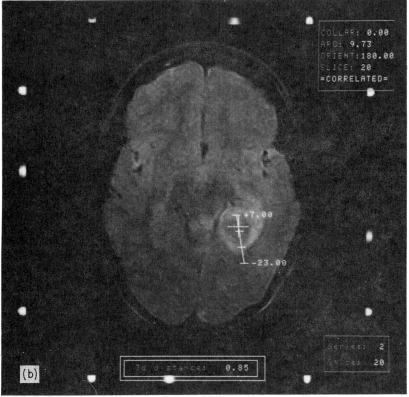

to manipulate a rubber-banding line. The surgeon deposits a series of vertices on the contour by depressing the mouse button. The system automatically connects the beginning and end points on the circumscribed contour. This process is repeated for each type of contour selected (e.g. contrast-enhancing, hypodense). When all contours are completed, a target point (usually within the volume) is then selected and saved as the reference point of the volume. (A previously saved target may be retrieved for this function.) While the physician performs other tasks with the software, the computer three-dimensionally reconstructs the volume(s).

Each of the digitized contours is suspended in stereotactic space in relationship to the target point. A single 3-D matrix is created, whose center corresponds to the focus of the stereotactic frame. The software interpolates contours inbetween every two adjacent outlines to generate a contour every 1 mm in the matrix. Adjacent contours vary in distance from one another, depending on the slice spacing and thickness from their derived imaging set. Usually they are 3–5 mm from one another. Each of the digitized and interpolated contours is then filled with millimeter cubes.

Each cube within the matrix contains eight bits, by means of which an algorithm is employed to encode which volume(s) each cube was filled from. This allows, for example, the combination of CT and MRI volumes into the common matrix, so that they can be statistically (volume measurements) and graphically analyzed (by gray levels display, for instance) for correlations (unions) and deviations (complements). The software may display this 3-D volume in two ways: cross-sections and 3-D renderings.

Cross-sections of the combined volume may be created and rapidly displayed at millimeter intervals perpendicular to any convenient surgical trajectory. CT and MRI-defined boundaries are indicated by different gray levels. This trajectory is communicated to the software by collar and arc settings on the stereotactic frame. The computer transforms this into a vector emanating from a tangent of the sphere passing through the origin of the matrix. Any cross-section along this viewline may then be created and displayed. Negative cross-section levels indicate slices proximal to the target, while positive levels indicate slices distal to the target. These cross-sections are useful in performing interstitial implants, radiosurgery, and especially computer-assisted CO_2 laser craniotomies. They are also useful when determining the surgical trajectory using angiography, as described earlier.

Stereotactic craniotomy

Cross-sections of a 3-D reconstructed tumor volume are used as a guide to resect the lesion. The software slices the volume perpendicular to any trajectory to preplan the optimal surgical approach (Fig. 16.4). This is often along the long axis of the lesion. The software initially calculates the range of the lesion along the proposed trajectory, and identifies the proximal and distal locations along the approach where the tumor resides. Cross-sections at every millimeter interval in this range are then calculated, and may be displayed on the imaging console. The surgeon then reviews these in relationship to the position of the surgical retractor that is annotated on each image.

The COMPASS™ system allows the removal of lesions even when their diameter is larger than the diameter of the retractor. The surgeon may identify small deviations in the primary trajectory to access edges outside the retractor. In most cases, the surgeon selects many small translations of the image in the orthogonal surgical coordinate system (x', y') to bring areas of the lesion under the retractor. The computer calculates the corresponding movements on the stereotactic positioner to move the patient in its x, y, z coordinate system to match the orthogonal movements desired. A combination of alterations in the trajectory and orthogonal translations may be rapidly and efficiently simulated to obtain the optimal combination.

Stereotactic interstitial irradiation

Lesion and radiation isodose volumes may be correlated for planning interstitial irradiation. A simulation program allows the surgeon to place and evaluate a number of source locations. The surgeon selects these locations on a series of

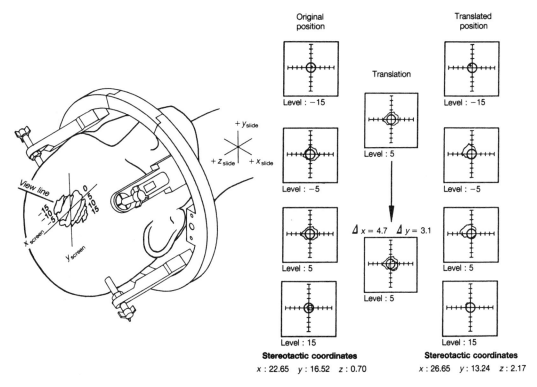

FIGURE 16.4 The 3-D reconstructed lesion volume (from CT and/or MRI) is sliced perpendicular to the surgical trajectory. Cross-sections of the volume may then be displayed on the operating room monitors, or within the intramicroscope display device. The circle represents the position of the cylindrical retractor. The surgeon selects translations along the orthogonal coordinate system (x_{screen}, y_{screen} — which is perpendicular to the viewline) to move areas of the lesion within the retractor. Corresponding x, y, z stereotactic coordinates for the stereotactic positioner (x_{slide}, y_{slide}, z_{slide}) are calculated to match the translated image. The stepper motor-controlled slide is then used to reposition the patient, directly by the physician or under computer control.

cross-sections along the intended surgical implantation trajectory. The software demonstrates the isodose configuration as percentages of the total dose. Locations of each source are retained, redisplayed, and revised on sequential cross-sections of the tumor. Individual sources may be added, deleted, and moved at any time. Proximal and distal levels for each source are identified.

The surgeon may not always be able to fit the isodose volume precisely onto the tumor. It is therefore a physician's decision to decide whether to deliver a subtherapeutic dose to portions of the tumor and augment it by external beam radiation.

The software ultimately determines x, y, z stereotactic coordinates and the length of each source to match the preplanned parameters. A double catheter afterloading technique is then used to implant the sources [34,35].

Radiosurgery planning

The COMPASS™ system can similarly overlay isodose volumes generated by the Gamma Knife Kula software onto the volumetric cross-sections. It can, furthermore, correlate this treatment volume onto the stereotactically collected CT, MR, and DSA images.

Two methods are currently available to plan these procedures. Typical single-shot dose volumes are precomputed for each helmet-collimator size, and are transferred from the Gamma Knife Microvax computer to the operative Sun–Vicom system by a network. These may then be placed by cursor interaction to fit the lesion volume identified on cross-sections, CT, MR, and DSA images. This "first pass" technique allows these single shots to be added, moved, deleted, weighted, and merged into a composite dose volume. The software auto-

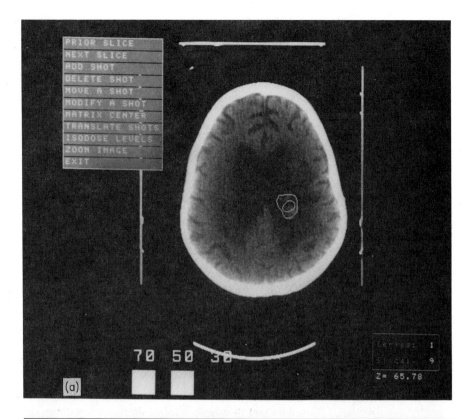

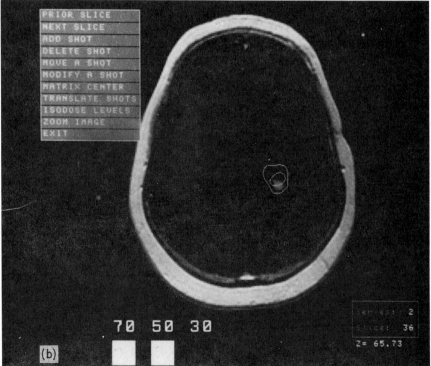

FIGURE 16.5 (a) CT image with a proposed isodose volume for a stereotactic radiosurgery procedure. (b) Proposed isodose volume for stereotactic radiosurgery reviewed on MR image.

matically scales and slices this composite dose matrix along appropriate angles, to match each image in the CT, MRI, and DSA examinations and cross-section images (Fig. 16.5a and b).

The "first-fit" locations are then entered into the Kula program to provide a new composite dose matrix generated by the manufacturer's software and is transferred into the operative computer system. It may then be reviewed on the CT, MRI, DSA, and cross-section images. The process may be repeated as many times as necessary until the treatment is determined to be optimal. The radiosurgery is then performed on the Gamma Knife unit.

We have found this technique to be quite useful. This procedure allows the surgeon, oncologist, and physicist to perform in minutes what takes several hours using the mechanisms provided by the manufacturer. Calculation of the integrated dose volume on the Sun-Vicom computer from the actual physics of the sources will obviate the need for the Kula program altogether once it is validated.

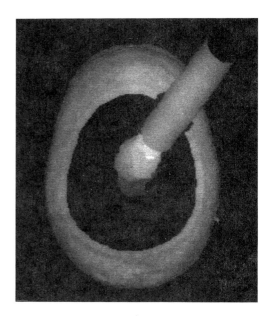

FIGURE 16.6 3-D rendering of the patient's skull, 3-D reconstructed lesion volume, and position of the stereotactic retractor.

Three-dimensional renderings

Stereotactic software has also been developed to automatically obtain skull outlines from the axial CT database by an intensity detection algorithm. These can then be combined with the lesional volume to display 3-D rendered images along a variety of static views as well as in a cine loop.

The axes of the stereotactic positioner are always noted for reference. The position of the stereotactic retractor may also be displayed at various levels along the surgical viewline, as well as a trephine opening and a skull cutaway to reveal the interior of the rendered image (Fig. 16.6). Three-dimensionally rendered stereoscopic pairs of the lesion volume may also be displayed.

Interactive surgery

Interactive computer-assisted stereotactic neurosurgery is performed in a stereotactic operating room and involves the "playback" of the surgical plan. The headframe is reapplied into the stereotactic headframe and the 3-D slide set to the preplanned target coordinates.

The surgeon utilizes the software in the operating room from a mouse or joystick held in a sterile wrapper, and a cursor and menus on the ceiling-mounted display screens, or within the intramicroscope display in the operating room. When the software first enters the surgical mode, the "active" target is recalculated (for redundancy) and displayed on the operating room monitors. The computer automatically reads the current position of the stereotactic frame from the digital display device to determine if the patient is positioned correctly. If not, the system will notify the surgeon and will then wait to reposition the patient when the surgeon depresses a foot pedal.

The entire operative plan is then manipulated in the operating room. This includes display of trajectories as well as cross-sections and 3-D rendered images. If any of the parameters need to be modified intraoperatively, the surgeon merely returns to the planning phase and instantly recalculates targets, trajectories, and volumes.

Fixed-tube teleradiography, using films or the interactive image intensifier-based X-ray acquisition system, may be used to confirm targeting, monitor the position of probes, and provide valuable feedback to the surgeon. Lateral and A/P reticules appear on each image, enabling the surgeon to perform measurements. Interactive image intensifier-based images appear instantaneously on the operating room monitors, and may also be windowed and leveled by the physician, allowing details to be enhanced which may otherwise be undetected using film imaging.

POINT-IN-SPACE PROCEDURES

Stereotactic point-in-space procedures usually entail playback of the preoperative plan. There are a variety of cases where the surgeon may need to determine several targets and/or trajectories, and may only select the appropriate parameters intraoperatively. The system is also used to monitor the position of probes and instruments, using the interactive image intensifier-based X-ray acquisition system described above.

VOLUMETRIC PROCEDURES

Volumetric resections are the most interactive procedure. Cross-sections of the CT/MRI volume are displayed on the operating room monitors, as well as within the intramicroscope display device correlated to the trajectory of the surgical cylindrical retractor. These cross-sections are provided perpendicular to this trajectory, at the depth at which the surgeon is operating. The cross-sections appear within the intramicroscope display as a shadow overlaid only the surgical field and are used as a template to identify the limits of the lesion and the location of normal brain tissue.

The surgeon removes the lesion by a stereotactically-directed CO_2 laser, sucker, or other means. When portions of the lesion lie outside the retractor, a modified trajectory is selected, or the images are translated, new stereotactic coordinates are calculated, and the motorized positioner is then utilized to move the patient to these new coordinates when the surgeon presses a foot pedal. Either of these techniques can be simulated preoperatively in order to provide the optimal surgical technique. In either scenario, the software provides immediate reformation of the three-dimensionally reconstructed lesion along the new trajectory or alternate translation.

Discussion

The COMPASS™ system is a state-of-the-art hardware and software system for planning and performing a variety of neurosurgical procedures. The procedures and methods have a wide range of applications, including functional procedures for movement disorders, biopsy, cyst aspirations, IIIrd ventriculostomy, placement of deep brain electrodes, radiation treatment, and the volumetric resection of brain tumors in deep and central locations. The system has been utilized in well over 2000 stereotactic procedures at the Mayo Clinic alone since mid-1984.

The instrumentation, computer hardware, and software have evolved over a 10-year period in order to reach the present level of technological sophistication. Furthermore, the system has been carefully tested in laboratory and clinical environments. A variety of "phantoms" have been developed that may be scanned on the various diagnostic units that allow the user to verify the performance of the system. Intra-operative teleradiographic procedures are also used to verify the system at any time.

The software has been developed at a busy educational institution in which a new resident is obliged to master the system every 3 months. Therefore, the software has been designed to be intuitive, easy to use, and easy to learn. We have found that the stand-up menu system, employed throughout the COMPASS™ software, is easier to master than pull-down or walking menus employed on Apple Macintosh- and UNIX-based workstations. This allows the computer-inexperienced novice, as well as experts, to use the system with a minimal amount of training.

The full COMPASS™ system comprises a stepper motor-controlled stereotactic positioning system, multimodality-compatible replaceable headframes with localization devices for each scanner, stereotactic retractors, intramicroscope display, a computer and imaging workstation, and support software. Scaled-down (unmotorized) manual versions of the system are used in non-stereotactic

operating rooms for conventional neurosurgical procedures performed stereotactically (e.g. removal of superficial lesions).

The support hardware and software allow the surgeon to plan various procedures accurately in a rapid, comprehensive, and efficient manner. This saves time for the surgeon and the operating room. The fact that the stereotactic headframe can be applied for CT, MR, and DSA imaging, and removed and reapplied for surgery, also helps in using the facilities efficiently. The database acquisition and surgical procedures can therefore be performed on two separate days. Furthermore, with the COMPASS™ system, it is possible to do complex procedures in less time than would normally be required using conventional manual means or other stereotactic systems.

The system is operated directly by the physician and does not necessarily require additional personnel to run it. Nevertheless, some additional part-time support is usually required to transfer data from radiology, turn the computer on and off and perform maintenance. Usually someone from the information system department or biomedical engineering who has an interest in computers is involved in this process. Vendor support is provided for the computer itself.

The Sun−Vicom-based system uses a standard UNIX-based operating system, and the central processing unit is scalable to provide faster computational speeds as the technology advances. The software has been developed in standard high-level languages, providing a high level of maintainability and portability to other imaging architectures as technology advances. The entire COMPASS™ system — computer hardware, software, and instrumentation — has been designed modularly, so that introducing new technological improvements is easy while the basic system remains intact.

There are a variety of backup mechanisms built directly into the system. Intraoperative X-ray and conventional techniques are the most important backup. Most, if not all, of the stereotactic procedures may be performed without the computer if necessary, once the planning is completed, using conventional stereotactic techniques. Furthermore, reapplication of the headframe is an alternative for diagnostic

scanner or intraoperative computer failures before the surgical case begins. The motors on the slide can be controlled by the computer or, alternatively, by push buttons on the control rack. All motors may be disengaged at any time and each axis may be moved by hand cranks. Vernier scales are attached to each axis as a backup for the optical encoders and digital display.

A variety of calculations are performed to quantitatively relate images from various modalities that have differing slice thicknesses, angulations, and fields of view. Geometric correction calculations are automatically performed to account, for example, for the distortion introduced by an image intensifier in a DSA unit. MRI distortion corrections are also possible, although in our experience with a General Electric Signa[R] MRI unit, these corrections have only infrequently been required. The quality of MRI-based computations should always be verified by multimodality target and volumetric reconstructions correlated to CT-based calculations.

There are a number of patients who would not be offered surgery at all by conventional means, or with other stereotactic systems, who can safely undergo these computer-assisted stereotactic procedures. Furthermore, hospital stay times are typically shorter for any of these procedures in comparison to conventional neurosurgical procedures.

References

1 Goerss, S., Kelly, P.J., Kall, B. & Alker, G.W. Jr. A computed tomographic stereotactic adaptation system. *Neurosurgery* **10**(3): 375−9 (1982).
2 Kelly, P.J., Goerss, S.J. & Kall, B.A. Modification of the Todd−Wells system for imaging data acquisition. In: Lunsford, L.D. (ed.) *Modern Stereotactic Neurosurgery*, pp. 79−97. Boston: Nijoff (1988).
3 Kall, B.A., Kelly, P.J. & Goerss, S.J. Comprehensive computer-assisted data collection treatment planning and interactive surgery. *Proceedings of the Society of Photo-optical Instrumentation Engineering* **767**: 509−14 (1987).
4 Kelly, P.J., Goerss, S.J. & Kall, B.A. The stereotaxic retractor in computer-assisted stereotaxic microsurgery. *J. Neurosurg.* **69**: 301−6 (1988).
5 Kelly, P.J. Stereotactic imaging, surgical planning and computer-assisted resection of intracranial lesions: methods and results. In: Symen, L. (ed.) *Advances and Technical Standards in Neurosurgery,*

Vol. 17, pp. 77−118. Vienna, New York: Springer-Verlag (1990).

6 Kelly, P.J., Kall, B. & Goerss, S. Stereotactic CT scanning for the biopsy of intracranial lesions and functional neurosurgery. *Appl. Neurosurg.* **46**: 193−9 (1983).

7 Kelly, P.J., Alker, G.J., Jr., Kall, B.A. & Goerss, S. Method of computed-tomography-based stereotactic biopsy with arteriographic control. *Neurosurgery* **14**: 172−7 (1984).

8 Kelly, P.J., Kall, B.A. & Goerss, S. Computer-assisted stereotactic biopsy utilizing CT and digitized angiographic data. *Acta Neurosurg.* (suppl.) **33**: 233−5 (1984).

9 Kall, B.A., Kelly, P.J., Goerss, S.J. & Earnest, F.IV. Cross-registration of points and lesion volumes from MR and CT. *Proceedings of the 7th Annual Conference of the Institute of Electronic and Electrical Engineers Engineering in Medicine and Biology Society, Chicago, September 27−30*, 1985, pp. 939−42.

10 Kelly, P.J., Earnest, F.IV, Kall, M.S., Goerss, S.J. & Scheithauer, B.W. Surgical options for patients with deep-seated brain tumors: computer-assisted stereotactic biopsy. *Mayo Clin. Proc.* **60**: 223−9 (1985).

11 Davis, D.H., Kelly, P.J., Marsh, W.R., Kall, B.A. & Goerss, S.J. Computer-assisted stereotactic biopsy of intracranial lesions. *Appl. Neurophysiol.* **50**: 172−7 (1987).

12 Davis, D.H., Kelly, P.J., Marsh, W.R., Kall, B.A. & Goerss, S.J. Computer-assisted stereotactic biopsy of intracranial lesions in pediatric patients. *Pediatr. Neurosci.* **14**: 33−6 (1988).

13 Kelly, P.J., Daumas−Duport, C., Scheithauer, B.W., Kall, B.A. & Kispert, D.B. Stereotactic histologic correlation of computed tomography and magnetic resonance imaging-defined abnormalities in patient with glial neoplasms. *Mayo Clin. Proc.* **62**: 450−9 (1987).

14 Earnest, F.IV, Kelly, P.J., Scheithauer, B.W., Kall, B.A., Cascine, T.L., Ehman, R.L., Forbes, G.S. & Axley, P.L. Cerebral astrocytomas: histopathologic correlation of MR and CT contrast enhancement with stereotactic biopsy. *Radiology* **166**: 823−7 (1988).

15 Kelly, P.J., Goerss, S., Kall, B.A. & Kispert, D.B. Computed tomography-based stereotactic third, ventriculostomy: technical note. *Neurosurgery* **18**(6): 791−4 (1986).

16 Kelly, P.J., Kall, B. & Goerss, S. Functional stereotactic surgery utilizing CT data and computer generated stereotactic atlas. *Acta Neurochir.* (suppl.) **33**: 577−83 (1984).

17 Kall, B.A., Kelly, P.J., Goerss, S. & Frieder, G. Methodology and clinical experience with computed tomography and a computer-resident stereotactic atlas. *Neurosurgery* **17**(3): 400−7 (1985).

18 Kelly, P.J. Applications and methodology for contemporary stereotactic surgery. *Neurol. Res.* **8**: 2−12 (1986).

19 Kelly, P.J., Ahlskog, J.E., Goerss, S.J., Daube, J.R., Duffy, J.R. & Kall, B.A. Computer-assisted stereotactic ventralis lateralis thalamotomy with microelectrode recording control in patients with Parkinson's disease. *Mayo Clin. Proc.* **62**: 655−64 (1987).

20 Kelly, P.J. & Alker, G.J. Jr. A stereotactic approach to deep-seated central nervous system neoplasms using the carbon dioxide laser. *Surg. Neurol.* **14**: 331−4 (1981).

21 Kelly, P.J., Alker, G.J. & Goerss, S. Computer-assisted stereotactic laser microsurgery for the treatment of intracranial neoplasms. *Neurosurgery* **10**: 324−31 (1981).

22 Kelly, P.J. Method of computer-assisted stereotactic implantation of ^{192}iridium into CNS neoplasms. In: Dyck, P., (ed.) *Stereotactic Biopsy and Brachytherapy of Brain Tumors.* Baltimore: University Park Press (1983).

23 Kelly, P.J., Alker, G.J. Jr & Goerss, S. Computer-assisted stereotactic laser microsurgery for the treatment of intracranial neoplasms. *Neurosurgery* **10**(3): 324−31 (1982).

24 Kelly, P.J., Kall, B.A. & Goerss, S. Precision resection of intra-axial CNS lesions by CT-based stereotactic craniotomy and computer-monitored CO_2 laser. *Acta Neurosurg.* **68**: 1−9 (1983).

25 Kelly, P.J., Kall, B.A. & Goerss, S. Transposition of volumetric information derived from computed tomography scanning into stereotactic space. *Surg. Neurol.* **21**: 465−71 (1984).

26 Kall, B.A., Kelly, P.J. & Goerss, S.J. Stereotactic computer-aided neurosurgery: CO_2 laser resection of CNS tumors. *Proceedings of the 7th Annual Conference of the Institute of Electronic and Electrical Engineers Engineering in Medicine and Biology Society, Chicago, IL,* pp. 692−5 (1985).

27 Kelly, P.J., Kall, B.A. & Goerss, S. Computer-assisted stereotactic resection of posterior fossa lesions. *Surg. Neurol.* **25**: 530−4 (1986).

28 Kelly, P.J., Kall, B.A., Goerss, S. & Earnest, F. IV. Computer-assisted stereotaxic laser resection of intra-axial brain neoplasms. *J. Neurosurg.* **64**: 427−39 (1986).

29 Kelly, P.J., Kall, B.A., Goerss, S. & Cascine, T.L. Results of computer-assisted stereotactic laser resection of deep-seated intracranial lesions. *Mayo Clin. Proc.* **61**: 20−27 (1986).

30 Kelly, P.J. Computer-assisted stereotaxis: new approaches for the management of intracranial intra-axial tumors. *Neurology* **36**(4): 535−41 (1986).

31 Kelly, P.J., Kall, B.A. & Goerss, S.J. Results of computed tomography-based computer-assisted stereotactic resection of metastatic intracranial tumors. *Neurosurgery* **22**(1): 7−17 (1988).

32 McGirr, S.J., Kelly, P.J. & Scheithauer, B.W. Stereotactic resection of juvenile pilocytic astrocytomas of the thalamus and basal ganglia. *Neurosurgery* **20**: 447−52 (1987).

33 Kelly, P.J., Sharbrough, F.W., Kall, B.A. & Goerss,

S.J. Magnetic resonance imaging-based computer-assisted stereotactic resection of the hippocampus and amygdala in patient with epilepsy, *Mayo Clin. Proc.* **62**: 103–8 (1987).

34 Kelly, P.J., Kall, B.A. & Goerss, S. Computer simulation for the stereotactic implantation of interstitial radionuclide sources into computed tomography-defined tumor volumes. *Neurosurgery* **14**: 442–7 (1984).

35 Kelly, P.J., Kall, B.A. & Goerss, S. Preoperative computer determination of interstitial ^{192}Iridium sources in CNS tumor volumes. *Acta Neurosurg.* (suppl.) **33**: 377–83 (1984).

36 Kelly, P.J., Kall, B.A. & Goerss, S. Computer simulation of interstitial radionuclide sources into computer-tomography-defined tumor volumes. *Neurosurgery* **14**: 422–8 (1984).

Computer Support for the Talairach System

Alim L. Benabid, Stéphane Lavallée, Dominique Hoffmann, Philippe Cinquin, Jean F. Le Bas, and Jacques Demongeot

Origins of stereotactic frames

It is generally agreed that stereotaxy was invented in 1905 by Horsley and Clark [1] who needed an accurate tool for electrode insertion and lesion making in laboratory animals. This laboratory equipment was later adapted for neurosurgical purposes by Spiegel and Wycis in 1947 [2], although the first human stereotactic apparatus was probably built in London around 1919 by Aubrey Mussen, who had worked with Clarke [3]. This made functional surgery possible at the level of deep brain structures, such as the basal ganglia and IIIrd ventricle. The introduction of pallidothalamotomy, following the accidental observation of Cooper, led to considerable development in stereotaxy as a conventional neurosurgical procedure [4]. The evident need for accuracy, reproducibility, safety, and minimal invasiveness is responsible for the design of several types of stereotactic frame, each of them addressing a specific concern [5]. Logically enough, the majority of frames during the first half of this century were mainly designed for procedures involving stereotactic lesions in the basal ganglia, which then represented the only surgical treatment of Parkinson's disease and of other types of dyskinesias. Apparently, the mathematic aspect of stereotaxy, implying calculations of target coordinates, made it unappealing to most neurosurgeons. Stereotaxy was therefore restricted to a narrow set of "mathematically-minded" neurosurgeons. The recent possibility of linking stereotactic frames and CT scanners, with adequate software to calculate target coordinates and frame parameter values required before surgery, has made this procedure available to a larger group of neurosurgeons. Although this constitutes a real improvement, this newly available simplicity has contributed to a tremendous increase in the practice of stereotactic neurosurgery, which could contribute to an increased risk of hemorrhagic complications. All stereotactic frames share a common goal, which is to establish rigid relationships between the patient's head and brain, and the external space which contains surgical tools, such as cannulae, probes, electrodes, or larger systems such as X-ray tubes, used either for neuroradiologic examination or for radiosurgery. To achieve this goal, the frames are always firmly anchored to the patient's skull by several pins, at least three and usually four, more or less deeply inserted into the bone. Less invasive relationships, such as fixation by ear plugs and nose and neck positioners, have been used, but they are not compatible with precise and stable positioning.

Advantages and drawbacks of frames

Two main types of frame can be considered, depending on how the target is reached:

1 The first type, which comprises the Leksell—Elekta, Riechert—Mundinger—Fischer, Olivier—Bertrand—Tipal (OBT), and similar frames, are mainly based on a center-of-arc system allowing double oblique trajectories aimed at central targets. Most of these frames are characterized by their light weight and rather small size, the small depth of pin penetration into the skull, and the subsequent impossibility of placing the frame in the same position during a second procedure. Their light weight makes ambulatory procedures possible, and facilitates transfer of the patient from the operating room to the neuroradiology department and changes in the patient's position during X-ray examination, mainly during ventriculography. Their relatively small size has permitted them to be redesigned with X-ray-transparent and amagnetic materials, making them compatible with CT scan and MRI systems. The visibility of the frame structures and fiducial markers on these imaging systems has been used to develop software providing easy calculation of the coordinates to be set up on the frame, in order to reach a given target designated on CT scan or MRI pictures. In the Leksell-type frames, an arc-goniometer is designed to reach the center of the arc with special (fixed length) probes: the center of the arc can be projected onto X-ray films and precisely placed in front of the anterior—posterior (A/P) and lateral projections of the target by displacements of the arc support on the frame. In other cases (Reichert—Mundinger—Fischer), arc system parameters are determined, using a specific paradigm, and are checked on a phantom. Therefore, all procedures aiming at central targets can be easily and quickly performed [6], provided that the coordinates are available, from ventriculography-based atlases or from direct X-ray (angiography for arteriovenous malformations, for instance) and/or CT scan examinations.

A two-dimensional moving side-bar, placed on any one of the four sides of the OBT frame, provides the possibility of positioning a probe carrier perpendicular to the anterior, posterior and lateral sides of the frame and allowing non-oblique, orthogonal penetrations. This is necessary in order to check that the chosen track is not colliding with a blood vessel, which obviously requires a stereotactic angiographic examination and the alignment of the central X-ray beam on the target area [7,8] as in the Talairach system. The development of computer software adapted to CT scan and MRI examinations has more recently provided the possibility of easily determining the coordinates and characteristics of the tracks, in bi-orthogonal or double-oblique approaches, from the target as visible on the image display. This is particularly convenient when the target is clearly defined, which is the case for brain tumors, the size of which is larger than the accuracy of the pixel size of the images.

The drawbacks of these frames are mainly due to their lack of placement reproducibility, which is a direct consequence of superficial pin penetration into the skull. This could be easily overcome by slight modifications in the systems. The availability of software introduces a problem which is not actually specific to the frames themselves. The simplicity of target determination due to direct communication between the image display and the stereotactician has increased the attractiveness of stereotactic procedures, and creates a tendency to forget security rules and perform penetrating tracks, such as biopsy sampling, without angiography. This is actually validated by experience, as most supratentorial tumors submitted to biopsy are large and superficial enough to allow reaching them without much risk of bleeding, especially when sampling is limited to the central core of the tumor. However, this apparent ease can induce a feeling of confidence which could be responsible for biopsying tumors situated in more dangerous regions, such as the peri-insular region, posterior fossa or hypothalamic area, without an adequate anatomic evaluation of functional structures and of vessel distribution. Forthcoming progress in MRI angiography, and the possibility of visualizing the vessels precisely and atraumatically, will make these computerized procedures safer and validate the absence of contrast angiography.

The last inconvenience of these "light" frames is the approximate orthogonality of the X-ray investigations, which makes difficult the correspondence of the z coordinates of a given point in the brain on the A/P and lateral X-ray views. This also can be easily overcome by specific set-ups of the systems in dedicated stereotactic operating rooms. The Brown—Roberts—Wells and Codman−Roberts−Wells frames have solved this problem. The frame is held on a solid base, which is fixed onto the floor of the operating room in a permanent position with respect to the X-ray tubes. The center-of-arc system is positioned so that its center and the target are matched, or the patient's head can be eventually moved in the space of the frame. This feature is similar to that used in the Talairach hypophysectomy frame.

2 The second type, represented by the Talairach frame [9−11] is mainly based on orthogonal (frontal or lateral) approaches.

The Talairach system

Description and specific features

The Talairach frame comprises:

1 *A frame*, featuring a rectangular base with four poles supporting calibrated screws holding the fixation pins.

2 *A system of double grids*, allowing orthogonal tool penetration into the brain along directions parallel to the X-ray beams used for neuroradiologic examination (angiography and ventriculography), performed as a first step in the stereotactic procedure.

3 *Accessories.* A sham frame can be used to simulate double oblique trajectories, similar to what is featured in other systems. A probe holder, with several joints and oblique grids, makes possible the performance of double oblique trajectories. These accessories are not well suited to these polar approaches, which are achieved in a much more practical manner using the above-described center-of-arc systems.

4 *Added sets of accessories.*

(a) Sedan's [12] and Scerratti's [13] goniometers. These have been conceived and designed to provide the Talairach system with the advantages and flexibility of the center-of-arc systems, allowing easy and precise access via oblique approaches to targets near the midline [12]. The Sedan's goniometer is made of a carrier moving back and forth and mounted on two lateral poles of the frame. This carrier holds an axis, allowed to rotate with a sagittal angle β and to move laterally. On the medial end of this axis is mounted a

sector on which the probe holder can be set up with a frontal (coronal) angle α. Correspondence between the x, y, z Cartesian coordinates of a point P, the α and θ angles of the ρ, α, θ spherical coordinates, the β and γ angles read on the X-rays, and the β and ε angles set up on the goniometer are given by the following simple equations (see also Fig. 17.1):

$$\rho = OP$$
$$x = \rho . \cos\alpha . \sin\theta$$
$$y = \rho . \cos\alpha . \cos\theta$$
$$z = \rho . \sin\alpha$$
$$\beta = \text{Arctan} (\tan\alpha / \cos\theta)$$
$$\gamma = \text{Arctan} (\sin\theta / \tan\alpha)$$
$$\varepsilon = \text{Arctan} (x / [x^2 + z^2]^{1/2})$$

The Scerratti's goniometer is a center-of-arc system [13]. Similarly, all calculations used for the center-of-arc system are applicable to this goniometer [6].

(b) Implantable devices adapted to the Talairach frame. The grids and grid hole diameter (2.3 mm) call for specifically adapted

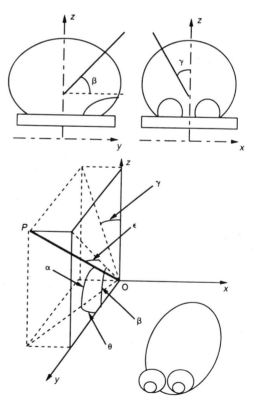

FIGURE 17.1 Spherical coordinates of a point P.

screws, tubes for after-loading brachytherapy [14,15], or electrodes for stereo-electro-encephalography (SEEG) [7,8,16,17].

5 *Talairach frame set-ups.* The frame by itself can be mounted, as other frames, in several different ways. Some are especially demonstrative:

(a) Sainte Anne set-up. This is an all mobile system, with a motorized table, two X-ray tubes mounted on a motorized ceiling arc, and a vertical lateral pole with a laser beam centering system.

(b) Rennes set-up. It is included in an iso-centric mobile seat, which is an ideal system for permanent centering of the frame and head, whatever the position of the patient.

(c) Grenoble set-up. It is an inexpensive and practical system, in which the frame is mounted on a rotating holder (Fig. 17.2), fixed on a solid base screwed onto the floor of the operating room at the focus point of a permanent bi-orthogonal X-ray system. The sitting position is not possible, and complete examination of the ventricular system is obtained by rotation of the patient around his longitudinal axis.

(d) Robot connection. This is described in Chapter 25 of this book.

Advantages and drawbacks

The Talairach frame is the result of an attempt to design a simple system, fulfilling the following prerequisites:

1 Reproducible placement of the patient. This is achieved by a heavy frame base, which cannot be distorted by current mechanical stresses, and by four strong pins which are inserted into burr holes drilled through the full depth of the skull,

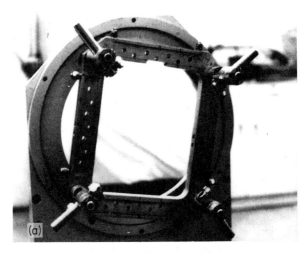

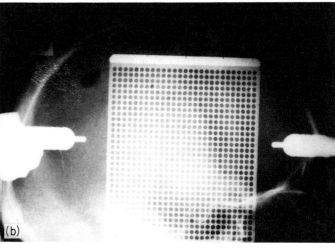

FIGURE 17.2 (a) The Talairach frame (without accessories) in a tilted position on the rotating holder. (b) Lateral X-ray of a grid fixed on the frame.

held by verniers, the graduations of which are recorded and can be replicated.

2 Perfect orthogonality of the X-ray beams in the A/P and lateral directions. This is achieved by a specific set-up in the operating room, and by repeated control of correct placement of the frame at the focus point of the X-ray set-up, using X-ray controls of the picture of double grids placed on both sides of the patient's head, or using laser beam reflection on mirrors attached to the sides of the frame.

3 Precise knowledge of the central X-ray beam, either placed on the area of interest, centered on the target, or used for exact correction of the parallax distortion due to a beam centered at a distance from the target.

However, this system had significant disadvantages which sometimes discouraged users and pushed them towards apparently easier systems. For example, positioning of the frame is rather time-consuming, but similar to that required by the first group of frames as soon as similar precision of placement is needed. The differences between frames are, however, more related to the industrial features than to the methodological principles, since a frame is nothing more than "sugar-tongs" holding the skull and the brain in a fixed position. Making frame positioning reproducible is easy to achieve with every type of frame, at the cost of very few changes. All of the specific features of each frame (such as goniometers) can be easily redesigned and adapted to the others, and in the end all stereotactic strategies can be universal. The Riechert–Mundinger–Fischer system, as well as the Codman–Roberts–Wells, feature a set of accessories and modifications (double grids, reproducible placement) which makes them "Talairach-like."

1 Superimposition of modalities. The pins inserted into the skull are in a fixed and reproducible position and their appearance is the same on every X-ray picture, taken during the same or different stereotactic sessions, provided that the pin-holding verniers are each time set at identical values. Therefore, by matching the pin projections on the X-ray pictures, the Talairach system has the major advantage of providing the possibility of superimposing different modalities, such as angiograms, ventriculograms, or any other kind of picture acquired in stereo-

tactic conditions (such as biopsy cannula or electrode placement controls).

2 Proportional anamorphosis. The ventricular system can therefore be superimposed on all other data (standard X-ray, angiograms) and a synthetic diagram can be drawn. Talairach has developed a proportional anamorphosis procedure [9,18], based on the IIIrd ventricle landmarks (anterior and posterior white commissures) and the inner skull contours, to normalize every individual brain on a standard scheme. Recognition of various structures (cortical sulci and lobes, white matter bundles, as well as basal ganglia substructures) can be done using this proportional anamorphosis, and this has recently been fully validated by comparison of the predicted location of cortical sulci with their actual position as shown by MRI [19].

Orthogonality of the X-ray beams

The Talairach frame is positioned at the focus of a two-directional X-ray system made of two tubes, the beams of which are orthogonal. A first tube is located at the ceiling of the operating room, with its axis in the vertical direction, and is used for A/P views of the patient's head in the supine position. The second tube has its axis horizontal and is located to the side of the room, for lateral X-ray views of the patient's head. Both tubes are at a distance from the head, depending on the room set-up, but always greater than 3 m. This achieves a low magnification ratio which is equal to 1.05 in our set-up, where the tubes are 3.75 m away from the center of the frame. This ratio is precisely determined by the respective positions of the tube, the patient's head and the film. Actually, the magnification ratio is different for each point of the brain, depending on its relative position with respect to the tubes and the X-ray film (Fig. 17.3). This involves special computations which are developed below.

The frame holds two sets of grids placed on the sides of the frame base and which are perpendicular two-by-two. Making calculation easier, and taking maximal advantage of the frame properties, requires orthogonality of the grids and of the corresponding X-ray beams. This is achieved by precise positioning of the frame at the beginning of the procedure. This

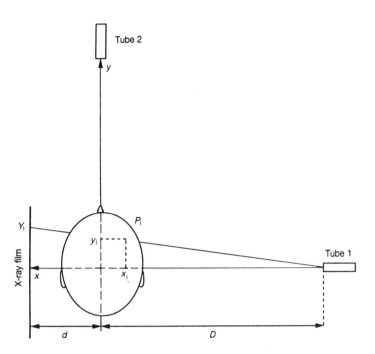

FIGURE 17.3 X-ray set-up. Any point of the brain with x_i, y_i, z_i coordinates will have X_i, Z_i radiologic coordinates, with a magnification coefficient $G(x_i)$ which depends on the geometry of the system.

can be done by using a laser beam coaxial with the X-ray beam and laser reflectors on the frame. Another method consists in mounting the Talairach frame on a solid base, strongly fixed to the floor of the room and initially positioned at the center of the X-ray system. In both cases, the X-ray system has to be perfectly perpendicular. As a consequence of this set-up, the altitude z of a given point in space in the brain with respect to the plane of the frame, which is named the "horizontal" plane of the brain, is the same on both A/P (frontal view) and lateral X-ray pictures. This is very useful in determining whether or not a point in the vascular bed, which appears to intersect the track of biopsies, actually does so. If so, this track must have the same z values of the projections of its suspected vascular intersection on both frontal and lateral projections, as explained below.

Computations of data in the Talairach system

Most computations are made possible by orthogonality of the X-ray beams, which provides for a given object the same z value on both lateral and frontal views. X-rays taken with two opposite grids mounted on the frame exhibit an interference pattern showing the exact location of the central axis of the X-ray beams. This can be used to displace either the frame or the tubes (mainly the horizontal lateral tube) in order to center the radiologic system on the area of interest. It is also possible, knowing the position of this central X-ray beam, to calculate the parallax error for any point in the brain, at a distance from this central beam.

CORRECTION OF PARALLAX ERRORS

As the X-ray beams are not parallel, the magnification coefficient depends on the position of a given point in the brain. When a structure is displaced to the right, its magnification ratio increases as $D/(D-d)$, where D is the distance between the X-ray tube and the film, and d the distance between the film and the structure in the brain. When this structure is placed on a beam other than the central beam, its projection on the film will correspond to a grid hole which is not in front of it (Fig. 17.4). Corrections must be made before performing the trajectory; these are easily calculated. Consider a point A, the projection (N) of which is situated between two points, O and M, corresponding to beams passing through two pairs of holes in coincidence. The maximal parallax error is therefore equal to the

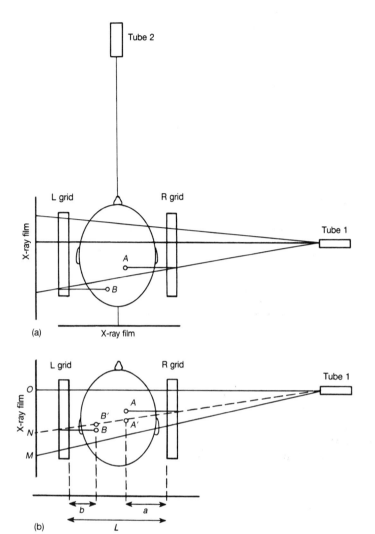

FIGURE 17.4 (a) X-rays are not parallel and the magnification coefficient depends on the position of a given point in the brain with respect to the X-ray film. As a consequence, two different points A and B may have similar X-ray projection. Using orthogonal trajectories through the grids will involve brain structures which are ahead or behind those actually projected on the film. (b) On the right side, if the trajectory is aimed at reaching point A', it will actually reach a point A, which is more anterior. The opposite is true on the left side. O is the projection of a beam passing through the aligned holes of the grid, and M the projection of the next beam passing through two holes, the left hole being one hole more posterior than the right one. As the space between two holes is 3 mm, the distance between A and A' is $3 \times (a/L)$ mm and is $3 \times (b/L)$ mm between B' and B.

distance between two grid holes, i.e. 3 mm. On the beam projecting on N, the maximal parallax error between the right and left grids is 3 mm $\times (ON/OM)$. The point A actually reached is then placed 3 mm $\times (ON/OM) \times a/L$ ahead of A' (the chosen point) on the film, and similarly, a point B on the left would be 3 mm $\times (ON/OM) \times b/L$ behind the chosen point B'. a and b are the distances of points A and B, respectively, from the inner faces of the grids, which are separated distance L.

DETECTION OF VASCULAR COLLISIONS ALONG A DOUBLE OBLIQUE BIOPSY TRACK

Vascular collision with a biopsy track must have the same z altitudes on frontal and lateral X-rays. However, intersection points between vessels and the track on frontal and lateral views may correspond to a false collision. Although this test leads to excess detection of collisions, it is safe and must be complemented by an expert surgeon's analysis in order to distinguish false and true collisions (Fig. 17.5). Any penetrating trajectory into the brain raises the question of vascular collision, which is of highest risk in the case of biopsies. Biopsy tracks which are aligned along the X-ray axes, i.e. either lateral or frontal approaches, provide the safest procedures, since it is possible to check on the corresponding X-ray images that the projected track which appears as a point does not correspond to any projection of a vessel. This is the most frequent circumstance in the Talairach

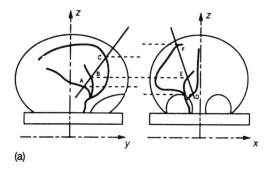

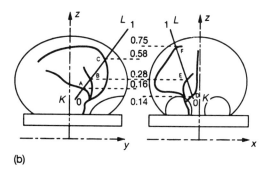

FIGURE 17.5 Vascular collision of a vessel with a track must have same z altitudes on frontal and lateral X-rays (a) or have similar index (varying from 0 to 1) between two given points K and L (b).

system, which is mainly set up for these orthogonal, frontal, or lateral, approaches. In the case of double oblique approaches, the problem of vascular collision detection is not easy to solve. Despite the fact that CT-guided stereotactic biopsies without angiographic control are becoming increasingly popular [6,20−23], the theoretical risk of hitting and damaging a vessel with the biopsy cannula persists, and is sometimes demonstrated by bleeding complications. Efficient solutions have to be found, and some of them have already been designed and used [24,25,26]. The intrinsic features of the Talairach system have led Szikla et al. [27,28] to a routine procedure, proven to be efficient, which is quite easy to perform without any computation, but which can be easily computerized and automated. Provided that the two X-ray beams are orthogonal, a given point in the brain appears on X-rays as two couples of coordinates (Fig. 17.3) (x, z) on the frontal view and (y, z) on the lateral view, z being the same in both couples. Therefore, the projections of the intersection of a putative track with a vessel must have the same z value (as measured on X-ray films from the base plate of the frame) on both lateral and frontal planes (Fig. 17.5a). Obviously, the reciprocal is not true, and it may happen that lateral and frontal intersections having a same z value do not correspond to the same vessel: in this case, the decision between true and false collision is made by the surgeon's expertise; this has proven to be satisfactory and is daily used in the routine practice of stereotacticians. This can easily be computerized on digitized angiograms, on which the theoretical track is projected by the computer, which can calculate the coincidence on both projections of the intersections between the track and the vessels and display, as hyperbrilliant points, the intersections with similar z values. These hyperbrilliant points will comprise all the true collisions but also false collisions, which, in a first phase, can be deleted by the surgeon's expertise.

A second way to achieve this [29] is to compute and display on the two orthogonal views the theoretical trajectory and two extreme points K and L (Fig. 17.5b), which will appear as (K', L') and (K'', L''). The intersection points between the vessels and the projected lines can be fully described using an index ranging from 0 to 1, 0 corresponding to K and 1 to L, for instance. Every true collision must have similar lateral and frontal index values. Obviously false collisions will be detected by this paradigm and will be deleted by the surgeon's "expert system" analysis as easily and efficiently as in the previous case. This is evidently less elegant than true collision detection, without false-positive points, which can be expected from real 3-D reconstruction of the vascular network, but is also much easier and faster to achieve.

Three-dimensional (3-D) evaluation of vessel position by stereoscopic analysis (double incidence angiography)

A first approach is provided by the "floating line" concept [30]. A specially built stereocomparator features two movable lines on transparent grids, applied on the two stereoscopic angiograms and representing the projections, on these tilted angiograms, of a theoretical line in the brain space. Observation of this line through the stereocomparator allows the surgeon to check the eventual collision of the line with vessels, and eventually to change it.

The Talairach system provides another approach which has been profitably used in routine practice [14] to recognize the in-depth position of the vessels, using small-angle−double-incidence angiograms (SADIA) taken under a 5° tilt angle, corresponding to the natural binocular angle. One may use a stereo-comparator or, with some training, it is possible to squint and obtain a 3-D perception of the vascular network. One may also superimpose the two angiograms and try to make the vessels correspond. From experience, it appears that coincidence of the two images of the vessels is only possible for those which are in the same plane perpendicular to the X-ray axis. Slightly sliding the films one over the other will change this "coincidence plane" and display another array of vessels situated in it. This is easily used in daily routine to evaluate the depth of vessels projecting on a proposed trajectory. This can be also more formally computed, as described below.

Attempt to design a paradigm for computerized 3-D vascular reconstruction

Obviously, the above-described approach can be formally demonstrated and could be used as a possible basis for 3-D reconstruction. Let us consider lateral views taken as SADIAs. Every point P of the brain is assigned a triplet of coordinates (x, y, z) in the brain space, a pair of coordinates (y, z) on the regular lateral view film, and (y', z') on the lateral view film of the 5° tilted head. Therefore, x corresponds to the "depth" of a point along an axis Ox perpendicular to the film plane. When the two films are superimposed with a given shift, with respect to an arbitrary reference $(y + \delta = y')$, two sets of points belonging to the two films are placed in coincidence. Is there any relationship between δ and x? Is this relationship independent of y? (See Fig. 17.6.)

1 *Coordinates of a point P in the referential of the X-ray system.* Any point P in the brain space can be described using either Cartesian coordinates x, y, z or spherical coordinates ρ, α, θ, where O is the origin of the coordinate system,

ρ is the modulus of the vector OP, α the angle between OP and the horizontal plane xOy, and θ the angle between OP and the vertical plane yOz.

$$x = \rho . \cos\alpha . \sin\theta$$
$$y = \rho . \cos\alpha . \cos\theta$$
$$z = \rho . \sin\alpha$$

If the frame is rotated along the body axis of the patient by an angle $\Delta\theta$, such as:

$$\theta' = \theta + \Delta\theta$$

then the point P has, in the X-ray referential, the new coordinates x', y', z'.

$$x' = \rho . \cos\alpha . \sin\theta'$$
$$y' = \rho . \cos\alpha . \cos\theta'$$
$$z' = \rho . \sin\alpha = z$$

This can be expressed by a rotation matrix:

$$\begin{bmatrix} x' \\ y' \\ z' \end{bmatrix} = \begin{bmatrix} \cos\Delta\theta & -\sin\Delta\theta & 0 \\ \sin\Delta\theta & \cos\Delta\theta & 0 \\ 0 & 0 & 1 \end{bmatrix} . \begin{bmatrix} x \\ y \\ z \end{bmatrix}$$

2 *Coordinates of projections of the point P on the X-ray film.* Due to the divergence of the X-ray beams, D being the distance from the X-ray tube to the center of the head and d the distance from this center to the X-ray film, the magnification coefficient G of the X-ray pictures is:

$$G = \frac{D + d}{D + x}$$

$G(x)$ depends on the value of x, which changes when the head is tilted.
Then:

$$Y = y . \frac{D + d}{D + x}$$

There is a similar relationship between Z and z, as well as when x is changed into x', then:

$$\left(\frac{Y}{Z}\right) = \left(\frac{D + d}{D + x}\right) . \left(\frac{y}{z}\right)$$

and

$$\left(\frac{Y'}{Z'}\right) = \left(\frac{D + d}{D + x'}\right) . \left(\frac{y'}{z'}\right)$$

3 *Relationship between x and δ.* When superimposition of the films is achieved, some structures, such as vessels, can be matched on both

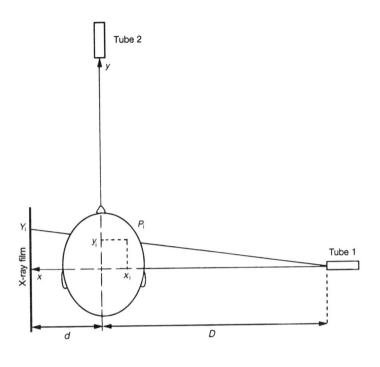

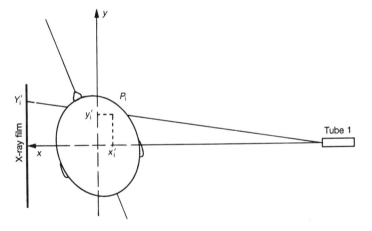

FIGURE 17.6 Stereoscopic angiography. Tilting the head by 5° does not change z_i, but changes x_i and y_i.

films when there is a shift equal to δ:

(a) Simple case of no magnification, with parallel X-rays:

$$G(x) = 1 \text{ or } dG(x)/dx = 0$$

Then:

$$
\begin{aligned}
\delta &= y - y' \\
&= \rho \cdot \cos\alpha \cdot [\cos\theta' - \cos\theta] \\
&= -2\rho \cdot \cos\alpha \cdot \sin\left[\frac{\theta + \theta'}{2}\right] \cdot \sin\left[\frac{\theta' - \theta}{2}\right]
\end{aligned}
$$

$$
= -2\rho \cdot \cos\alpha \cdot \sin\left[\theta + \frac{\Delta\theta}{2}\right] \cdot \sin\frac{\Delta\theta}{2}
$$

$$
= -2\rho \cdot \cos\alpha \cdot \sin\frac{\Delta\theta}{2}\left[\sin\theta \cdot \cos\frac{\Delta\theta}{2} + \cos\theta \cdot \sin\frac{\Delta\theta}{2}\right]
$$

$$
= -2\sin\frac{\Delta\theta}{2}\left[x \cdot \cos\frac{\Delta\theta}{2} + y \cdot \sin\frac{\Delta\theta}{2}\right]
$$

$$\Delta\theta = 5°$$

Let's call

$$b = \cos\frac{\Delta\theta}{2} = 0.999048$$

which is not significantly different from $b = 1$.

$$a = \sin\frac{\Delta\theta}{2} = 0.0436$$

$$a = 0.04$$

Then

$$x = -\frac{1}{2ab}.[\delta + y.a^2]$$

and, in our set-up

$$x = -12.5\,\delta - 0.02\,y$$

(b) Regular case with non-parallel X-rays, where magnification $G(x)$ depends on x, i.e.:

$$dG(x)/dx \neq 0$$

Then, in our set-up

$$\Delta\theta = 5°$$

then

$$x' = x.\cos\Delta\theta - y.\sin\Delta\theta$$
$$x' = x - y.\sin\Delta\theta$$
$$\sin\Delta\theta = 0.08715$$
$$\cos\Delta\theta = 0.99619 \equiv 1$$
$$|x - x'| = |y|.(0.09)$$

The A/P diameter of the head is about 20 cm

$$|y| < 20 \text{ cm}$$

$$|x - x'| = 18 \text{ mm}$$

which is negligible ($< 1/200°$), as compared to

$$|D + x| = 3750 \text{ mm}$$

Then

$$\delta = Y - Y'$$

$$= \frac{D + d}{D + x}.(y - y')$$

$$= -2a.\frac{D + d}{D + x}.(ay + bx)$$

It becomes:

$$x = \frac{-2a^2(D + d).y - \delta D}{\delta + 2ab.(D + d)}$$

$$x = \frac{-2a^2\left(1 + \dfrac{d}{D}\right).y - \delta}{\dfrac{\delta}{D} + 2ab.\left(1 + \dfrac{d}{D}\right)}$$

δ/D varies from $1/1000$ to $2/1000$ and can be neglected.

$$1 + \frac{d}{D} = G(0) = 1.05$$

which is the average magnification at the center of the brain. Then:

$$x = -\frac{\delta}{2ab.\left(1 + \dfrac{d}{D}\right)} - \frac{a}{b}.y$$

$$x = -11.9\,\delta - 0.04\,y$$

The depth x can therefore be calculated, for all points of the film which are situated at the coordinate y, and coincident to their homologous projection on the tilted film when the shift is equal to δ. A paradigm can be derived from this procedure, in several steps:

1 Digitization of the regular angiogram, attributing a set of coordinates (Y_i, Z_1) to the points P_i of the vascular network projection.
2 Digitization of the tilted angiogram, attributing a new set of coordinates (Y'_i, Z'_i) to the points P_i of the vascular network projection.
3 Application to the set of coordinates (Y_i, Z_i) a shift δ along the y axis and detection of the points P_i, verifying the relationship:

$$(Y_i + \delta, Z_i) = (Y'_i, Z'_i).$$

For these points, according to the previously demonstrated equations, once the corresponding values of x_i, and therefore of:

$$G = \frac{D + d}{D + x}$$

are calculated, y_i and z_i may be calculated from Y_i and Z_i. A complete set of coordinates (x_i, y_i, z_i) is therefore generated and, when displayed, provides a 3-D reconstruction of the vascular network.

CONNECTION OF A STEREOTACTIC FRAME WITH COMPUTERIZED IMAGING SYSTEMS

The Talairach frame does not have localizers designed for MRI or CT scan examinations in stereotactic conditions. Several solutions have been proposed to overcome this problem.

CT scan

1 Adapters. Specific adapters have been designed to enable CT scan examinations of patients held in a Talairach frame, provided that the diameter of the gantry is large enough, which is currently achieved in whole-body systems. Sedan has adapted the Leksell frame system. The patient is initially set up with the Leksell frame, and CT scan examination is performed using the localizers and software developed for this system. The patient is then transferred to the Talairach frame, on which the Leksell frame is mounted, using a specifically designed adapter. The stereotactic procedure is performed, taking advantage of the Talairach frame features as well as of the calculations derived from the Leksell software and localizers.

2 Data transfer. When the CT scan examination has been obtained under regular circumstances, several methods still make possible the use of this information for stereotactic procedures: the simplest one consists, when vertical slice reconstruction is available, of displaying a sagittal pattern of the lesion on the scout-view. When this is enlarged to the scale of the lateral stereotactic X-ray view, superimposition of these two pictures allows report of the lesion profile obtained from CT scan in the stereotactic coordinates.

Nguyen *et al.* [31] have reported another way of doing this when vertical slice reconstruction is not available: the head of the patient is envisaged as comprising a cube, which is sliced perpendicularly to its frontal face. Therefore, any point on a given CT slice can be reported in the 3-D space, according to its position on the slice with respect to its distance from each side of the CT picture, and to its altitude as given by the number of the slice and the space distance between two adjacent slices. Pictures can therefore be redrawn as lateral and frontal projections of the skull and of the lesion, and matched to

the corresponding stereotactic X-rays. We used a similar, and even simpler, procedure: on each slice, remarkable anatomic features are recognized and pointed on the stereotactic X-rays (sella turcica, various features of the ventricles, choroid plexuses, calcified pineal gland, etc.). This helps to position the CT slices on the lateral X-ray [32]. The internal length of each slice is measured on the X-ray as well as on the CT slice, and the average ratio of all the slices provides the value of the stereotactic : CT scan magnification ratio. On each CT slice, the distances to the inner table of the skull of the anterior, posterior, and lateral limits of the lesion are measured, multiplied by the magnification ratio and reported on the corresponding line of the stereotactic X-ray. It is therefore possible to outline the profile of the lesion (Fig. 17.7).

MRI

1 The problem of the magnetic components of the surgical tools. The adapters made for CT

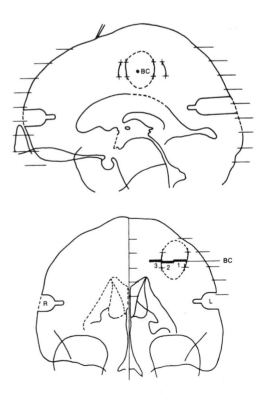

FIGURE 17.7 Grenoble's method for CT scan data transfer. BC = biopsy core.

scan must be used, as the Talairach frame is currently built using magnetic components. Therefore, there is no other possibility of performing stereotactic MRI with this type of frame. Another method is to reconstruct the lesion profile from the MR images in a similar manner to that used for CT scan. It is better to display sagittal MRI pictures enlarged at the same magnification as that of the stereotactic pictures and featuring a common landmark (cross or $x-y$ calibration scale), allowing precisely matched superimposition of these sagittal parallel slices. The midline slice showing the IIIrd ventricle structures can be matched to the stereotactic ventriculograms. The lesion contours are then easily reported onto the stereotactic maps.

2 Linearity of the MRI data. It is a commonly accepted statement that MRI has in its basic principle the sin of non-linearity and that, as a consequence, a precise spatial localization cannot be expected from it [33,34]. This is actually wrong: spatial localization in MRI is due to the frequency coding of the space, which is achieved by applying a linear magnetic gradient which locally changes the main B_0 field of the magnet, and therefore locally changes the resonance frequency of the protons in a space-dependent manner. The linearity of the gradients on the three axes x, y and z may be not properly tuned, and the magnification may be different along these three directions. This is a matter of correctly tuning the system. In the

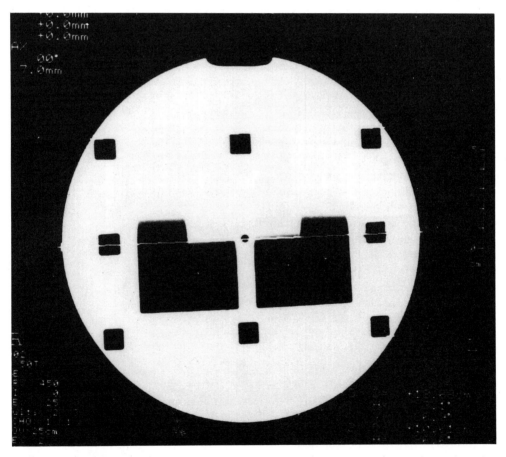

FIGURE 17.8 Linearity of the MRI data. The picture shown corresponds to an axial slice of a plexiglass phantom filled with CuSO$_4$, 20 cm in diameter, in which eight square tubes (1 cm side) build a rectangle, the size of which is 150 × 186 mm. On the image, which is enlarged by a ratio of 1.04, one may verify that the length of the large side is 156 mm, which is 150 × 1.04, and that the small side is 110 mm, which corresponds to 106 × 1.04. This can also be checked in a perpendicular direction. One may also verify that the section of the cylinder is actually a circle and is not distorted. This type of control allows a millimetric precise measurement of the accuracy of the imaging.

same manner, a wrong tuning of the x and y displays on the TV screen, or on the photographic reprograph, would lead to a distorted final picture.

The system has to be regularly checked and eventually corrected, using a calibrated phantom (Fig. 17.8). The statement that MRI measurements are inaccurate due to distortions can be right for whole-body sections, where it is known that the homogeneity of the magnetic field B_0, and the linearity of the gradients, are not correctly achieved near the walls of the gantry due to inhomogeneity and to the eddy currents. For a brain MRI examination, centered on the axis of the magnet, these distortions can be efficiently avoided. This has to be stressed, as MR imaging in the coming decade will be the principal source of spatial imaging of the brain, and will be used for 3-D reconstruction, as well as for designation of targets in the brain for computer-assisted systems such as robots.

3 Transfer of data. As far as the Talairach system is concerned, in its present commercial availability, its direct use in MRI systems is impossible. New methods of transfer of the MRI data to the stereotactic space must be designed. The easiest way is to enlarge the images at the scale of the stereotactic pictures, and to match them on similarly visible features and anatomic structures.

Sedan *et al.* [35] designed a TV-based system which could pick up the MRI parasagittal views and redisplay them, using a variable gain along the x and y axis. This had the advantage of correcting the distortion of MR images, but was rather difficult to use and required special, although inexpensive, equipment. The recent MRI system can actually display the pictures on the reprograph at any desired magnification. Provided that the MRI gradients are properly checked and adjusted if needed, stereotactic-compatible MR images are easily available if the neuroradiologist adds to the pictures a calibration grid positioned identically on each picture. By superimposition of these grids, one may draw a composite picture featuring all relevant data, principally the inner contour of the skull, the coronal suture, depression of the torcular, the ventricular system and essentially the IIIrd ventricle, aqueduct of Sylvius and the IVth ventricle, the rostrum and splenium of the corpus callosum, and sometimes the siphon of the carotid artery. All these structures can be equally drawn on a stereotactic scheme, which can therefore be matched to the MRI scheme, and the data are transfered (Fig. 17.9). This procedure could be computerized.

Digitized angiography

Digitized subtraction angiography (DSA) has been used in the OBT frame [8] in a manner similar to that in the Talairach system. Matching of either DSA or MRI pictures has been developed and is perfectly applicable to Talairach frame usage.

Conclusions

The stereotactic Talairach frame is suited for connection with spatially guided and computer-assisted robots, as it provides a basic spatial reference, easy to integrate in a routine to drive a robot towards a spatially defined target. Until recently, the Talairach system has been the basis of a rational approach, taking advantage of the orthogonality of the X-ray incidences to

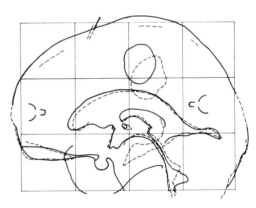

FIGURE 17.9 Transfer of MRI data on a stereotactic scheme: the grid which is displayed on the MRI parasagittal pictures, enlarged at the size of the stereotactic diagram, allows superimposition of the various images. The final drawing (dotted line), which comprises all MRI information including the IIIrd ventricle structures, can be matched with the corresponding structures of the stereotactic diagram (continuous line). In the present case, the position of the parietal lesion, as shown by MRI (dotted line), is different from the less precise position recalculated from CT scan (continuous line).

define precisely the position of the targets and vascular structures within the brain with respect to the frame referential. These features have been used to develop methods of computation accessible to surgical teams with little or no computational means, but also applicable to automated software.

References

1 Horsley, V.A. & Clarke, R.H. On the intrinsic fibers of the cerebellum, its nuclei and its effect tracts. *Brain* 28: 12−29 (1905).

2 Spiegel, E.A., Wycis, H.T., Marks, M. & Lee, A. Stereotactic apparatus for operations on the human brain. *Science* 106: 349−50 (1947).

3 Picard, C., Olivier, A. & Bertrand, G. The first human stereotaxic apparatus. The contribution of Aubrey Mussen to the field of stereotaxis. *J. Neurosurg.* 59: 673−6 (1983).

4 Gildenberg, P.L. Whatever happened to stereotactic surgery? *Neurosurgery* 20(6): 983−7 (1987).

5 Munari, C. & Betti, O.O. The stereotactic biopsy of brain lesions: a critical review. In: Broggi, G. & Gerosa, M.A. (eds) *Cerebral Gliomas*, pp. 179−206. Amsterdam: Elsevier (1989).

6 Colombo, F., Angrilli, F., Zanardo, A., Pinna, V., Alexandre, A. & Benedetti, A. A universal method to employ CT scanner spatial information in stereotactic surgery. *Appl. Neurophysiol.* 45: 352−4 (1982).

7 Olivier, A. Double-headed stereotaxic carrier apparatus for insertion of depth electrodes. *J. Neurosurg.* 65: 258−9 (1986).

8 Peters, T.M., Clark, J.A., Olivier, A. *et al.* Integrated stereotaxic imaging with CT, MR imaging, and digital subtraction angiography. *Radiology* 161: 821−6.

9 Talairach, J., David, M., Tournoux, P., Corredor, H. & Kvasina, T. *Atlas d'Anatomie Stéreotaxique des Noyaux gris Centraux.* Paris: Masson (1957).

10 Talairach, J., de Ajuriaguerra J. & David, M. A propos des coagulations therapeutiques sous-corticales. Etude topographique du systeme ventriculaire en function des nogaux guis centraux. *Presse Médicale* 58: 697−701 (1950).

11 Talairach, J., de Ajuriaguerra J. & David, M. Études stereotaxiques des structures encéphaliques profondes chez l'Homme. Technique, intérêt physiologique et thérapeutique. *Presse Médicale* 60: 605−9 (1952).

12 Sedan, R. & Duparet, R. Stéréomètre adaptable au cadre stéréotaxique de J. Talairach. *Neurochirurgie* 14: 577−82 (1968).

13 Scerrati, M., Fiorentino, A., Fiorentino, M. & Pola, P. Stereotaxic device for polar approaches in orthogonal systems. Technical note. *J. Neurosurg.* 61: 1146−7 (1984).

14 Szikla, G. & Peragut, J.C. Irradiation interstitielle des gliomes. In: Constans, J.P. & Schlienger, M. (eds) *Radiothérapie des Tumeurs du Système Nerveux Central. Neurochirurgie* (suppl.). Paris: Masson (1975) 21: 187−228.

15 Benabid, A.L., Chirossel, J.P., Mercier, C. *et al.* Removable, adjustable and reusable implants for stereotactic interstitial radiosurgery of brain tumors. *Appl. Neurophysiol.* 50: 278−80 (1987).

16 Bouvier, G., Saint Hilaire, J.M., Giard, N., Lesage, J., Cloutier, L. & Beique, R. Depth electrode implantation at Hospital Notre-Dame, Montreal. In: Engel, J. Jr. (ed) *Surgical Treatment of the Epilepsies*, pp. 589−94. New York: Raven Press (1987).

17 Bancaud, J., Talairach, J., Bonis, A., *et al.* La *Stéreo-électro-encéphalographie dans l'Épilepsie.* Paris: Masson (1965).

18 Talairach, J., Szikla, G., Tournoux, P., *et al.* Atlas *d'Anatomie Stereotaxique du Télencéphale.* Paris: Masson (1967).

19 Steinmetz, H., Fürst, G. & Freund, H.J. Cerebral cortical localization: application and validation of the proportional grid system in MR imaging. *J. Comput. Assist. Tomogr.* 13(1): 10−19 (1989).

20 Brown, R.A. A computerized tomography−computer graphics approach to stereotactic localization. *J. Neurosurg.* 50: 715−20 (1979).

21 Gildenberg, P.L., Kaufmann, H.H. & Krishna Murthy, K.S. Calculation of stereotactic coordinates from the computed tomographic scan. *Appl. Neurophysiol.* 45: 443−8 (1982).

22 Kelly, P.J., Alker, G., Kall, B. & Goerss, S. Method of computed-tomography-based stereotactic biopsy with arteriographic control. *Neurosurgery* 14: 172−7 (1984).

23 Mundinger, F., Birg, W. & Klar, M. Computer-assisted stereotactic brain operations by means including computerized axial tomography. *Appl. Neurophysiol.* 41: 169−82 (1978).

24 Perry, J.H., Rosenbaum, A.E., Junsford, L.D., Swink, C.A. & Zorub, D.S. Computed tomography-guided stereotactic surgery; conception and development of a new stereotactic methodology. *Neurosurgery* 7: 376−81 (1980).

25 Kelly, P.J., Kall, B.A. & Goerss, S. Computer-assisted stereotactic biopsy utilizing CT and digitized angiographic data. *Acta Neurochir.* (suppl.) 33: 233−5 (1984).

26 Kelly, P.J., Earnest, F. IV, Kall, B.A., Goerss, S.J. & Scheithauer, B.W. Surgical options for patients with deep-seated brain tumors: computer-assisted stereotactic biopsy. *Mayo Clin. Proc.* 60: 223−9 (1985).

27 Szikla, G., Bouvier, G. & Hori, T. Localization of brain sulci and convolutions by arteriography. A stereotactic anatomo-radiological study. *Brain Res.* 95: 497−502 (1975).

28 Szikla, G., Bouvier, G., Hori, T. & Petrov, V. *Angiography of the Human Brain Cortex.* Berlin, Heidelberg, New York: Springer Verlag (1977).

29 Lavallée, S. Gestes médico-chirurgicaux assistés par ordinateur. Thèse Sciences Mathématiques,

Université Joseph Fourier, Grenoble (1989).

30 Cloutier, L., Nguyen, D.N. & Ghosh, S. Simulator allowing spatial viewing of cerebral probes by using a floating line concept. Symposium on Optical and Electro-optical Applied Science and Engineering, Cannes, France (1985).

31 Nguyen, J.P., van Effentere, R., Fohanno, D., Robert, G., Sichez, J.F. & Gardeur, D. Méthode pratique de repérage spatial des petites néoformations intracrâniennes à partir des données de la tomo-densitométrie. *Neurochirurgie* **26**: 333−9 (1980).

32 Mussolino, A., Munari, C., Betti, O. *et al.* Interet et technique du transfert des données tomo-densitométriques dans les coordonnées stéréotaxiques du systeme Talairach. *Rev. EEG Neurophysiol. Clin.* **17**: 11−25 (1987).

33 Schad, L., Lott, S., Schmitt, F., Sturm, V. & Lorenz, W.J. Correction of spatial distortion in MR imaging: a prerequisite for accurate stereotaxy. *J. Comput. Assist. Tomogr.* **11**: 499−505 (1987).

34 Wyper, D.J., Turner, J.W., Patterson, J., *et al.* Accuracy of stereotactic localisation using MRI and CT. *J. Neurol. Neurosurg. Psychiatr.* **49**: 1445−8 (1986).

35 Sedan, R., Peragut, J.C., Farnarier, Ph. & Vallicioni, P.A. Imagerie moderne et stéréotaxie. *Neurochirurgie* **33**: 29−32 (1987).

Stereotactic Imaging-based Surgical Planning

18

Stereotactic Arteriography and Biopsy Simulation with the Brown–Roberts–Wells (BRW) System

Paul Suetens, Dirk Vandermeulen, Jan M. Gybels, Guy Marchal, and Guy Wilms

Introduction

Stereotactic biopsy planning is a decision-making process that is largely based on a number of separate images from different sources. Despite the wide variety of digital imaging techniques, such as computed tomography (CT), magnetic resonance imaging (MRI), positron emission tomography (PET), digital subtraction angiography (DSA), and ultrasound (US), there are still serious difficulties in obtaining an overall three-dimensional (3-D) image that integrates the information from different imaging modalities. The main problems are the lack of a common spatial reference frame and the difficulty in displaying 3-D volumetric data.

In the work of Suetens *et al.* [1] angiograms, CT scans, and a simulated biopsy needle are combined into a single 3-D image by generating and integrating three stereoscopic image pairs, one of the blood vessels, one of the CT lesion, and one of the trajectory. The geometric registration problem is solved by putting three small platinum markers in the cranial bone. These markers are visible on both X-rays and CT scans. The geometric relationship between the angiographic, CT, and stereotactic coordinate space can then easily be calculated. The lesion boundary is manually delineated on the CT scans, and the 3-D lesion surface is displayed as a wireframe or as a transparent object based on standard surface shading techniques. The

stereoscopic images of the blood vessels, lesion, and simulated trajectory are finally added into one integrated image. If only film angiograms are available, the lesion and trajectory can be represented as line drawings on transparency sheets, which are superposed onto the film. Although the system can be used in practice, it has some drawbacks. The procedure of introducing metal markers into the skull is uncomfortable to the patient. The use of transparency sheets is tedious and, at the time the paper [1] was written (1983), graphics workstations were expensive, the resolution was too low for displaying X-rays, user interactivity was very limited, and digital image networks were almost non-existent.

The problem of geometric registration has been approached by several authors. Limited success has been obtained with internal anatomic reference features [2–4], because corresponding features on different imaging modalities are hard to detect or match accurately. When using external markers for the registration, it is more comfortable to the patient to use non-invasive fixation devices, such as individually made molds [5–7], or an adapter mounted to the patient's head by means of two ear plugs and a nasion support [8]. For stereotactic purposes, however, the external markers can simply be fixed to the stereotactic frame. CT and MR images are usually registered by using commercially available adapters with N-shaped rods. For registering angiograms, a number of different methods have been described [9–14]. The SGV Angiographic Localizer [14] is the system we currently use in our hospital. It is very similar to the systems developed by Siddon and Barth [12] and Peters *et al.* [13], which do not require the position of the central X-ray beam on the image to be known, or that the image be parallel to the frame that contains the markers. More details follow below.

Graphics and image processing workstations are increasingly being used in the hospital environment. Recent developments in PACS (picture archiving and communication systems) make it possible to integrate these workstations into the digital image network of the radiology department. Images from different modalities, such as CT, PET, MR, and DSA, can now easily be transmitted and stored in the workstation for further processing. Stereotactic neurosurgery planning is one of the applications that benefits by this technical evolution. Stereotactic trajectories can now be simulated in an overall 3-D image that integrates the information from CT, MR, and DSA. The Montreal Neurological Institute, for example, developed a commercially available stereotactic workstation [13] for use with the Olivier–Bertrand–Tipal (OBT) and Leksell stereotactic frames. At the Mayo Clinic, Kelly *et al.* [11] developed an operating room computer system for use with a modified Todd–Wells frame. Our system works in combination with the Brown–Roberts–Wells (BRW)

frame, and consists of a 3-D graphics workstation connected to the digital image network of the radiology department, a stereoscopic imaging system for depth perception, and two 3-D cursors for 3-D interactive measurements. It is further described below.

Current limitations of the 3-D integrated images for stereotactic planning are due to the lack of real 3-D vascular data and the difficulty of automatically outlining low-contrast tissue structures to be displayed. Magnetic resonance angiography (MRA) may be a way to overcome the first problem. The second problem is a fundamental problem of object recognition, yet some progress is being made by using volume rendering techniques [15], instead of the surface rendering procedures that are traditionally used in the computer graphics community. As discussed below, we expect that the improved methods of 3-D vascular imaging and volume rendering will soon be introduced in stereotactic neurosurgery.

The SGV angiographic localizer for the BRW system

The SGV (Suetens–Gybels–Vandermeulen) Angiographic Localizer [14] (Radionics Boston, MA) (Fig. 18.1) fits onto the BRW base ring and contains four sets of four metal reference pellets with known BRW stereotactic frame coordinates. Each set of four markers is embedded in an acrylic plate. Eight (mathematically at least

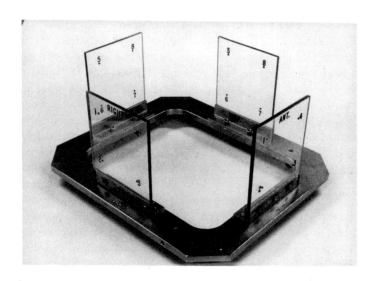

FIGURE 18.1 SGV Angiographic Localizer.

six) markers must be visible on each angiogram (Fig. 18.2) in order to calculate the geometric transformation between stereotactic frame coordinates and angiographic image coordinates. The SGV system does not impose any restriction on the position of the X-ray tube and cassette. It can be used in two different modes, the projection mode and the reconstruction mode.

Projection mode

The projection mode is used for stereotactic neurosurgery planning. In this mode any point with known BRW coordinates, such as a stereotactic target point, can be projected onto an arbitrary X-ray or angiogram. BRW coordinates of a target point can, for example, be obtained from a CT scan by using the standard BRW software package. Digital X-rays or DSA images are directly transmitted to the stereotactic workstation via the Ethernet digital network of the radiology department. The X-ray coordinates of the eight reference points (Fig. 18.2) are then entered into the workstation with a mouse-driven cursor. If only film X-rays or angiograms are available, these coordinates can be read into the BRW microcomputer by means of a digitizing tablet. The workstation or BRW microcomputer then calculates the mathematical transformation between BRW-coordinates and X-ray coordinates. The X-ray coordinates of each point with known BRW coordinates can subsequently be computed.

Reconstruction mode

The reconstruction mode is used for stereotactic planning, but it can also be used for stereotactic radiosurgery and for functional neurosurgery. In this mode, the BRW coordinates of any point visible on two X-rays or angiograms, e.g. an anterior—posterior (A/P) and a lateral X-ray or a stereoscopic pair of angiograms, can be calculated. Note that this requirement may be too strong for functional neurosurgery, since a single target point cannot always be clearly indicated on both X-rays. The SGV procedure is inappropriate for this particular case. By applying the method to stereotactic planning, the surgeon is able to select an appropriate entry point and, as a result, the stereotactic trajectory, on a stereoscopic pair of angiograms.

The SGV system was tested on a few thousand simulated points, randomly located within

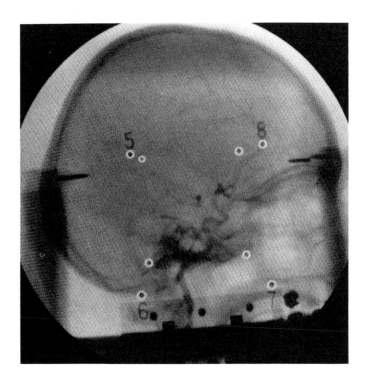

FIGURE 18.2 Angiographic reference markers, numbered from 1 through 8.

the stereotactic space. A maximum displacement error of 0.5 mm was superimposed on the X-ray coordinates of the markers. The maximal error in the projection mode was less than 0.5 mm. In the reconstruction mode, the maximal error was less than 0.5 mm for orthogonal X-rays, and less than 5 mm for stereoscopic images with a visual angle of 6°. Because of the limited accuracy for stereoscopic images, it is recommended not to rely completely on the position of the entry point and the stereotactic trajectory chosen in a stereoscopic pair of angiograms. A verification on a third angiogram, perpendicular to the stereo pair, may be required.

The pseudo-holographic display system

Our workstation [16] (Fig. 18.3) consists of a Silicon Graphics IRIS 2400T 3-D graphics workstation with 8 Mbytes of random access memory (RAM), a Stereographics stereoscopic imaging system employing electro-optical shutters in glasses, and two Polhemus 3-D cursors with six degrees of freedom, one in style form and one in block form. Based on low frequency magnetic field technology, these cursors transmit their relative position (x, y, z) and orientation (azimuth, elevation, roll) at a rate of 40 times s^{-1}. Instead of the electro-optical shutters, polarized

glasses in combination with a liquid crystal polarizing plate (e.g. the Tektronix SGA system) can be used. In this case more than one observer can simultaneously perceive the stereoscopic depth effect.

Active stereoparallax

The 3-D display technique is based on the principle of active stereoparallax, a combination of stereopsis and movement parallax. We also call this principle pseudo-holography because it offers a visual perception similar to that obtained with real holography. Stereopsis is based on retinal disparity, and is still regarded by many as the primary mechanism of space perception. Parallax effects can be caused by a change of the observer's position (movement parallax), or by a shift of the positions of objects relative to each other (motion parallax). Passive stereoparallax systems are, for example, 3-D movies, in which the parallax effect is caused by the dynamic scene and by the camera movements, and 3-D computer animation, where artificially created objects are rotated. Active stereoparallax systems, on the other hand, require the observer's movements to be coupled to the shifts in the image, as in natural vision.

In our 3-D display system, active parallax is obtained by attaching the 3-D cursor in block form to the stereoscopic glasses, and transmit-

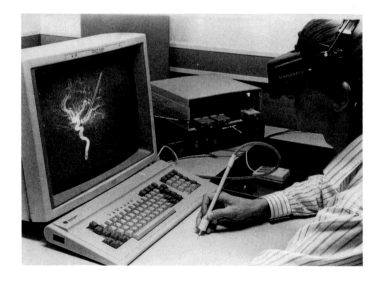

FIGURE 18.3 Stereotactic workstation.

ting the position (x, y, z coordinates) of the observer's head to the graphics workstation. A projection of the 3-D object onto the display screen is then performed, choosing the head position as the focal point. We note that the head position is also used to adjust the disparity angle between both images of the stereoscopic pair if the observer moves back and forth. Besides the position, the orientation of the stereoscopic glasses is transmitted to the graphics workstation. In this way, the orientation of the disparity, which is normally horizontal, can be adapted if the observer's head is tilted or even upside-down.

Active parallax requires the calculation of projections to be synchronized with the speed of the observer's movement. Our current computer system is not powerful enough to calculate projections of complex objects in real-time. Furthermore, vascular image data are projections themselves, and are therefore not available as real 3-D data sets. Consequently, the observer's view direction is usually restricted to lateral or frontal, defined by the geometry of the X-ray equipment. Nevertheless, we expect that faster hardware and new vascular imaging modalities, such as MR angiography, will soon make active stereoparallax an attractive feature for stereotactic planning.

3-D interaction

Two-dimensional cursors, such as a mouse or trackball, are impractical to select an appropriate 3-D stereotactic trajectory on a stereoscopic pair of angiograms. In our system, the 3-D cursor in style form is used as a natural simulation of the trajectory (Fig. 18.3). By transmitting the position and orientation of the style to the workstation, the observer is able to move a floating line with the same orientation through the stereoscopic image of the blood vessels. Below, our procedure for stereotactic neurosurgery planning is described in more detail.

Volume rendering

Most commercial graphics systems represent 3-D shape information by displaying the surface as a shaded object. The necessary surface segmentation schemes are based on an all-or-none classification into surface and non-surface points. However, for low-contrast tissue this approach is mostly inappropriate. Intrinsic intensity variations within the object, partial volume phenomena, system inhomogeneities, and noise introduced during image acquisition and reconstruction require the use of complex model knowledge to obtain the correct segmentation. This complex segmentation prevents us from routinely integrating shaded tumor boundaries into a 3-D image of the blood vessels.

To some extent this problem can be overcome by volume rendering, which is based on probabilistic segmentation. Instead of a yes/no classification, the voxels are ranked by assigning to each of them a probability value that expresses the likelihood of belonging to the object of interest. In spite of its inadequacy to solve the fundamental problem of recognizing complex objects in ambiguous image data, and its computationally expensive display approach, which is different from surface rendering [15], volume rendering is expected to become increasingly important for 3-D medical image display.

Stereotactic biopsy planning

Our stereotactic workstation is connected to the Ethernet digital image network of the radiology department (Fig. 18.4). Images from different modalities, such as CT (Somatom Plus), MR (Magnetom), DSA (Polytron), and PET can easily be transmitted in ACR−NEMA format to our stereotactic workstation (IRIS).

The procedure for stereotactic biopsy planning [17] works as follows.

First, the operator identifies the reference markers on the available images, such as CT scans, MR scans, and/or DSA images, with the mouse. The computer then corrects these positions with subpixel precision. Using this information, the necessary geometric transformations of image coordinates to BRW stereotactic coordinates are calculated, and the stereoscopic angiograms are made epipolar, i.e. corresponding object points lie on the same horizontal image in both images. The geometric correction into epipolar images improves the 3-D depth perception. When planning a biopsy, the surgeon then uses the mouse to indicate a target point on the series of CT or MR

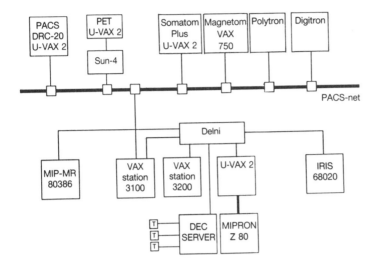

FIGURE 18.4 Diagram of the Ethernet network of our Radiological Imaging Unit. The stereotactic workstation is connected to CT (Somatom Plus), MR (Magnetom), DSA (Polytron) and PET.

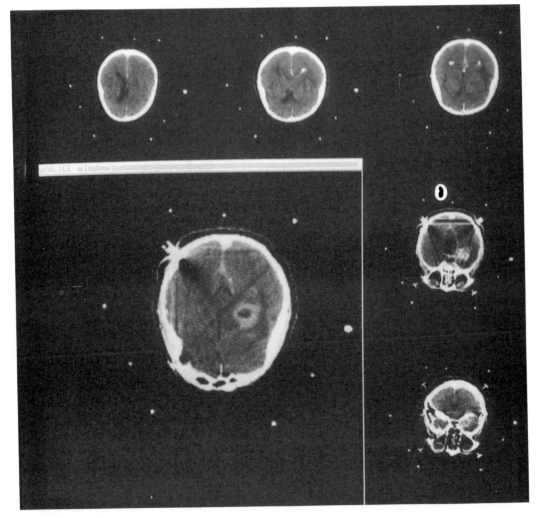

FIGURE 18.5 Identification of CT reference markers and stereotactic target point with the mouse. The computer corrects these positions with submillimeter accuracy.

scans (Fig. 18.5). The BRW coordinates of this point are automatically and instantaneously calculated.

Once the target point is fixed, it is projected onto the available angiograms. Typically, a stereoscopic pair of lateral angiograms is displayed, together with a simulated biopsy trajectory (Fig. 18.6) that can be rotated in real-time by means of the 3-D cursor in style form, in order to select an appropriate entry point. The operator can easily switch between the arterial and venous phase. Because of the limited depth accuracy it is recommended to verify the position of the trajectory on a frontal angiogram. Another interesting feature is shown in Fig. 18.7. The intersection of the selected trajectory is shown in the subsequent CT (or MR) slices. The angiographic and CT images are physically stored in separate image buffers. This allows the user to switch from one image to the other without any delay.

The stereotactic workstation is physically located in the Radiological Imaging Unit because it is integrated into the existing digital network. However, as soon as the images from the differ-ent modalities have been collected, it can be disconnected from the network and moved to the operation room. In this way, the surgeon can follow the stereotactic procedure on the available images and if necessary he can start a new biopsy simulation.

Future directions in 3-D vascular imaging

Current MR angiography (MRA) is a safe and non-invasive imaging technique that has the potential of producing real 3-D vascular images (Fig. 18.8). Numerous methods have been proposed. One class of methods approaches MRA, as does DSA. Two sets of images are produced, a first set of flow-refocused images, in which the moving blood produces high intensity signal, and a second set with defocusing gradients, in which flowing blood causes signal void. Since both rephasing and dephasing gradients do not affect stationary tissues, subtraction of these two sets will produce an MR angiogram corre-sponding to the high intensity moving blood. In

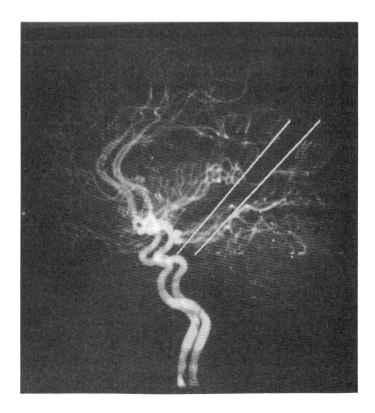

FIGURE 18.6 Stereoscopic angiogram with simulated stereotactic trajectory. The image was taken without using polarized glasses. The left and right images of the stereo pair are therefore projected onto each other.

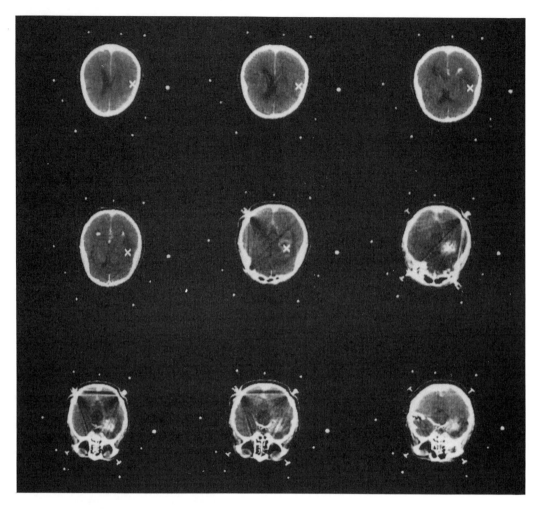

FIGURE 18.7 Subsequent CT slices showing the intersection of the selected stereotactic trajectory.

general only uniform coherent flow will yield a high intensity signal. Turbulent flow, frequently associated with vascular pathology, causes phase cancellation and reduces the signal in the affected areas. For this reason, hyperdynamic vessels are frequently poorly visualized, whereas stenotic lesions are generally overestimated.

A second class of techniques is based on 3-D gradient echo sequences, in combination with phase refocusing gradients. In this set-up, the inflow of unsaturated spins produces higher signal in the vessels than the more saturated spins of the stationary tissues, which are in steady state. Here also, turbulent flow causes signal drop-out.

Besides the problems of signal drop-out mentioned above, current state-of-the-art MR angiography still compares unfavorably with DSA images. It generates lower resolution images and requires expensive equipment. Furthermore, MR images have to be corrected for geometric distortions due to inhomogeneities of the main magnetic field and non-linearities of the orthogonal field gradients. Uncorrected images can contain displacement errors of the order of a few millimeters. Current procedures for assessment and correction of these errors are based on phantom measurements. In spite of these limitations, MRA is rapidly making progress, and we expect that it will soon be introduced in stereotactic neurosurgery.

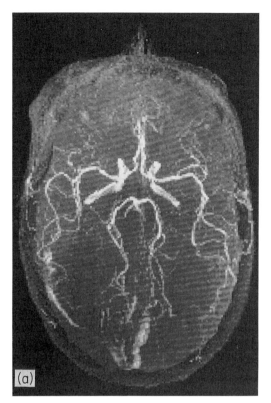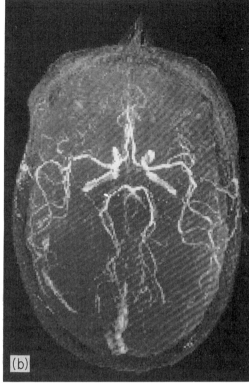

FIGURE 18.8 Stereoscopic inflow MR angiogram. Since MRA is a true 3-D imaging technique, the view direction can be chosen arbitrarily. (a) Left; (b) right.

Discussion

Our procedure for stereotactic biopsy planning takes advantage of the latest developments in digital imaging and communication systems. The images are all digital and they are transmitted via the digital image network of the radiology department to the workstation. Data from different imaging modalities, including DSA, are integrated with submillimeter precision into a 3-D image, and visualized on a graphics workstation with stereoscopic display capabilities and true 3-D interactivity.

The active parallax feature of the display system is not used because the DSA images are acquired stereoscopically and cannot be rotated. It will be useful as soon as MR angiography replaces DSA. It should be noted that displaying a dynamic sequence of images in real-time requires a larger and faster image buffer than the one that we have currently available.

We do not make full use of the graphics capabilities of the workstation. The reason is that the representation of a soft tissue structure as a shaded object is usually not satisfactory, mainly because the segmentation process requires complex model knowledge, which is not available. Volume rendering based on probabilistic segmentation overcomes this problem to some extent.

In summary, our stereotactic biopsy planning procedure is fully computerized and satisfactorily used in practice. The computer system is based on advanced but proven technology. The usefulness of MR angiography and of volume rendering have still to be explored.

References

1 Suetens, P., Baert, A.L., Gybels, J., *et al.* An integrated 3-D image of cerebral blood vessels and CT view of tumor. *Frontiers Eur. Radiol.* **3**: 81–100 (1984).

2 Pelizarri, C.A., Chen, G.T.Y., Spelbring, D.R., Weichselbaum, R.R. & Chen, C.T. Accurate three-dimensional registration of CT, PET, and/or MR images of the brain. *J. Comput. Assist. Tomogr.* **13**(1): 20−6 (1989).

3 Marrett, S., Evans, A.C., Collins, L. & Peters, T.M. A volume of interest (VOI) atlas for the analysis of neurophysiological image data. *Society of Photo-optical Instrumentation Engineers* **1092**: 467−77 (1989).

4 Apicella, A., Kippenhan, J.S. & Nagel, J.H. Fast multi-modality image matching. *Society of Photo-optical Instrumentation Engineers* **1092**: 252−63 (1989).

5 Evans, A.C., Beil, C., Marrett, S., Thompson, C.J. & Hakim, A. Anatomical−functional correlation using an adjustable MRI-based region of interest atlas with positron emission tomography. *J. Cerebr. Blood Flow Metab.* **8**: 513−30 (1988).

6 Greitz, T., Bergstroem, M., Boethius, J., Kingsley, D. & Ribbe, T. Head fixation system for integration of radiodiagnostic and therapeutic procedures. *Neuroradiology* **19**: 1−6 (1980).

7 Schad, L.R., Boesecke, R., Schlegel, W., *et al.* Three-dimensional image correlation of CT, MR and PET studies in radiotherapy treatment planning of brain tumors. *J. Comput. Assist. Tomogr.* **11**(6): 948−54 (1987).

8 Laitinen, L.V., Liliequist, B., Fagerlund, M. & Eriksson, A.T. An adapter for computed tomography-guided stereotaxis. *Surg. Neurol.* **23**: 559−66 (1985).

9 Bergstroem, M., Greitz, T. & Ribbe, T. A method of stereotaxic localization adopted for conventional and digital radiography. *Neuroradiology* **28**: 100−4 (1986).

10 Lunsford, L.D. & Leksell, D. The Leksell system. In: Lunsford, L.D. (ed.) *Modern Stereotactic Neurosurgery*, pp. 27−46. Boston: Martinus Nijhoff (1988).

11 Kelly, P.J., Goerss, S.J. & Kall, B.A. Modification of Todd-Wells system for imaging data acquisition. In: Lunsford, L.D. (ed.) *Modern Stereotactic Neurosurgery*. pp. 79−97. Boston: Martinus Nijhoff (1988).

12 Siddon, R. & Barth, N.H. Stereotaxic localization of intracranial targets. *Int. J. Radiat. Oncol. Biol. Phys.* **13**: 1241−6 (1987).

13 Peters, T.M., Clarck, J.A., Pike, G.B., *et al.* Stereotactic neurosurgery planning on a personal-computer-based work station. *J. Dig. Imag.* **2**(2): 75−81 (1989).

14 Vandermeulen, D., Suetens, P., Gybels, J., Oosterlinck, A., Cosman, E.R. & Wells, T.H. Jr. Angiographic localizer for the BRW stereotactic system. *Appl. Neurophysiol.* **50**: 87−91 (1987).

15 Levoy, M. Volume rendering − display of surfaces from volume data. *Institute of Electrical and Electronic Engineers Comp. Graphics Appl.* **6**(3): 29−37 (1988).

16 Suetens, P., Vandermeulen, D., Oosterlinck, A., Gybels, J. & Marchal, G. A 3-D display system with stereoscopic, movement parallax and real-time rotation capabilities. *Society of Photo-optical Instrumentation Engineers* **914**: 855−61 (1988).

17 Vandermeulen, D., Suetens, P., Gybels, J., Oosterlinck, A. & Marchal, G. A prototype medical workstation for computer-assisted stereotactic neurosurgery. *Comput. Assist. Radiol. CAR '89* 386−9 (1989).

19

Stereotactic Neurosurgery Planning using Integrated Three-dimensional Stereoscopic Images

Terry M. Peters, Christopher J. Henri, D. Louis Collins,
Louis Lemieux, G. Bruce Pike, and André Olivier

Introduction

The personal computer AT-based stereotactic planning system, developed at the Montreal Neurological Institute (MNI) has been in clinical use for the past 6 years (see Chapter 15) [1–3]. With this system, images acquired stereotactically from computed tomography (CT), magnetic resonance imaging (MRI), and digital subtraction angiography (DSA) are analyzed together in a common environment, allowing the neurosurgeon to determine the stereotactic coordinates of any target he identifies on the screen with a mouse-driven cursor. Similarly, a user-defined point with coordinates x, y, z may be displayed upon request at the appropriate position in an image. Additional facilities allow the neurosurgeon to plan the trajectory of a probe and to see where it passes through each slice of a tomographic data-set, or to view it with respect to the vessels displayed in DSA images.

The stereotactic apparatus consists of a rigid frame that is fixed to the patient's head during both imaging and surgery. The frame and associated fiducial marker plates (described in Chapter 15) provide a consistent coordinate system in which to localize targets appearing in the images acquired from each modality, and provide the basis for determining coordinate transformations between the stereotactic frame and image plane. The methodology behind target localization in tomographic data, based on fiducial markers in the images, is well known [4,5].

A different approach is required to obtain the three-dimensional (3-D) coordinates of a target appearing in a pair of biplane projections, as in DSA [6]. The process usually begins with the neurosurgeon identifying the desired target in one image, using a cursor. He then enters a likely depth coordinate, providing the system with an initial estimate of the target's true 3-D position. The tentative x, y, z coordinates are then reprojected into the other biplane image and compared with the target's location as seen in this alternate view. A slight refinement may be required before the reprojected coordinates correspond to the position of the target in each image. This iterative process is performed until the neurosurgeon is satisfied that the chosen target does indeed correspond to the structure of interest in both images. Difficulties arise, however, when there is some ambiguity in uniquely identifying the target, or when it is obscured in either of the images due to vessel superposition or foreshortening. Measurement accuracy, as a result, may be compromised.

While the target points are often determined on the basis of stereotactic analysis of CT or MR images [3], the role played by DSA is to ensure that the approach to the target is vascular-free. In order to plan probe trajectories using biplane projections, the neurosurgeon must draw upon his knowledge of vascular anatomy to assess the proximity of vessels along the path of the probe in each view. Conceivably, he could determine a clear path by iteratively comparing the position of each point along the trajectory with the positions of nearby vessels, but such an approach is impractical.

This limitation, along with the desire to utilize the inherently 3-D data from each imaging modality, has prompted us to investigate alternative methods of visualizing the data in 3-D for the purpose of planning stereotactic surgery procedures.

The material presented here describes a number of developments toward this goal. We begin with a discussion of a stereoscopically-based enhancement to the computer system described in Chapter 15 of this volume. This is followed by an outline of the procedures used for creating volume-rendered images from CT and MR data. We then introduce the notion of using magnetic resonance angiography (MRA) techniques to acquire the vascular data in a true 3-D format, and discuss how MRA images may be utilized in stereotactic surgery planning. Finally, we discuss the techniques used to combine volume-rendered data with DSA images in a manner that permits a composite 3-D image to be viewed stereoscopically.

Materials and methods

Data acquisition — CT and MRI

Tomographic data for 3-D visualization are acquired on the CT scanner using standard techniques, with up to 30 contiguous 2.5 mm slices. MR data-sets generally comprise 64 3 mm slices overlapped by 1 mm. In-plane pixel dimensions are typically 0.6×0.6 mm for CT and 1.1×1.1 mm for MR.

Data acquisition — DSA

Stereoscopic angiography has been employed for many years at the Montreal Neurological Institute by both radiologists and surgeons for diagnosis and surgery planning [7]. Recently we have begun to use stereoscopically acquired DSA projections in a quantitative manner, to plan stereotactic neurosurgery (for target localization, etc.).

We acquire stereoscopic DSA projections using one of two techniques. Currently, the preferred method employs an isocentric C-arm gantry rotation with a nominal 7° angulation. This approach yields stereo-pairs with greater disparity than the alternative method, which until now employed a dual-focus X-ray tube whose effective lateral shift was only 25 mm. We have recently upgraded the system, and now employ a 65 mm separation between the two foci. This is expected to eliminate the requirement of gantry angulation. For stereotactic purposes, a 270 mm field-of-view is employed for lateral projections, while 170 mm is used for anterior–posterior (A/P) views. Object magnification is constrained in order to maintain the fiducial markers within these limits, so that we are unable to benefit fully from a magnification stereoscopic technique [8, 9]. We find typical magnifications for lateral and A/P projections to be 1.8 and 1.1, respectively.

Data acquisition — MRA

MRA images are typically acquired using a fast gradient echo sequence with a short echo time to suppress the magnetically saturated static tissue in a selected thin slice, while imaging the fresh blood that has flowed into the slice. Vascularity in the head and neck may be imaged in 3-D by stacking up to 64 of these slices and viewing them using projection, cine-loop, and stereoscopic techniques.

STEREOSCOPIC WORKSTATION

Image display

The analysis of stereoscopic images is performed on a system similar to the one we describe in Chapter 15. The main additional component required for stereoscopic viewing is a specialized graphics card (Tektronix Stereo Graphics Adapter), which controls output to a high performance color monitor capable of displaying $512 \times 512 \times 8$ bit images, non-interlaced, with a refresh rate of 120 Hz. This device also controls a liquid-crystal polarizing shutter, attached to the front of the monitor, which circularly polarizes alternate images (right- and left-eye views) at the frame rate. A stereoscopic effect is achieved when the monitor is viewed with an appropriate pair of polarized glasses. Since each eye receives an image at 60 Hz, the observer perceives no flicker.

The new stereoscopic DSA system, described below, offers the ability not only to display the images in 3-D, but allows interaction with them as part of the stereotactic planning process. This new approach is more natural for planning many procedures, and is easily integrated with traditional methods of analyzing tomographic data.

Stereoscopic/stereotactic planning facilities

This system offers an alternate approach to planning stereotactic neurosurgery on the basis of DSA images. The primary difference with respect to the conventional technique lies in the ability of the stereoscopic system to derive 3-D coordinates directly from a stereoscopic pair of images. Although measurement accuracy is subject to various limitations [10,11], it is nevertheless a more convenient approach and more enlightening in terms of appreciating the overall structure, since the operator perceives the 3-D vasculature floating within the imaged volume during the entire planning procedure. Figure 19.1 illustrates a typical stereoscopic angiogram, where the arteries are displayed in white and the veins in black.

Stereotactic analysis begins with the user identifying the fiducial markers in the unsubtracted images of each view. The program uses this information to calculate a transformation matrix that relates actual 3-D locations within the stereotactic frame to their projected positions in each image [6].

The information contained in two such matrices obtained from different views is sufficient to calculate a target's 3-D coordinates via triangulation [6]. Mathematically, this is accomplished by solving an overdetermined system of equations, using a least-squares technique, and is equivalent to finding the point where the rays between the X-ray source and target in each image come closest to intersecting. The details of this approach are given in the Appendix of Chapter 15 of this book.

Since we routinely acquire lateral and A/P stereoscopic projections, it is often useful to load each stereopair into the frame buffer of the display system, which may store up to four separate images at one time. Although only one stereopair may be viewed at a time using this mode, the operator may switch between lateral and A/P projections instantly, to obtain an alternate view of the vasculature along with a cursor and/or a probe that has been placed within the 3-D volume. While the cursor is manipulated, its 3-D frame coordinates, calculated via the transformation matrices, are

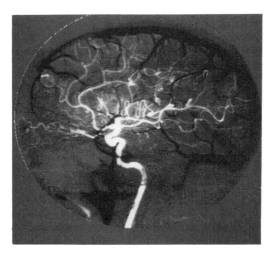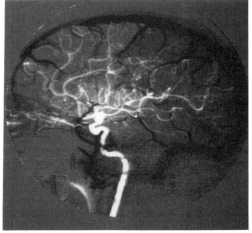

FIGURE 19.1 A typical stereoscopic angiogram pair. The composite arterial/venous image was created by subtracting the appropriate images in the acquired sequence of projections. This image, and other stereoscopic images presented in this chapter, may be perceived in 3-D using a crossed-eye viewing technique.

continuously updated and presented on the screen. This facility is useful to assess the proposed path for a biopsy needle or depth electrode, and may be used to resolve any visual ambiguities that may arise.

Interaction with the image is achieved via a stereoscopic cursor controlled by a conventional 3-button mouse. The cursor is active at all times and may be moved anywhere within the 3-D volume defined by the stereoscopic images. The illusion of depth is achieved by introducing a disparity between the position of the cursor in the left- and right-eye images. Movement of the cursor in depth is accomplished by depressing the center button on the mouse and moving it away from or towards the operator, moving the perceived position of the cursor into or out of the screen, respectively. The operator has the option of viewing the A/P and lateral stereoscopic images separately or, alternatively, using a split-screen to display rectangular regions-of-interest from each image simultaneously (Fig. 19.2).

A major strength of this stereoscopic/stereotactic image analysis package is its capacity for drawing and manipulating arbitrary vectors within the 3-D space defined by the stereotactic frame. In this respect, it bears a resemblance to the mechanical "floating-line" system described by Cloutier *et al.* [13]. With our approach, the neurosurgeon is able quickly to assess possible trajectories toward a target, which previously were tedious to evaluate using two-dimensional (2-D) images. In particular, he is able to place the probe within an appropriate vascular-free region, ensuring the approach to the target does not encroach on major blood vessels in the brain. In the process of defining a 3-D vector in space, the azimuthal and declination angles of the line related to an isocentric arc system are also made available to the user. This approach has already allowed us to consider unorthodox probe trajectories which could not otherwise have been planned with confidence.

DSA/CT display

In addition to stereoscopic A/P and/or lateral images being available to the user, the system also permits a reduced-size version of the appropriate CT or MR slices to be displayed simultaneously. A window containing the tomographic data, typically less than a quarter of the screen in size, is displayed within a full-size stereoscopic DSA image (see Fig. 19.3). In this manner, images from the separate modalities can be analyzed together. The position of the cursor may be followed simultaneously in each image; i.e. a change in cursor depth within the lateral DSA image is reflected as a lateral shift of the corresponding pointer in the tomographic image. Likewise, a vertical movement of the cursor within the DSA image results in a new tomographic slice being displayed.

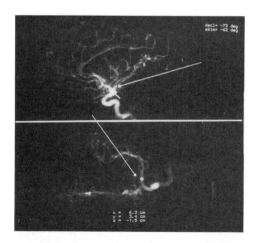 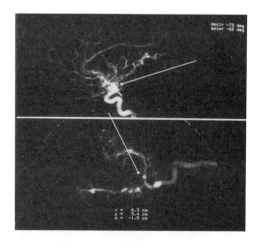

FIGURE 19.2 A split-screen display of lateral (top) and anterior–posterior (bottom) stereoscopic angiograms of a patient undergoing planning for a stereotactic procedure. Note that the displayed 3-D probe, which is placed interactively by the operator, is seen in each view.

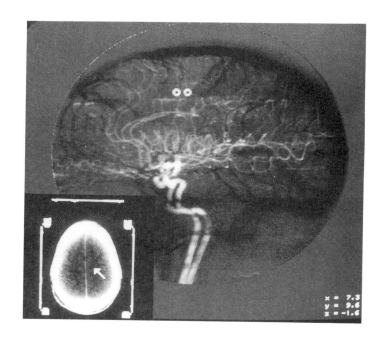

FIGURE 19.3 A stereoscopic image showing the position of a 3-D cursor in both the angiogram and the corresponding CT slice. The double image presented here is what is seen when it is viewed without the polarized glasses.

VOLUME-RENDERING

Standard technique

As previously mentioned, we have chosen to explore the use of a volume-rendering technique to display 3-D images for our applications. We employ a specialized image-processing computer (PIXAR, San Raphael, CA) to accomplish this task [14]. Within the PIXAR, the data are stored as 48-bit pixels, where 12 bits are ascribed to each of the red, green, and blue (r, g, b) channels, and a further 12 bits to the α channel to represent transparency. Each voxel, therefore, has a four-element coloropacity vector associated with it. Using this formulation, it is possible to represent the volume as a 3-D gel-like substance, each element of which has an associated luminous color intensity (the r, g, b values) as well as an opacity (the α value). If the voxel is opaque ($\alpha = 1$), a simulated light-ray will not pass through it. However, if it is completely transparent, the incident ray will be appropriately colored but not attenuated.

The standard technique employed by the PIXAR to form 3-D images employs a projection method that accounts for the colors and opacities of each voxel, using a simple recursive compositing scheme known as *opacity-weighted*

integration. Placing one voxel over another, the projection begins at the back of the volume and ends at the front. The result of the opacity-weighted integral for each ray is displayed as a colored pixel with the appropriate intensity in the image plane.

Hidden surface removal is achieved by careful selection of the traversal order of the data. Since orthographic projections are used, this order must simply ensure that the columns of data (one column per pixel) are traversed from back to front. Thus voxels deeper within the volume are hidden by opaque voxels in the front.

In order to improve the visualization of internal structures, information on surfaces (boundaries between regions of different MR signal intensities within the volume) is incorporated. This is achieved by enhancing the edges of regions within the 3-D volume using a *gradient* operator, and incorporating this information in the projection of the volume to the image plane.

Modified technique

The highly transparent images formed using the PIXAR method described above are not particularly appropriate for surgical planning. While the rendered images share some characteristics with radiographic images, they do not model the organs as they are seen during a surgical procedure. The human brain is opaque and, during surgery, it is illuminated both by direct and ambient light, usually from the same side as the surgeon. We therefore attempt to model the brain as if viewed under similar conditions. The necessary modifications to the algorithm are described presently.

The surface normals estimated in the PIXAR technique are calculated from the voxel values in the classified volume, so there is a potential that errors in the classification could lead to errors in the estimation of the surface normals. Our modified technique computes the classification and the gradient volumes independently, similar to the approach described by Levoy [15].

Rather than illuminate the volume from the rear, we place our light-source model in front of the object, in line with the viewing direction. Depth cues are achieved by allowing some reflected light from deep surfaces to be com-

bined with the light reflected from the front of the object. "Surfaces" defined by the gradient operator, described above, are emphasized by introducing a maximum degree of light reflection for voxels with associated surface normals parallel to the lighting direction.

The original PIXAR rendering algorithm assigns the same range of relatively low opacities to both interior and surface voxels. Features that appear to lie on the rendered surface may actually be just above or just below it. Assigning a higher opacity to the surface voxels eliminates this error, at the risk of hiding subsurface structures that one may wish to visualize.

The result of applying this algorithm to a set of 64 T1-weighted MR slices, which have been preprocessed by removing a wedge-shaped section to better visualize the region of interest, is shown in Fig. 19.4. This is one frame of a cine-loop that displays the 3-D reconstruction from multiple viewpoints. In practice, we find that color is useful in displaying images of this nature, and we have found a "hot-metal" display (black through shades of red and orange to

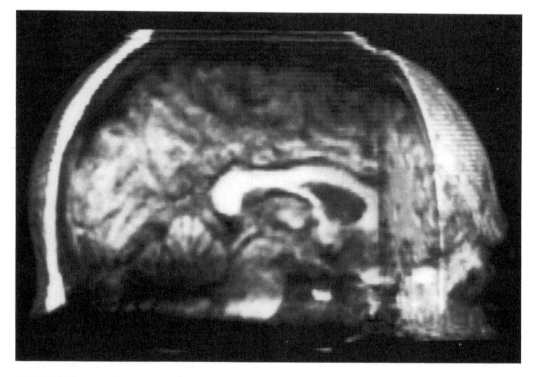

FIGURE 19.4 A "volume-rendered" MR image, after processing by the PIXAR image computer. The original data-set is 64 T1-weighted MR slices, which have been preprocessed by the removal of a wedge-shaped section in order to visualize the region of interest.

white) to be particularly effective for the display of 3-D volume-rendered images. This color scale appears to present a wider dynamic range of intensities to the observer than is possible with a black and white scale, and without the false contours introduced by other color scales. We believe that the use of color is almost mandatory when displaying combined images from different modalities. Unfortunately it is not possible to reproduce these images in color here.

Combining tomographic and projection data

Encouraging results have been obtained recently that demonstrate the ability of MRI to image blood-flow as well as soft tissue [16], and we demonstrate the potential use of MR angiography in stereotaxy later in this chapter. However, this is still an evolving technology, and the technique currently lacks the fine resolution required to visualize many of the smaller intracranial vessels. Because of these present limitations, we are continuing with our efforts to combine data acquired from separate modalities. Below, we describe an approach based on the stereoscopic technique described earlier that allows volume-rendered images (either CT or MR) to be combined with projection DSA.

While past techniques for combining angiograms with tomographic data have required that the vasculature be reconstructed in 3-D [17], the approach described here is less complicated, and requires only the information ordinarily employed to analyze the images stereotactically. In order to combine the two types of data, we generate a volume-rendered image of the tomographic data-set (using the method described previously) that precisely matches the viewing geometry used to acquire the projection angiogram, allowing the two to be superimposed. In so doing, we take advantage of the high resolution available with DSA, while relying on the rendering algorithm to create a realistic 3-D image of the tomographic volume. This process is performed for each image of the DSA stereopair, allowing the resulting images to be analyzed using the facilities described earlier.

The procedure relies on the stereotactic frame to provide a common coordinate system between each data-set. Since the frame is employed during the acquisition of images from each modality, every image possesses its own frame-to-image transformation which fully characterizes the imaging geometry used. Similarly, a frame-to-volume transformation exists when the tomographic data are loaded into PIXAR memory.

By decomposing a DSA-associated transformation matrix into its components (translation, rotation, perspective, scaling, and cropping), sufficient information is provided to generate the desired matching 3-D volume-rendered image. While the matrix decomposition may be accomplished analytically [18], we employ a modified version of the technique described by Strat [12] which is geometrically based. Amongst other parameters, we obtain three angles specifying the orientation of the image plane with respect to the frame in the DSA projection. A separate calculation is performed to determine the frame's orientation within the tomographic volume. The individual rotations which must be applied to the volume in order to match the DSA projection geometry are determined, then applied to the data using the PIXAR.

The PIXAR operates only on rows and columns of data to perform a projection operation. Thus, in order to simulate a perspective projection, the volume must be reshaped prior to rendering to give the desired view when projected orthographically. Reshaping requires that successive planes perpendicular to the projection axis be progressively resized from front to back. Since the resizing must be centered along the principal ray (assuming the volume has been correctly oriented), it is first necessary to determine where that ray intersects the volume. This is accomplished by locating any voxel whose stereotactic coordinates are "projected" (via the DSA transformation matrix) to the piercing point in the image plane. Such voxels constitute points on the principal ray. The resizing necessary for each plane is determined by comparing an object's size in the plane to its size in the DSA projection. Each plane within the volume is then rescaled accordingly. At the same time, the data are translated to align the piercing point through the volume with its position in the DSA image.

It is sometimes useful to remove a portion of data from the volume (at least the stereotactic plates) to prevent an underlying area of interest from being obscured. The angiogram is overlaid on the rendered image, using the image compositing utility on the PIXAR. Transparency may be varied between the two images to prevent the vessels from completely occluding the underlying rendered data, or vice versa. The procedure is repeated for each image of the stereopair before they are transferred to the stereoscopic workstation.

The result of a patient study, in which the above procedure was used to combine stereoscopic DSA images with an MR volume, is shown in Fig. 19.5. In this example, the left- and right-eye views of the arterial phase angiogram were overlaid on the 3-D MR volume-rendered image computed for the appropriate viewing geometries. Note the strong correspondence between the fissures in the anatomic image and the vessels in the angiogram. While the image in Fig. 19.5 is necessarily black and white, in practice the vessels are displayed in a color distinct from the background anatomy.

MR angiographic imaging

For true 3-D analysis of the cerebral vasculature within a stereotactic environment, the vasculature image data-set must itself be three-dimensional. The fact that DSA images are only two-dimensional (2-D) projections therefore limits their usefulness in stereotactic surgery planning. As discussed above, this problem can be partially solved through stereoscopic analysis, which aids in the visualization of the 3-D objects but does produce a true 3-D data-set. This problem has been overcome in recent years with the advent of a variety of magnetic resonance angiography (MRA) methods which allow true 3-D imaging of the vasculature [16, 21]. We use one such method to produce 3-D MRAs of the cerebral vessels for stereotactic analysis.

This technique employs an *inflow*-based MRA technique [19–21] in which a gradient echo sequence is used to acquire multiple thin 2-D slices or a 3-D volume. In this method the stationary material within the imaged volume produces a low signal intensity due to the short repetition times and high flip angles, which produce a saturation effect, whereas flowing blood produces a high signal intensity due to the *inflow* of unsaturated spins. Typical acquisition parameters are: repetition time (50 ms), echo time (10–15 ms), excitation pulse angle (45–90°), and slice thickness (1–3 mm). This method thus allows $256 \times 256 \times 64$ voxel data-sets to be acquired in under 15 minutes. Because the data-set is truly 3-D, the vasculature may be viewed retrospectively in a variety of formats. Figure 19.6 shows a stereoscopic pair of views

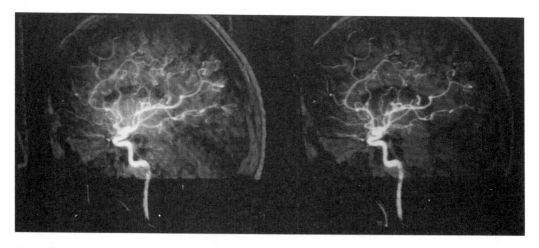

FIGURE 19.5 A multimodality stereoscopic image pair, obtained by combining a volume-rendered MR image with a pair of digitally subtracted angiograms. Here the 3-D MR image is projected to the viewing screen in such a manner as to exactly match the stereoscopic angiographic projections.

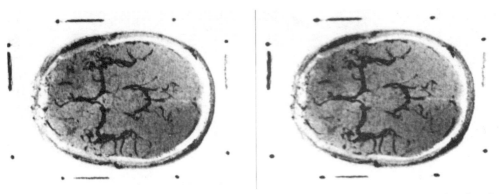

FIGURE 19.6 A stereoscopic MR angiographic image made under stereotactic conditions. The fiducial markers seen at the sides of the image consist of a copper sulfate solution embedded in a plexiglass plate. In spite of being stationary tissue, they show up brightly in the image, due to the short T1 characteristic of this solution.

of a cerebral MRA displayed as an orthogonal maximum intensity projection along the cranial–caudal axis.

We have investigated two methods of MRA data display for surgical planning. In the first, individual slices through the data volume are analyzed, using the stereotactic software described in Chapter 15. This approach allows the surgeon to assess a proposed trajectory, planned on standard MR or CT images, simply by moving through the MRA volume slice-by-slice and observing the intersection points of the probe with each slice as it is automatically displayed by the software. In this manner a vascular-free path to the target may be directly verified. By optimizing the MRA acquisition parameters, we may also produce a data-set in which we obtain both a reasonable quality stationary tissue and a flowing blood image.

The second display method for MRA-based surgical planning is volume-rendering. The simplest approach is to project the 3-D MRA volume to produce images such as those seen in Fig. 19.6. We may also employ two data volumes, one of stationary tissue for MRI and one of the vascularity using MRA. These volumes are then color coded and volume-rendered, using standard PIXAR-based methods [14] modified for this application [15]. An example of this technique is shown in Fig. 19.7, in which the scalp has been retrospectively segmented to expose the cortical surface and the superficial vasculature.

A significant advantage of MRA techniques over conventional radiographic approaches is that the resulting image is fundamentally 3-D in nature. Thus the data volume may be imaged from any viewpoint, viewed in stereo, and integrated readily with any other 3-D data-set of the same patient. For this reason, we believe that MRA will play a major role in stereotactic surgery planning.

Discussion

To date, we have used the stereoscopic angiographic analysis system in several types of clinical situations. With the system of stereotactic angiography, used since 1984 [1], it was simple to perform twist drill stereotactic biopsies, knowing the exact positions of both arteries and veins when an approach orthogonal to the side of the frame was used. It was also possible to use the twist drill technique based on DSA for other angles of approach, but this was only based on bi-plane angiograms. The procedure lacked the precision of the orthogonal approach, although it provided the delineation of the essential avascular zone of entry, and determination of the probe track. The new stereoscopic system, described earlier, may now be used routinely for tumor biopsies, implantation of depth electrodes, and craniotomy planning.

The main advantage of this system is that it reveals the 3-D appearance of the arteries and

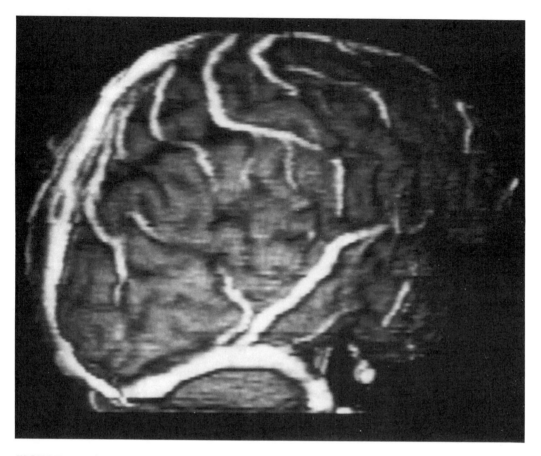

FIGURE 19.7 This Figure demonstrates the cortical vascularity on top of the reconstructed cortex, achieved by volume-rendering a 3-D MR data-set containing both vascular and anatomic information.

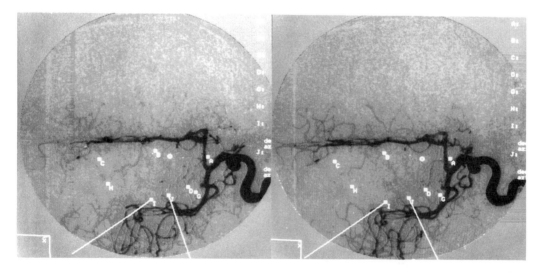

FIGURE 19.8 A stereoscopic DSA image pair, showing the location of electrode targets and the placement of two electrodes during a depth electrode implantation procedure.

veins with such clarity that the surface top-ography of the brain can be recognized with accuracy. The technique thus serves two main purposes: not only does it reveal the anatomy by the configuration of the arteries and veins, it also clearly displays the optimal vascular route to a specific target, itself determined by DSA and/or other modalities. This entails the zone of entry at the level of the cortex, the full extent of the tract in relationship to the sulci and main vascular trunks, and the target zone itself. An example of a stereoscopic angiogram with marked target points and trajectories is shown in Fig. 19.8.

Such a technique has been particularly useful for the placement of intracranial recording electrodes for recording in cases of intractable epilepsy. The relatively large number of elec-trodes used, the diversity of angle desired and the need to know the position of each recording site along an electrode array represent problems that have been solved with this technique. The stereoscopic workstation is taken to the oper-ation room and, prior to the final insertion of each electrode, the preselected pathway is dis-played on the image screen for final angular adjustment if needed. Each recording site (typically eight or nine along each electrode array) may be identified by markers at 5 mm intervals representing the interelectrode distance. The exact position of each of these sites can be easily retrieved and correlated with other modalities as well.

This workstation is also useful in the planning of standard or stereotactically guided crani-otomy procedures, since it is able to demonstrate the surface arteriovenous anatomy that is visualized at surgery. This aspect will be even further enhanced when we begin to use the integrated anatomic and vascular images described earlier, at surgery.

Conclusions

The technique described here for combining data from different modalities is new, and constitutes the first step towards the realization of a true 3-D workstation for the planning of stereotactic surgical procedures. In addition to the DSA image acquired explicitly in stereo, any image that has been reconstructed in 3-D

can be displayed in this mode also. It is envisaged that in its ultimate form, the surgeon will interact with such images, using a hand-held 3-D localizing probe to simulate the intended direction of approach.

Stereotactic localization demands a high degree of measurement accuracy, and we have made an extensive study of this issue with respect to the raw images obtained from each of the modalities. We have demonstrated that we may rely on the measured values to within an accuracy of ± 1 mm in DSA, transverse CT, and MRI. Volume-rendering involves several interpolation and rotation steps, each of which degrades the modulation transfer function of the imaging operation to some extent. For this reason, we have studied the global accuracy of this system as it compares to measurements made on the basis of the original images alone. Our initial experience, along with the enthusi-asm of our neurosurgical colleagues, leads us to believe that such a system will be a valued addition to the tools used by the neurosurgical community.

When dealing with MR images (either 2-D or 3-D) for stereotactic surgery planning, we must be aware of the extent of the distortion intro-duced by the characteristics of the scanner (see Discussion in Chapter 15). There remains much work to be done to characterize and fully correct such artifacts.

Some of the techniques described here have matured to the point where they are used regularly in a clinical setting by neurosurgeons, both prior to and during the procedures itself. Such is the case for the routine stereotactic and radiosurgery planning described in Chapter 15, and the stereoscopic system described here. While the other approaches are also used in the planning of surgical procedures, they are still in the developmental stage awaiting effective user-interfaces.

In clinical practice the surgeon must be able to quickly retrieve the data-sets from the relevant imaging systems, interact readily with the images in 3-D using simple spatial pointing systems, refer any operation back to the original 2-D images for confirmation purposes, and quickly manipulate the 3-D image (e.g. gen-eration of arbitrary views, interactive 'dis-section' of the images, etc.). In our opinion, this aspect of the development of imaging tasks is as important as the development of image processing algorithms themselves.

References

1 Peters, T.M., Clark, J.A., Olivier, A., *et al.* Integrated stereotaxic imaging with CT/MR imaging and digital subtraction angiography. *Radiology* **161**: 821−6 (1986).

2 Peters, T.M., Clark, J.A., Pike, B., *et al.* Stereotactic surgical planning with magnetic resonance imaging, digital subtraction angiography and computed tomography. *Appl. Neurophysiol.* **50**: 33−8 (1987).

3 Peters, T.M., Clark, J. & Pike, B. A personal-computer based workstation for the planning of stereotactic neurosurgical procedures. In: Kelly, P.J. & Kall, B.A. (eds), *Computers in Stereotactic Neurosurgery.* Oxford: Blackwell Scientific Publications (1992). (Chapter 15, this volume.)

4 Brown, R.A. A stereotactic head frame for use with CT body scanners. *Invest. Radiol.* **14**: 300−4 (1979).

5 Brown, R.A., Roberts, T.S. & Osborne, A.G. Stereotactic frame and computer software for CT-directed neurosurgical localization. *Invest. Radiol.* **15**: 308−12 (1980).

6 Sutherland, I.E. Three-dimensional data input by tablet. *Proceedings of the Institute of Electrical and Electronic Engineers.* **62**: 453−71 (1974).

7 Worthington, C., Peters, T.M., Ethier, R., *et al.* Stereoscopic digital subtraction angiography in neurological assessment. *Am. J. Neuroradiol.* **6**: 802−8 (1985).

8 Doi, K., Rossmann, K. & Duda, E.E. Application of longitudinal magnification effect to magnification stereoscopic angiography: a new method of cerebral angiography. *Radiology* **124**: 395−401 (1977).

9 Takahashi, M., Ozawa, Y. & Takemoto, H. Focal spot separation in stereoscopic magnification radiography. *Radiology* **140**: 227−9 (1981).

10 Mawko, G.M. Three-dimensional analysis of digital subtraction angiograms for stereotactic surgical planning. PhD Thesis, McGill University (1989).

11 Henri, C.J., Collins, D.L. & Peters, T.M. Multi-modality image integration for stereotactic surgical planning. *Med. Phys.* **18**: 167−177 (1991).

12 Strat, T.M. Recovering the camera parameters from a transformation matrix. In: Fischler, M.A. & Firschen, O. (eds) *Readings in Computer Vision: Issues, Problems, Principles and Paradigms.* Los Altos: Morgan Kaufmann (1987).

13 Cloutier, L., Nguyen, D.N., Ghosh, S.K., *et al.* Simulator allowing spatial viewing of cerebral probes by using a floating line concept. *Proceedings of the Society of Photo-optical Instrumentation Engineers: Medical Imaging* **602**: 315−9 (1985).

14 PIXAR *Image Computer Programmers Manual*, 2nd edn. San Rafael, CA: PIXAR (1987).

15 Levoy, M. Direct visualization of surfaces from computed tomography data. *Proceedings of the Society of Photo-optical Instrumentation Engineers: Medical Imaging II* 828−41 (1988).

16 Henri, C.J., Pike, G.B., Collins, D.L. & Peters, T.M. Three-dimensional display of cortical anatomy and vasculature: MR angiography versus multi-modality integration. *J. Dig. Imag.* **4**: 21−7 (1991).

17 Rubin, J.M. & Sayre, R.E. A computer-aided technique for overlaying cerebral angiograms onto computed tomograms. *Invest. Radiol.* **13**: 362−7 (1978).

18 Ganapathy, S. Decomposition of transformation matricies for robot vision. *Proceedings of the Institute of Electrical and Electronics Engineers Computer Vision and Pattern Recognition.* Los Alamitos, CA. 130−9 (1984).

19 Dumoulin, C.L., Cline, H.E., Souza, S.P., *et al.* Three-dimensional time-of-flight magnetic resonance angiography using spin saturation. *Magnetic Resonance in Medicine* **11**: 35−46 (1989).

20 Laub, G.A. & Kaiser, W.A. MR angiography with gradient motion refocusing. *J. Comp. Assist. Tomogr.* **12**: 377−82 (1988).

21 Keller, P.J., Drayer, B.P., Fram, E.K., *et al.* MR angiography with two-dimensional acquisition and three-dimensional display. *Radiology* **173**: 527−32 (1989).

20

Surgical Simulation for Stereotactic Biopsy

Dudley H. Davis

Introduction

Stereotactic biopsy has become the diagnostic procedure of choice for many intracerebral lesions [1−3]. Although human stereotactic techniques have been available for decades [4], the computer has been instrumental in the development of the image-based stereotactic biopsy capability. Computed tomography (CT) visualized the intracranial contents by acquiring imaging data in three dimensions and storing it in computer memory. The grayscale value assigned to the three-dimensional (3-D) imaging element is determined by the tissue X-ray attenuation coefficient. A similar concept was applied in magnetic resonance imaging (MRI). Tissue grayscale values in MRI are determined by a complex interaction of a variety of unique physical properties, the most basic of which are T1 and T2 relaxation times and proton density. The data processing of these imaging modalities could only be performed by modern computers. Subsequent improvements in software and hardware have permitted imaging in axial, coronal, and sagittal planes. By placing anatomic structures in a defined, 3-D space, imaging and stereotaxy had a common ground that allowed their integration. The result has been the rapid development and utilization of image-based stereotactic neurosurgery.

Patient selection

Stereotactic biopsy is indicated to make a histologic diagnosis in patients with intracerebral lesions, particularly lesions that are deep and relatively inaccessible by conventional craniotomy. Also, lesions that are located in eloquent brain, where there is a high risk of neurologic deficit with conventional craniotomy, are best biopsied stereotactically. Neoplasms are the most common lesions requiring stereotactic biopsy, but other pathologic processes such as infection, inflammation, or infarct may require a histologic diagnosis [1−3]. An accurate diagnosis then guides further therapy, which may include surgical resection, irradiation, chemotherapy or antimicrobials.

Data acquisition

The first step in stereotactic biopsy is data acquisition. This consists of a stereotactic CT, angiogram, and/or MR. The head is fixed in a stereotactic headframe. A reference or localization system is fixed to the headframe, which creates fiducial artifacts on CT or MR images. These artifacts define the "stereotactic space" in which the head is fixed and the center of this space is the common reference point for all studies. Most stereotactic systems employ a reference device shaped like the letter "N" [5,6]. By digitizing the fiducial artifacts on the display screen, the computer can calculate the stereotactic coordinates of any target selected on the imaging studies. The multiplanar capability of MRI creates stereotactic images in axial, coronal, or sagittal planes. Software has been developed that allows the computer to automatically digitize the fiducial artifacts [5].

For stereotactic angiography a different reference system is fixed to the headframe. This consists of reference fiducials located bilaterally and anteriorly and posteriorly [7]. Angiograms are obtained in orthogonal and oblique projections. Again, by digitizing the fiducial artifacts the computer can perform the complicated calculations necessary to place the digital subtraction angiogram in stereotactic space [8]. Placing the angiographic data in the same three-dimensional space as the CT and/or MRI allows for the display of the target point selected from CT or MRI on the angiographic study [5]. The display of the vascular anatomy related to a target enhances the safety of stereotactic biopsy [2,5].

Data manipulation by the computer allows any area of the brain to be accessed stereotactically. Conventional placement of a headframe may exclude the posterior fossa contents from the stereotactic space defined by the reference system. Also, the headframe precludes surgical access to the suboccipital region. This problem is overcome by placing the headframe in an inverted position [9]. Once informed that the headframe is inverted, the computer can calculate the correct target coordinates from the fiducial artifacts.

Surgical planning

Following the acquisition and storage of stereotactic data, surgical planning is performed. This is done at a computer console which simultaneously displays the stereotactic imaging studies (Fig. 20.1). The computer system employed at the Mayo Clinic includes a Vicom VME image processor and a Sun SPARC System 370. Since the data are stored on a disk, surgical planning can be done electively. The biopsy does not have to be performed the same day as

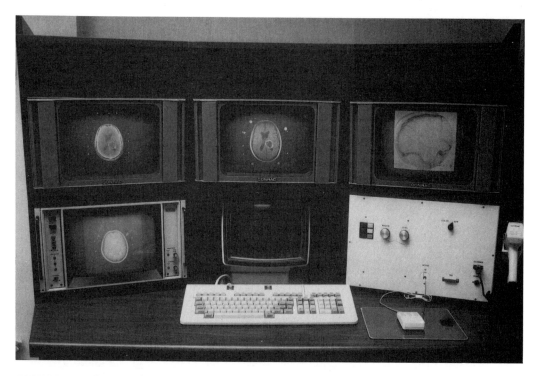

FIGURE 20.1 The surgical planning console which simultaneously displays the imaging studies and allows for computer simulation of the biopsy.

data acquisition if the headframe can be accurately replaced [10]. This feature, provided by data storage, creates flexibility in scheduling and allows planning and the biopsy to proceed in an unhurried fashion.

The first step in surgical planning is the selection of a target point for the stereotactic biopsy. The target may be selected from the stereotactic CT or MRI or both, by placing a cursor over the point selected on the imaging studies. The computer immediately calculates the stereotactic coordinates (Fig. 20.2). The most pathologic, and thus most diagnostic, tissue is found in areas of contrast enhancement [11–14]. Low attenuation on CT, or increased T2 signal on

MRI, surrounding an area of contrast enhancement may represent edema or parenchyma infiltrated by tumor cells [10]. When dealing with a cystic or centrally necrotic lesion, the center of the lesion may be targeted for biopsy or aspiration and drainage. Serial biopsies along a trajectory traversing the target permit sampling of all abnormal areas.

The computer display of the images and calculation of stereotactic coordinates offer distinct advantages in target selection. First, the selected target can be displayed on the stereotactic angiogram (Fig. 20.2). This permits visualization of the vascular anatomy relative to the target, and may influence target selection. Second, the

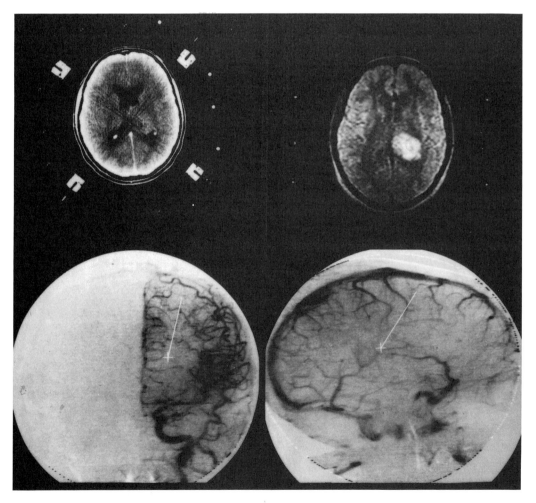

FIGURE 20.2 A target may be selected from the stereotactic CT or MRI by placing a cursor over the area of interest. Digitizing the fiducial artifacts allows calculation of the stereotactic coordinates of the target. The computer places the selected target on the stereotactic angiogram and various collar and arc angles can simulate the trajectory to the target.

rapid calculation of stereotactic coordinates permits the target to be changed and reviewed on the angiogram without delay. Lastly, the rapid calculation and storage of target coordinates allows the selection and retrieval of multiple targets. This can be useful in patients with multiple lesions, or patients who require a therapeutic intervention (such as IIIrd ventriculostomy [15]) in addition to biopsy (Figs 20.3 and 20.4).

Once a target for stereotactic biopsy has been selected, the trajectory, or surgical approach, to the target is planned. In planning a trajectory, consideration must be given to the nature of the brain tissue to be traversed, the vascular structures that may be encountered, and the

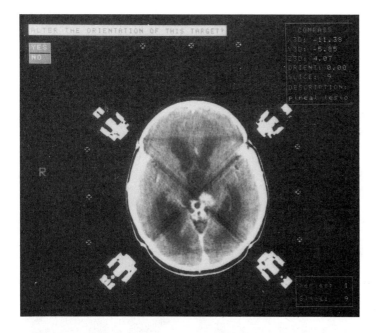

FIGURE 20.3 Biopsy target in a patient with a pineal region tumor and hydrocephalus.

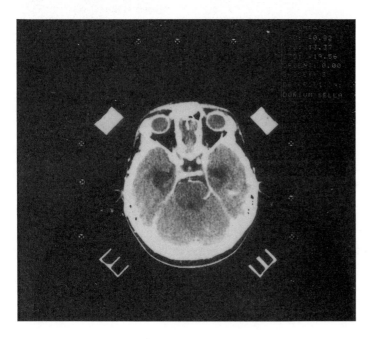

FIGURE 20.4 A second target is selected behind the dorsum sellae for a IIIrd ventriculostomy (same patient as Fig. 20.3).

location of the ventricular system. Although the biopsy probe creates little parenchymal injury *per se*, a trajectory through eloquent cortex is best avoided if at all possible. Major vascular structures must be avoided to prevent an intracerebral hemorrhage. Traversing a ventricle carries the risk of intraventricular hemorrhage from disruption of ependymal veins. Also, biopsying near a ventricle may lead to the selective aspiration of cerebrospinal fluid rather than tissue.

Computer simulation plays a critical role in trajectory planning. The target is visualized on the stereotactic angiogram and an infinite num-

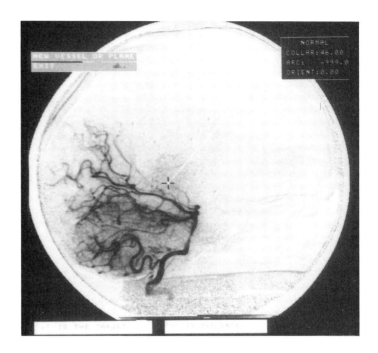

FIGURE 20.5 The trajectory for the biopsy is simulated and stored (same patient as Fig. 20.3).

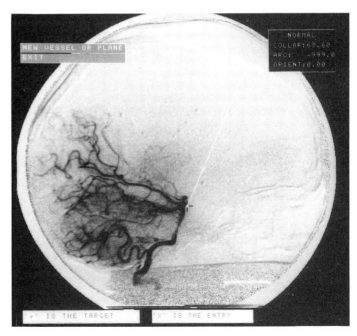

FIGURE 20.6 The IIIrd ventriculostomy trajectory is simulated and stored (same patient as Fig. 20.3).

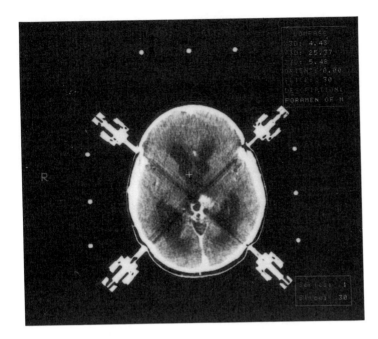

FIGURE 20.7 A second target point is digitized at the foramen of Monro for stereotactic IIIrd ventriculostomy.

ber of approach angles (collar and arc) can be visualized (Fig. 20.2). The trajectory is displayed on the angiogram and its relationship to critical arterial and venous structures viewed directly [7]. This permits the use of a twist drill opening and blind perforation of the dura and cortex, avoiding a burr hole. The computer simulation allows multiple trajectories to be previewed quickly and an appropriate trajectory selected. If multiple targets are to be accessed, the computer will store the trajectories that are selected for each target (Figs 20.5 and 20.6).

The storage and processing of stereotactic data by a computer also permits calculation of a trajectory from two points. An entry point may be selected from the stereotactic CT or MRI and the computer will calculate the corresponding collar and arc angles to traverse the two points [5]. In the case of IIIrd ventriculostomy, a target is selected behind the dorsum sellae and a second target is selected at the foramen of Monro (Figs 20.4 and 20.7). The computer calculates the appropriate collar and arc angles of a trajectory through these two points [15] (Fig. 20.8).

After a particular trajectory has been selected, the computer can display the trajectory on the stereotactic CT or MRI as well as the angiogram. This is done on serial images if the trajectory traverses multiple image planes, or on a single image if the trajectory lies within the plane of the image. The computer also calculates and displays the distance to the target from any point on the trajectory. This information permits precise selection of biopsy sites along the trajectory (Figs 20.9 and 20.10). With this information it is possible to correlate radiographic findings with histologic findings [11,12]. The simultaneous display of the trajectory on the stereotactic angiogram, CT, and/or MRI permits the surgeon to be confident that appropriate biopsies can be obtained, while avoiding vascular and ventricular structures.

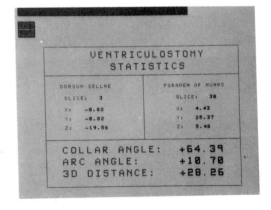

FIGURE 20.8 The computer will calculate the appropriate collar and arc angles for a trajectory to pass through the foramen of Monro to the target behind the dorsum sellae.

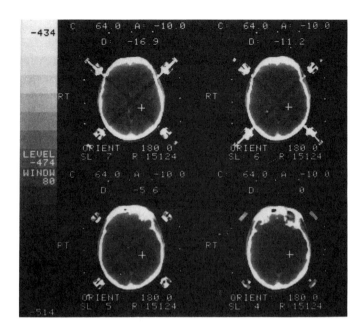

FIGURE 20.9 Serial CT images demonstrating the simulated trajectory and the distance to the target.

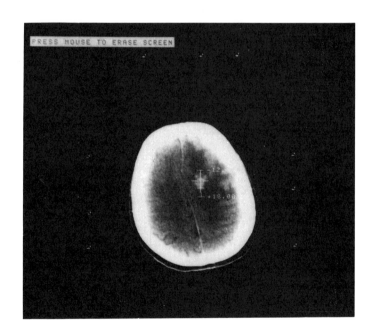

FIGURE 20.10 CT image with a simulated trajectory and distances for biopsy locations.

Conclusions

The computer is a critical element in image-based stereotactic biopsy of intracranial lesions. The non-invasive imaging of the intracranial contents by CT or MRI is dependent on computers, as is the acquisition of stereotactic images. Stereotactic angiography, which adds a new dimension to stereotactic biopsy, could not be accomplished without computerization. Computer simulation allows for the rapid selection of targets and calculation of their stereotactic coordinates. The trajectory of the biopsy probe can be previewed on the angiogram, CT, and/or MRI, permitting a rehearsal of the biopsy procedure that is planned. Changes in the target or trajectory can be made preoperatively as dictated by vascular or ventricular anatomy. Biopsy sites can be planned to include any radiographic abnormality with precision. The net result is a safer and more diagnostic procedure for the patient. Improvements in diagnosis can hopefully be paralleled by improvements in treatment.

References

1 Apuzzo, M.L.J., Chandrasoma, P.T., Cohen, D., Zee, C. & Zelman, V. Computed imaging stereotaxy: experience and perspective related to 500 procedures applied to brain masses. *Neurosurgery* **20**: 930−7 (1987).

2 Davis, D.H., Kelly, P.J., Marsh, W.R., Kall, B.A. & Goerss, S.J. Computer-assisted stereotactic biopsy of intracranial lesions. *Appl. Neurophys.* **50**: 172−7 (1987).

3 Lunsford, L.D. & Martinez, A.J. Stereotactic exploration of the brain in the era of computed tomography. *Surg. Neurol.* **2**: 222−30 (1984).

4 Spiegel, E.A., Wycis, H.T. & Lu, A.J. Stereotaxic apparatus for operations on the human brain. *Science* **106**: 349−50 (1947).

5 Kelly, P.J., Earnest, F. IV, Kall, B.A., Goerss, S.J. & Scheithauer, B. Surgical options for patients with deep-seated brain tumors: computer-assisted stereotactic biopsy. *Mayo Clin. Proc.* **60**: 223−9 (1985).

6 Heilbrun, M.P., Roberts, T.S., Apuzzo, M.L.J., Wells, T.R. Jr, & Sabshin, J.K. Preliminary experience with Brown−Roberts−Wells (BRW) computerized tomography stereotaxic guidance system. *J. Neurosurg.* **59**: 217−22 (1983).

7 Kelly, P.J. Computer-assisted stereotaxis: new approaches for the management of intracranial intra-axial tumors. *Neurology* **36** (4): 535−41 (1986).

8 Kelly, P.J., Alker, G.J. Jr, Kall, B.A. & Goerss, S. Method of computed tomography-based stereotactic biopsy with arteriographic control. *Neurosurgery* **14**: 172−7 (1984).

9 Kelly, P.J., Kall, B.A. & Goerss, S. Computer-assisted stereotactic resection of posterior fossa lesions. *Surg. Neurol.* **25**: 530−4 (1986).

10 Kelly, P.J., Goerss, S.J. & Kall, B.A. Modification of Todd-Wells stereotactic system for imaging data acquisition. In: Lundsford, L.D. (ed.) *Modern Stereotactic Surgery*, pp. 79−97. Boston: Martinus Nijhoff (1988).

11 Kelly, P.J., Daumas-Duport, C., Scheithauer, B.W., Kall, B.A. & Kispert, D.B. Stereotactic histologic correlations of computed tomography and magnetic resonance imaging-defined abnormalities in patients with glial neoplasms. *Mayo Clin. Proc.* **62**: 450−9 (1987).

12 Kelly, P.J., Daumas-Duport, C., Kispert, D.B., Kall, B.A., Scheithauer, B.W. & Illig, J.J. Imaging-based stereotaxic serial biopsies in untreated intracranial glial neoplasms. *J. Neurosurg.* **66**: 865−74 (1987).

13 Heilbrun, M.P. *Stereotactic Neurosurgery, Vol. 2. Concepts in Neurosurgery*. Baltimore: Williams & Wilkins (1988).

14 Chandrasoma, P.T. & Apuzzo, M.L.J. *Stereotactic Brain Biopsy*. New York: Igaku-Shoin Medical Publishers (1989).

15 Kelly, P.J., Goerss, S., Kall, B.A. & Kospert, D.B. Computed tomography-based stereotactic third ventriculostomy: technical note. *Neurosurgery* **18** (6): 791−4 (1986).

21

Dose Planning for Interstitial Irradiation

*Lucia Zamorano, Bernhard Bauer-Kirpes,
Manuel Dujovny, and Daniel Yakar*

Introduction

Intratumoral implantation of radioactive sources constitutes a radiobiologically effective model of treatment of malignant tumors [1–8]. The aim is to achieve a high intratumoral radiation dose without damaging the surrounding healthy brain tissue. This highly localized treatment requires a three-dimensional (3-D) configuration of the isodose distribution curves adjusted to tumoral volume and shape. Computer processing of image data allows an accurate definition of the target volume in three dimensions [9]. Computer dose calculations for interstitial implants of radioactive seeds are based on the knowledge of the spatial coordinates for each seed. To avoid migration of seeds, and to allow their removal if the patient develops undesired effects, we place them into coaxial catheters.

High speed computation and graphic capabilities of modern workstations have allowed the implementation of 3-D planning systems for interstitial radiotherapy; its main advantage is the display of the dose distribution within and outside the target volume. The goal is to find the optimal irradiation parameters, such as number and position of catheters, and number, activity, and spacing of seeds. These parameters can be optimized by using either a trial-and-error method or some automatic optimization computational technique. These must be chosen in such a way that a therapeutically sufficient dose reaches the target without damaging healthy tissue or critical structures. Technical aspects of 3-D planning, fundamentals of dose planning for interstitial radiotherapy, and implantation methodology are presented.

Performance of 3-D image-guided stereotactic interstitial radiotherapy involves three steps:

1 Image data acquisition.
2 3-D dose planning.
3 Intraoperative stereotactic procedures.

Stereotactic image data acquisition

Since treatment planning requires exact knowledge of the anatomy of the patient, the planning system uses a series of axial CT or MRI scans as a 3-D tissue model. Stereotactic image data acquisition generally requires an imaging modality, which can be basically tomographic — such as computed tomography (CT) or magnetic resonance imaging (MRI) — or projective — such as digital subtraction angiography (DSA), a fixed reference system, and a method of interfacing both of them.

To provide a stereotactic reference, images are acquired with a base ring (Riechert–Mundinger; Zamorano–Dujovny, Fisher, Freiburg, Germany) fixed to the patient's skull (Fig. 21.1) [10]. The stereotactic ring defines the stereotactic coordinate system. The origin is the center of the ring and coordinates are

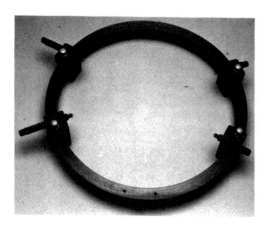

FIGURE 21.1 Z–D (Zamorano–Dujovny) base ring made of carbon fiber to allow compatibility with CT, MRI, and angiography.

defined as x (right–left), y (anterior–posterior), and z (superior–inferior) to this origin (Fig. 21.2).

To interface the image data with the reference system, different approaches can be used, depending upon the type of image modality, i.e. tomographic versus projective.

TOMOGRAPHIC IMAGING (CT, MRI)

An alternative is the use of the isocentric re-lationship of the ring with the CT gantry or MRI coiler. Advantages of this methodology include the direct measurement of coordinates in mul-tiple planes using available software; disadvan-tages are that very accurate movement of the operating table is required, and the isocentric relationship needs to be assessed at the begin-ning of every procedure [11].

The other alternative (the two are not ex-clusive) is the use of CT- or MRI-compatible localizers attached to the ring, which provides landmarks for stereotactic target localization in the scans [12,13]. This can be a very cumber-some method if done manually, but by using computer graphics capabilities these landmarks can be measured automatically as a background task. The tomographic image acquisition needs to include the volume of interest with equi-distant slices. The scan parameters, e.g. pixel size, image matrix, must not be changed be-tween the individual slices. The spatial resol-ution (pixel size and slice distance) is chosen according to the required stereotactic accuracy. A slice thickness of between 1.5 and 3.0 mm is considered as appropriate. The CT or MRI data are then stored on a magnetic tape which can be used to transfer the data to the work-station, or a direct transfer can be done using networking capabilities.

PROJECTIVE IMAGE (CONVENTIONAL ANGIOGRAPHY) OR DSA

Although vessels can be seen in contrasted CT scans and using special sequences on MRI, it is sometimes desirable to determine precisely the vascular anatomy surrounding the target vol-ume using conventional or DSA data. In this case, X-ray localization can be used to measure stereotactic coordinates of a point found in two orthogonal radiographs. This is particularly use-ful for verification of the target and entry point of a catheter before the dosimetric planning. The opposite is also possible: a trajectory, which has been defined in the tomographic images and is therefore known in stereotactic coordi-nates, can be projected into the two radio-graphs. With this procedure critical intersections of a catheter's trajectory with vascular structures can be detected, and the trajectory changed, if necessary.

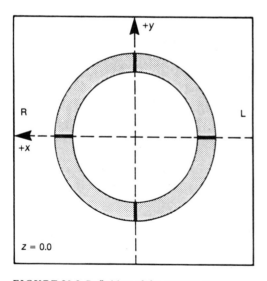

FIGURE 21.2 Definition of the stereotactic coordinates system. The origin is in the center of the ring plane.

For stereotactic localization in X-rays, the classical teleradiography or an angiolocalizer can be used. The classical teleradiography uses two orthogonal far distant X-ray tubes which are perfectly aligned with the stereotactic x and y axes. If the source–image and source–target distances, and thus the magnification factors, are known, the stereotactic coordinates of a target can be measured from anterior–posterior (A/P) and lateral films [13].

Teleradiography implies a high cost; if the equipment is not available, an angiolocalizer alone with computer calculations can be used for stereotactic target localization [13]. The localizer consists of four radiolucent plates that rigidly attach to the stereotactic base ring. A rectangle made of steel wires is embedded in each plate. The coordinates of the rectangle corners are precisely known with respect to the stereotactic coordinate system. The X-ray information can be processed in two ways:

1 Markers and target points can be digitized from the films with a digitizing table.

2 To display X-ray images on the computer screen, the X-ray films can be digitized with a video camera or grabbed directly from the video signal going to the monitor of a digital angiography unit. In the lateral and A/P images, the corners must be digitized. A mathematic analysis of the projected corners establishes the relationship between the film orientation and the stereotactic coordinates system. By knowing this relationship, target points can be digitized in the films and translated into stereotactic coordinates, and information from the CT images, such as target and entry points defining catheter trajectories, volumes of interest, etc., can be projected onto the angiographic films.

Three-dimensional and multiplanar stereotactic dosimetry for interstitial radiotherapy using CT data

The stereotactic planning system presented (STP, Fisher, Freiburg, Germany) uses a VAX GPX-II workstation, VMS operating system, and specially developed software (Fig. 21.3). The first step is the transfer of CT data to the workstation: tapes are read by the planning system which stores the CT data in an appropriate format on the hard disk. Since CT images are

stored in Hounsfield units, the CT scans can be displayed with appropriate gray level window settings on the graphics monitor during the course of the treatment planning. Furthermore, sections can be reformatted through the stack of CT scans in sagittal, coronal, and oblique directions. For the treatment planning, graphic information is superimposed on these axial and reformatted CT scans, such as stereotactic trajectories of the catheters or isodoses. This makes it possible to evaluate a particular plan on the basis of the CT information. Thus stereotactic trajectories or dose distributions can be related to the underlying tissue structures.

TARGET VOLUME DEFINITION

Target volume can be defined by the neurosurgeon, drawing contours on each tomographic slice using the pointer device ("mouse") of the workstation. Contours need to be digitized on a series of tomographic images to define several regions (areas) of interest, such as the tumor borders or certain organs at risk. The neurosurgeon and radiotherapist define the regions to be treated and, depending on clinical factors, this may correspond to borders of lesion, or borders with a margin if considered safe. Computer interpolation transforms this series of areas (pixels) into a target volume (voxels). Although cumbersome, there are several reasons to define volumes of interest through contours:

1 During the course of the planning these contours are plotted in axial images and in reformatted sections (coronal, sagittal, para-axial planes), which is helpful in defining the catheter's trajectory, or checking the intersection of catheters with critical structures, or in assessing the isodoses.

2 These objects can also be measured (length, volume), which will be helpful in the quantitative analysis of the planning.

3 To elucidate the spatial relationship between the various objects or between the target volume and isodoses, the objects can be displayed as solid 3-D models.

4 The automatic source optimization of the seed implantation program needs the target volume to be described by a set of contours.

5 Dose–volume histograms can be generated

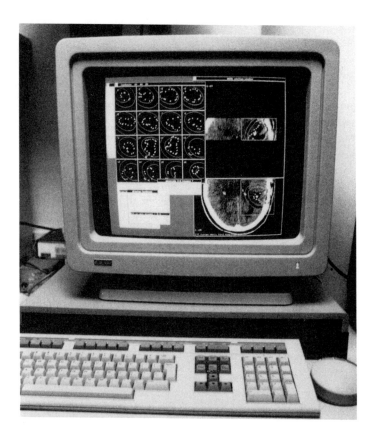

FIGURE 21.3 Three-dimensional and multiplanar stereotactic dose planning system.

to describe the dose distribution within a volume of interest.

Contours can be defined manually or automatically. Contours which should be digitized manually, such as the target volume, are outlined in the slices on the screen using the mouse. Objects of significant contrast can be segmented automatically, using a threshold technique. The user selects a threshold CT value and a starting point inside the volume of interest. A program then traces the contour along this threshold until a closed loop has been formed. This process can be checked visually to provide a possibility of rejecting incorrect contours. Additionally, a 3-D wireframe of the contours can be displayed which allows an easy detection of faulty contours. These contours can be deleted and manually digitized.

STEREOTACTIC COORDINATES MEASUREMENT

As mentioned, the images have been acquired under stereotactic conditions using a base ring

as reference. To define a catheter's trajectory, two points are necessary: one can be the target point and another the entry point. The relationship of these points to the target volume is arbitrary, but we have found it useful to define the first point ("target") in the lower border of tumor and the second point ("entry") in the superior margins. If there are no anatomic contraindications, the catheters will usually follow the main axis of the tumor. Of course the line can be extended up to the skull to visualize in multiple planes the relationship to surrounding anatomy. Any point defined on the images can be correlated to x, y, and z coordinates.

The computer allows automatic computation of stereotactic coordinates, using either the isocentric relationship or the localizers. The wires of the localizer appear as reference points in the tomographic slices. The position of the reference points in these images is automatically determined, and from this the position of the stereotactic coordinates system is calculated relative to the CT coordinates system. Since the position of the reference points cannot be determined any better than the spatial resolution of a CT scan (pixel size, slice distance), the landmarks of the localizer wires are searched in a series of tomographic slices. With the assumption that the landmarks are distributed statistically around their "true" position, a straight line is fitted into the measured points. With this mechanism the accuracy of the stereotactic coordinate transformation can be better than the CT voxel size [13]. The program detects any tilts of the stereotactic system, which are accounted for in the transformation of the coordinates. This makes it possible to calculate the stereotactic coordinates of any point in the image. Once the relationship between the CT and the stereotactic coordinate system is established, a stereotactic target point obtained from other imaging modalities, such as MRI or DSI, can be displayed in the appropriate tomographic slice.

CATHETER DEFINITION: PLANNING STEREOTACTIC TRAJECTORIES

Stereotactic localization makes it possible to simulate and optimize the catheter's trajectory. As mentioned, two points are necessary to define a trajectory. This can be done directly by defining the points in the axial images with the mouse, and then calculating its stereotactic coordinates or, by defining a point, entering stereotactic coordinates taken from another image modality, such as angiography, and then drawing it in the CT scans.

Once a stereotactic trajectory is defined by two points, for example the proximal and distal ends on the longitudinal axis of a lesion, the relationship of the catheter to the target volume and surrounding anatomic and vascular structures can be displayed and interactively optimized on axial and reformatted images. Useful features in catheter planning are:

1 The projection and the intersection point of the defined catheter with the displayed CT slice is marked.

2 The intersection point of the catheter with any reformatted coronal or sagittal section is marked.

3 An oblique section in the plane of the catheter is reconstructed showing the entire "real" pathway of the catheter.

4 A 3-D image of the target volume, critical

structures, and the catheter's trajectories can be displayed and presented as movie loops.

This makes it possible for the neurosurgeon to examine the trajectory and to make sure, for example, that no critical structures are in the pathway of the catheter, in which case the position can be corrected. To measure the length of a given catheter inside the target volume, an oblique section in the direction of the trajectory is reconstructed and the length can be measured in this image. This information is useful to determine the number of seeds which can be placed in this catheter.

DOSE PLANNING FOR SEED IMPLANTATION

Three-dimensional and multiplanar dosimetric programs allow computerized simulation of planning, interactive changes in implantation parameters, and interactive or automatic optimization. The dose planning is finalized once the optimal seed configuration for achieving a certain dose distribution is determined.

The stereotactic implantation of catheters can be simulated by defining catheters, as previously mentioned. These catheters are then loaded with seeds, which are positioned within the catheter. Seed parameters include the seed activity, time of implantation, and spacing between seeds. This latter feature, one of the advantages of this 3-D dosimetric system, allows different distances between seeds to provide a better adjustment to tumoral shape. For the same seed configuration, different times can be entered to study the dose distribution at different times. This specific program accepts implantation times from 1 hour (dose rate) up to permanent implantation.

Seed data input

The seed configuration is determined by stereotactically defined catheters and by the seeds they contain having different activities and positions within the catheters. The catheters can be defined either by digitization of two points directly into the tomographic images or by entering the stereotactic coordinates. The planned trajectories are automatically stored on a disk file. The seeds are "loaded" into the catheter by assigning them an initial activity, an implantation time, a seed type, and the position in the catheter relative to the target point.

Dose calculation

For the entered seed configuration, the dose distribution is calculated in a 3-D grid. Its size and location can be set interactively to cover any region of interest. The dose that has accumulated during the entire implantation time can then be calculated at all matrix points, using measured and published dose data [14–16]. The program needs to consider the decrease of activity due to radioactive decay over the implantation time. The dose rate can be calculated by specifying a 1 hour implantation time. At our Institution we have used mainly ^{125}I seeds. The dose calculation for ^{125}I seeds is based on measurements that have been published by numerous authors [14–16]. There is a dose table for each seed type, to which the calculation algorithm has access. The dose distributions can be described by means of formulae adapted to the measured values. This also allows simple manual calculation at individual test points. A calculation point is expressed in spherical coordinates relative to the seed (Fig. 21.4). The dose is broken down into a radial and an angle-dependent part. These are calculated by polynomials and multiplied for the dose.

The accumulated dose at point *P* is a function of the seed activity, implantation time, and the polar coordinates of *P* relative to the seed:

$$D(r,a) = act . tf . DR(r,a)$$

where D = accumulated dose at P (cGy); act = apparent activity of seed (mCi); tf = time factor; and $DR(r,a)$ = dose rate (cGy hour^{-1} mCi^{-1}).

The time factor, *tf*, is given by:

$$tf = \lambda^{-1} (1 - \exp(-t . \lambda))$$

where t = implantation time (hour); and λ = decay constant = ln 2 $T_{1/2}^{-1}$ (hour^{-1}) ($T_{1/2}$ is the half life).

The dose rate per milliCurie (mCi) at point *P* is approximated by a product of factor *B*, which is radius-dependent, and factor *W*, which is angle-dependent:

$$DR(r,a) = B(r) . W(a)$$

For a fast dose calculation, the *B* and *W* factors can be precalculated and stored in dose tables for the individual seed types:

B factors are stored for $0 < r \leqslant 200$ mm in steps of 0.1 mm.
W factors are stored for $0 < = \cos(a) \leqslant 1$ in steps of 0.0001 mm.

These tables are calculated for 6701, 6702, and 6711 seeds (3M Company) using polynomial parameters obtained from published data [14–16]. Dose tables for other source types such as ^{192}Ir can also be generated from published or measured data.

Planning optimization: interactive and automatic

To accelerate the trial-and-error method of conventional treatment planning, computers offer the possibility of automatic optimizing procedures [17]. Its objective is to change the source configuration in such a way that a selected isodose surface can be adjusted as close as possible to the target volume surface. The program then moves the catheters and varies the seed activities until the optimal seed configuration has been found. The resulting dose distribution can then be analyzed with the various isodose displays. If some changes of the seed configuration are still necessary, the operator can change the seed configuration interactively

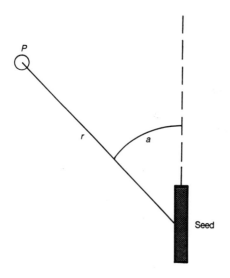

FIGURE 21.4 Seed dose calculation. r = radius; a = angle; P = point.

using the trial-and-error method. A trial-and-error method of seed dose planning is laborious and time-consuming. Therefore, an automatic optimization for a manually defined seed configuration is an important contribution of a planning system. To be able to optimize a seed plan, three variables need to be defined:

1 What is the definition of an optimum dose distribution? How can this criterion be expressed in a mathematic formula (called an objective function)? Can the objective function be calculated in a reasonable time?

2 Which parameters of a seed configuration may be modified and which are parts of a clinical decision and may therefore not be changed by software?

3 Which is the best mathematic algorithm to minimize the objective function?

Objective function For small brain tumors, homogeneity of dose is less important than the choice of an appropriate surface dose and steep dose fall-off beyond the target surface. This is reflected in the objective function, which gives a measurement of how well a given isodose surface is adjusted to the target surface. With "real" targets, often very asymmetrically shaped, and due to the limitations of a restricted number of planes (catheters) as well as isotope characteristics, a compromise always must be found. This is reflected in the so-called weight factor which "weights" the influence of underdosed surface points into the objective function. The objective function Q is then defined as:

$$Q(b) = \Sigma_i \, W_i \cdot (N - D_i(b))^2$$

where $i =$ the index for all surface points; $b =$ the vector of optimization variables; $N =$ dose required at tumor periphery; $D_i =$ calculated dose at point i; and $W_i =$ weight factor, with:

$W_i = w$, if $D_i < N$
$W_i = l$, if $D_i <\, = N$

Optimization parameters The direction of the catheter is determined mainly by the choice of the trephination point. This is a clinical decision and therefore should not be changed by the program. The trajectory was defined interactively by the neurosurgeon on the basis of image and anatomic information, as described

earlier. The implantation time is another clinical decision, which is determined by radiobiologic considerations and practical aspects. If, for example, a dose of 60 Gy should be administered (with an average dose of 50 cGy $hour^{-1}$), an implantation time of 6 days must be chosen. Thus the target point of the catheters and the activity of the seeds are the variables for an automatic optimization process. If only selected activities are available, the optimization can be performed in two steps. At first an optimum is searched for, without restrictions on the activities. Then those activities from the seed pool are chosen which are closest to the optimum values. Then optimization is repeated, allowing the variation of the target points of the catheter in such a way that the optimal trajectory is defined for the specific seed configuration.

Optimization procedure Optimization is carried out with an algorithm which modifies the set of variables in several iteration steps, so that the objective function decreases. The variation of the parameter vector b is a step in an n-dimensional space, which is uniquely defined by direction and length:

1 The direction of the step is given by the negative gradient of the objective function at the actual position. This direction is then modified to accelerate convergence by being rotated in the direction of the anticipated minimum.

2 The length of the step in this direction is determined by a linear minimizing procedure, which searches for the minimum of the objective function along the previously determined direction.

This algorithm provides, after only a few iteration steps, an optimum seed configuration. The optimization loop is finished either if the maximum number of iteration steps is reached, or when no further improvement on the objective function can be obtained.

Isodose display: qualitative analysis

The dose distribution can be visualized by isodoses of any value. Isodoses can be superimposed on any axial CT scan (Fig. 21.5) or reformatted section (Fig. 21.6). The 3-D dose distribution, together with the total volume, can be visualized by displaying simultaneously a series of target contours with selected isodoses (Fig. 21.7). Finally, a solid 3-D model with an isodose as wireframes can be generated and rotated to analyze the planning [18] (Fig. 21.8).

Dose—volume histogram: quantitative analysis

To evaluate the dose distribution in any volume of interest, such as the target volume or critical structures, dose—volume histograms can be generated (Fig. 21.9). They give easy access to statistical data such as the minimum or maximum dose in a given volume, how much of a volume receives a determined radiation dose or more, and the median dose in a volume.

Protocol output

An implantation protocol can be printed when the dose distribution has met the requirements. It contains the catheters' stereotactic coordinates and catheter loading in terms of seed activities and spacer length.

Calculation of aiming device parameters

The setting parameters of the stereotactic aiming device are automatically calculated by the computer. In the case of the Riechert—Mundinger, which is a polar coordinates system, four angles and a depth are calculated. With the Zamorano—Dujovny, a semiarc localizing sys-

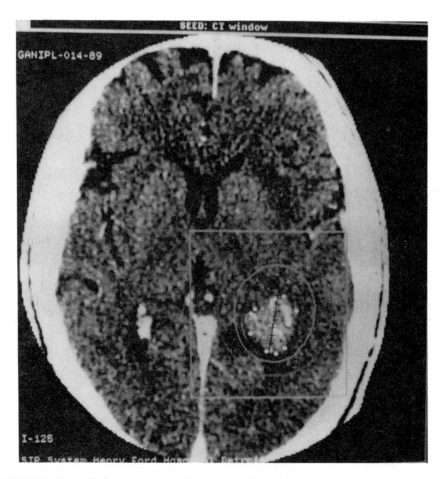

FIGURE 21.5 Patient with deep temporal glioblastoma multiforme diagnosed by stereotactic biopsy. Postoperatively the patient received external radiation therapy (50 Gy) at a dose rate of 200 cGy day^{-1}. Two weeks later planning is done for local boost with ^{125}I brachytherapy. Axial CT scan showing target, projection of catheter, and 60, 40, and 20 Gy isodose lines, representing total dose after 10 days of implant.

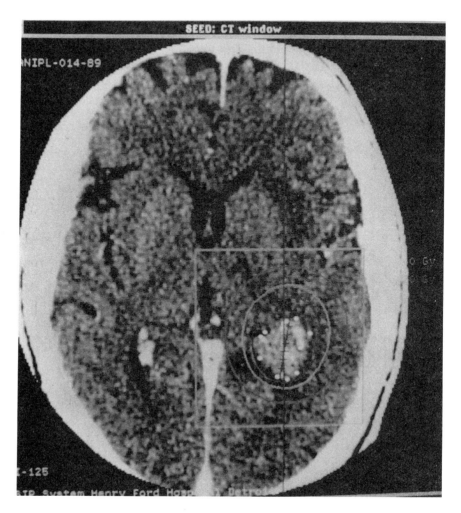

FIGURE 21.6 Same patient as Fig. 21.5. Sagittal reformation showing target volume, catheter projection, and 60, 40, and 20 Gy isodose lines.

tem, the target point is set up directly in the aiming device and two angles define the trajectory [19].

Intraoperative stereotactic procedure

The stereotactic catheter placement is generally done under local anesthesia and completely sterile conditions. The aiming device is set up and the entry level is marked with a rigid needle. A small incision is made and a 1 cm burr hole is made. The dura is coagulated and incised in a cruciate fashion. We prefer direct visualization of the cortical surface in order to avoid damage to cortical vessels (Fig. 21.10). Usually, serial biopsies at different levels are taken to confirm diagnosis and/or to correlate

the histologic extent of lesion with the image data [20]. The catheters are inserted using the calculated aiming device parameters. Different catheters can be inserted through the same or different burr holes, according to the optimized preplanned trajectories. The intraoperative procedure will continue according to the type of implant, whether temporary or permanent, which ultimately means high versus low dose rate.

In the case of low dose rate or permanent implants, catheters are loaded intraoperatively with a coaxial catheter containing the seeds in the precalculated configuration; this approach is used when sources are less than 5 mCi. The preloaded coaxial catheters are brought from the Radiation Therapy Department in a pro-

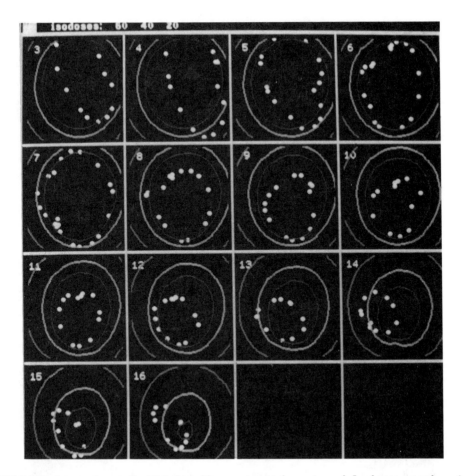

FIGURE 21.7 Same patient as Fig. 21.5. Dotted lines represent the contours defined as target volume in the axial CT scans. The 60, 40, and 20 Gy isodose lines are superimposed on each contour.

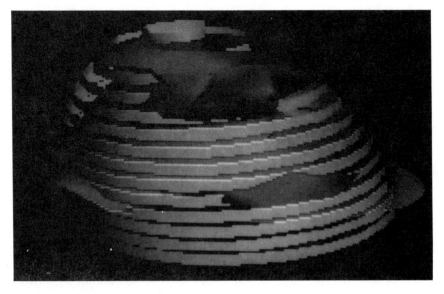

FIGURE 21.8 Same patient as Fig. 21.5. The tumor is shown on a 3-D solid model and the wire lines represent the 60 Gy isodose. Under- and overdosed regions can be visualized.

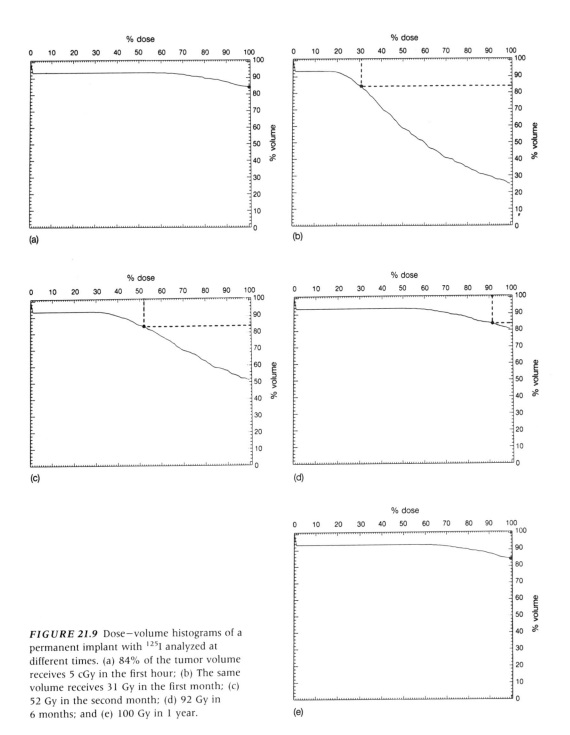

FIGURE 21.9 Dose−volume histograms of a permanent implant with ^{125}I analyzed at different times. (a) 84% of the tumor volume receives 5 cGy in the first hour; (b) The same volume receives 31 Gy in the first month; (c) 52 Gy in the second month; (d) 92 Gy in 6 months; and (e) 100 Gy in 1 year.

tected container and are sterilized. Once loaded into the stereotactically placed catheter, a button is used to keep the distal end of the catheters in position by means of glue. The excess catheter length is cut off and the wound is closed. Radiation is measured, and usually in these cases is in the range of maximum permissible dose. In some cases, where we intend to achieve a higher dose rate and the catheters need to be implanted more than 7 days, we prefer to load the catheters intraoperatively and close the wound to limit the risk of infection. If radiation measure-

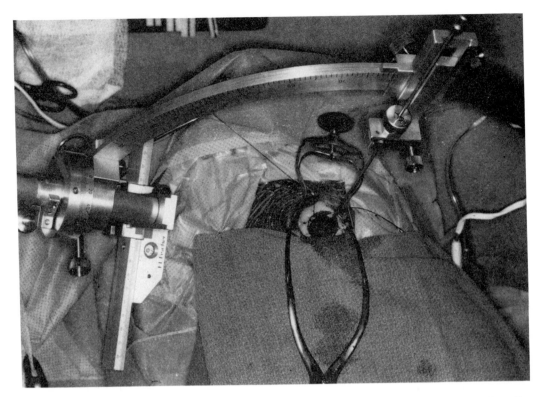

FIGURE 21.10 Intraoperative view. The Z−D aiming device parameters have been set up and a rigid needle is used to take biopsies from the lesion at different levels. Posteriorly the needle will be removed and replaced by the catheter.

ments are greater than the maximum permissible dose, a shielding device is applied. On the planned day of removal, the patient is brought to the operating room and the catheters are taken out under local anesthesia.

In the case of temporary implants of 7 days or less, catheters are stereotactically implanted, the wound is closed, and the catheters are secured externally to a button sutured to the skin. Catheters are loaded with dummy seeds and a postoperative CT scan is performed to confirm the position of the catheters in the desired location. The catheters will be loaded in a protected room where the patient will remain under radiation protection guidelines until the time of removal of the catheters in the same room.

Conclusions

Computer calculations and graphic capabilities contribute to optimized dosimetry for interstitial radiotherapy. The capability of quantitative and qualitative analysis of a specific plan in three dimensions enormously enhances the possibilities of understanding the *in vivo* radiobiology of tumors and normal brain tissue. From the dosimetric point of view, improvements in automatic optimization, including seed spacing, are necessary. From the clinical point of view, interstitial radiotherapy represents a very promising technique that improves survival in the case of brain tumors [3,5,6]. Refinements in surgical techniques for decrease of tumor volume [21,22] may lead to an increase in the number of patients considered for local delivery of high-dose radiation. Many questions need to be answered, such as necessary total minimal dose according to the histologic type of tumor, optimal dose rate, temporary versus permanent implants, relationship between external and interstitial radiotherapy in the management of malignant lesions, response of normal surrounding structures, maximum volume to be implanted, etc. [1−8]. In addition, combined use of hyperthermia and radiosensitizers needs to be evaluated. Clearly, additional clinical experience as well as basic research are necessary to answer these fundamental questions. 3-D dosimetry under stereotactic conditions offers an accurate procedure for optimization of the distribution of radiation to the target volume and minimizing the risk of normal brain damage, as well as providing an important research tool to evaluate tumor and brain tissue responses.

References

1 Findlay, P., Wright, D., Rosenow, U., Harrington, F. & Miller R. [125]I interstitial brachytherapy for primary malignant brain tumors: technical aspects of treatment planning and implantation methods. *Int. J. Radiat. Oncol. Biol. Phys.* **11**: 2021−6 (1985).

2 Gutin, P., Phillips, T., Hosobuchi, Y., *et al.* Permanent and removable implants for the brachytherapy of brain tumors. *Int. J. Radiat. Oncol. Biol. Phys.* **7**: 1371−81 (1981).

3 Gutin, P., Leibel, S. & Wara W. Recurrent malignant gliomas: survival following interstitial brachytherapy with high activity ^{125}I sources. *J. Neurosurg.* **67**: 864−73 (1987).

4 Mundinger, F. & Weigel, K. Long-term results of stereotactic interstitial curietherapy. *Acta Neurochir.* (suppl.) **33**: 367−71 (1984).

5 Mundinger, F. Dosimetry in imaging-stereotactic interstitial curietherapy (brachycurietherapy) with ^{192}Ir and [125]I: application in non-resectable brain tumors and recurrences. *Neurosurgery: State of the Art Reviews* **4** (suppl.). Philadelphia: Hanley & Belfus (1989).

6 Yakar, D., Zamorano, L., Dujovny, M., *et al.* Interstitial temporary implantation of high activity [125]iodine sources for malignant glioma and brain metastases. *Int. J. Radiat. Oncol. Biol. Phys.* (suppl.) **17**: 228 (1989).

7 Zamorano, L., Dujovny, M., Malik, G., Mehta, B. & Yakar, D. Multiplanar CT-guided stereotaxia and ^{125}I interstitial radiotherapy: image-guided tumor volume assessment, planning, dosimetric calculations, stereotactic biopsy and implantation of removable catheters. *Appl. Neurophysiol.* **50**: 281−6 (1987).

8 Zamorano, L., Dujovny, M., Yakar, D., Malik, G., Chavantes, C. & Mehta, B. Multiplanar image-guided stereotactic brachytherapy with [125]iodine. *Neurosurgery: State of the Art Reviews* **4** (suppl.): 95−103. Philadelphia: Hanley & Belfus (1989).

9 Zamorano, L., Dujovny, M., Flynn, M. & Ausman,

J. 3D−2D multiplanar workstation for neurosurgical stereotactic planning. Presented at 9th International Congress of Neurological Surgery, New Delhi, India, October 8−13, 1989.

10 Zamorano, L., Dujovny, M., Chavantes, C., Block, R. & Flynn, M. 2−D multipurpose neurosurgical image-guided localizing unit. Presented at Xth Meeting of the World Society for Stereotactic and Functional Neurosurgery, October 2−5, 1989.

11 Zamorano, L., Dujovny, M., Malik, G. & Mehta, B. Factors affecting measurements in computed tomography-guided stereotactic procedures. *Appl. Neurophysiol.* **50**: 53−6 (1987).

12 Sturm, V., Pastyr, O., Schlegel, W., *et al.* Stereotactic computer tomography with a modified Reichert−Mundinger device as the basis for integrated stereotactic neuroradiological investigations. *Acta Neurochir.* **68**: 11−17 (1983).

13 Siddon, R. & Barth, N. Stereotaxic localization of intercranial targets. *Int. J. Radiat. Oncol. Biol. Phys.* **13**: 1241−6 (1987).

14 Hartmann, G.H., Schlegel, W. & Scharfenberg, H. The third dimensional dose distribution of ^{125}I seeds in tissue. *Phys. Med. Biol.* **28**: 693−9 (1983).

15 Ling, C., Schell, M., Yorke, E., Palos, B. & Kibuiatowicz, D. Two-dimensional dose distribution of ^{125}I seeds. *Med. Phys.* **12**: 652−5 (1985).

16 Schell, M., Ling, C., Gromadzki, Z. & Working, K. Dose distribution of model 6702 ^{125}I seed in water. *Int. J. Radiat. Oncol. Biol. Phys.* **13**: 795−9 (1987).

17 Bauer-Kirpes, B., Sturm, V., Schlegel, W. & Lorenz W. Computerized optimization of ^{125}I implants in brain tumors. *Int. J. Radiation Oncol. Biol. Phys.* **14**: 1013−23 (1988).

18 Bauer-Kirpes, B., Schlegel, W., Boesecke, R. & Lorenz, W. Display of organs and isodoses as shaded 3-D objects for 3-D therapy planning. *Int. J. Radiat. Oncol. Biol. Phys.* **13**: 135−40 (1987).

19 Zamorano, L., Martinez-Coll, A. & Dujovny, M. Transposition of image-defined trajectories into arc-quadrant centered stereotactic systems. *Acta Neurochir.* (suppl.) **46**: 95−103 (1989).

20 Zamorano, L., Katanick, D., Dujovny, M., Yakar, D., Malik, G. & Ausman, J. Tumor recurrence vs. radionecrosis: an indication for multitrajectory serial stereotactic biopsies. *Acta Neurochir.* (suppl.) **46**: 90−3 (1989).

21 Kelly, P., Kall, B., Goerss S. & Cascino T. Results of computer-assisted stereotactic laser resection of deep-seated intracranial lesions. *Mayo Clin. Proc.* **61**: 20−7 (1986).

22 Zamorano, L., Chavantes, C., Dujovny, M. & Malik, G. Image-guided stereotactic resection of intracranial lesions: endoscopic and laser technique. *Neurosurgery: State of the Art Reviews* **4** (suppl.): 105−18. Philadelphia: Hanley & Belfus (1989).

part V

Interactive Intraoperative Applications

chapter 22

Computer Interactive Volumetric Stereotactic Resection of Brain Mass Lesions

Patrick J. Kelly

Introduction

Computed tomography (CT) and magnetic resonance imaging (MRI) indicate the boundaries of most intracranial lesions. Computer-assisted reconstruction of these CT- and MRI-defined contours allows the interpolation of a three-dimensionally (3-D) derived volume. If these imaging studies are performed in stereotactic conditions, that interpolated volume can be suspended in stereotactic space and resected, utilizing stereotactic methods. Precision resection of a tumor volume by computer-assisted and interactive stereotactic craniotomy presents one application of "volumetric stereotaxis."

This interactive computer procedure has been discussed at presentations in numerous meetings and in many publications over the past 8 years [1–9]. Time and space constraints usually limit the discussion of the procedure to the bare bones technological descriptions of what is being done now. The usual reaction from colleagues has been: "That's too complicated. We need something simpler."

Other centers are now beginning to do and report stereotactic craniotomies with commercially available stereotactic frames. Simplicity and low cost are cited as the major advantages of their methods over those reported by us [10]. However, our procedures started as simple procedures [11,12]. We soon found that without a computer these procedures were neither time-efficient nor practical. We acquired a computer

and began developing the software and necessary technology for computer-assisted volumetric resection. As clinical experience was acquired, technical innovations increased the facility and accuracy with which these operations were performed.

Historical aspects

Manual methods for stereotactic tumor resection

Our group began performing CT-based stereotactic resections of deep-seated intracranial lesions in 1979 [11,12]. Our first attempts at volumetric stereotactic procedures evolved from radiographically-based functional neuroablative procedures [11,12]. Axial CT information was transferred to collimated anterior–posterior (A/P) and lateral radiographs, obtained with the patient's head in the stereotactic frame. In the older generation CT scanners, we found that an X-ray film, attached to the side of the "water bag" during CT scanning, was exposed, and demonstrated a skull radiograph with horizontal artifacts in the precise location and inclination of each CT slice [13]. These A/P and lateral X-ray scatter films, obtained during non-stereotactic CT scanning, were then enlarged by opaque projector to the precise magnification of, and superimposed onto, the stereotactic radiographs.

Measurements taken from the outer table of the skull to anterior and posterior margins of a tumor on each CT slice were marked on the stereotactic radiographs at the appropriate CT slice level. Connecting the points from the various CT slice level lines produced a CT-defined contour on the lateral stereotactic radiograph. For the A/P projection, measurements were taken from the midline.

Newer generation CT scanning units provided the capability for sagittal and coronal reconstructions which could also be projected onto stereotactic radiographs [14]. Briefly, the midline sagittal reconstruction was projected to proper magnification onto the lateral stereotactic radiograph by an opaque projector. Various landmarks of the bony calvarium and skull base, identified on the CT reconstruction, were aligned to their counterparts on the lateral stereotactic radiograph. The image data window (the four corners of the image display) was transferred to the radiograph by four marks at each corner. Then sagittal reconstructions through the tumor were projected onto the radiograph, the data window aligned to the marks, and the tumor contours were traced onto the radiograph.

Surgical trajectory

A hole was drilled in the skull by means of a drill directed by the stereotactic frame. Then a hollow biopsy cannula was directed through the axis of the tumor. A small amount of methylene blue was injected as the cannula was withdrawn. This marked the surgical tract in the brain. A trephine craniotomy was done and, after dural opening, a cortical and subcortical incision was made and deepened, following the methylene blue tract to the tumor.

Resection procedures

In stereotactic resections, tumor removal by carbon dioxide (CO_2) laser was monitored by intraoperative A/P and lateral radiographs. The surgical cavity was filled with a Hypaque^R-soaked fluffy cotton ball, which resulted in excellent visualization of the cavity [12].

The object of the procedure, stated as simply as possible, was to produce a hole in the brain having the same location, size, and configuration as the CT-defined lesion. However, this method only helped us to *find* the tumor. It did not provide a conceptualization of the 3-D tumor volume, did not orient the surgeon within that volume, and did not demonstrate where tumor stopped and normal brain began.

Stereotactic laser procedures

The CO_2 laser was, and is still, used in the stereotactic resection of deep tumors [11,12, 15]. There are several reasons for this: (1) it is a convenient tool for removing tissue from within a deep cavity; (2) it is relatively hemostatic; and (3) the position of the laser beam focus in space can be determined by computer and appropriate interfacing, and its position displayed on a monitor [1,3]. However, for this last feature to be realized, the laser beam must be directed from a known point in space. Therefore we developed a 400-mm radius arc-quadrant, which fits onto the base unit of the Todd-Wells frame. A microscope and laser micro-manipulator (microslad) were fixed to this arc-quadrant, which directed the central focus of the microscope and the central axis of the laser beam to the focal point of the arc-quadrant [1−3,12]. The laser beam was deflected from its central axis by means of a mirror, which was manipulated by a joystick on the microslad.

Computer monitoring of laser position

The CO_2 and He−Ne laser aiming beams are delivered by articulated optical arm to a microslad fixed to the operating microscope. The beams pass through a variable focus lens system (which changes the focal length and spot size) and, in the microslad, are reflected by a mirror into the surgical field. The pitch of the mirror which deflects the laser beam is controlled by joystick, which is manipulated by the surgeon. The joystick can pass through a double gimble, the axes of which are connected to potentiometers or optical encoders. Signals from the potentiometers or optical encoders are transmitted to the computer which, from the position of the joystick and the focal working length (from mirror to surgical field), calculates the position of the laser beam in the surgical field.

The computer can then display the correct position of the laser beam as a cursor in relationship to an *x, y* grid centered on the surgical viewline. Reconstructions of the CT- and MRI-defined tumor volumes, sliced perpendicular to the viewline, are also displayed. However, for calculation of the beam's position, the precise position of the microslad's mirror system in space must be known. It was for this reason that we originally mounted the microscope on the 400 mm diameter arc-quadrant system in the so-called Kelly–Goerss system.

Computer-assisted interactive stereotaxis

BACKGROUND EXPERIENCE

Our group has used several computer systems for volumetric stereotaxis. Upgrades were necessary as we found the limitations of the system which we were using.

Initially we acquired a Data General Eclipse S140 minicomputer, with 128 Kbyte main memory, 25 Mbyte disk storage (Data General Corporation, Watertown, MA), and Tektronix 4014 vector display unit [1]. CT scan stereotactic fiducials and tumor outlines were entered by means of a digitizing tablet. The position of a surgical laser in the stereotactic operating field was inputted by means of an $x-y$ gimbal on the microslad joystick corrected to x and y potentiometers. The output of the potentiometers led to the game paddle ports of an Apple II microprocessor PC in the operating room. This was connected to the minicomputer by data link. By means of a Tektronix simulator board, the Apple II displayed the position of the laser, represented by a cursor on the displayed tumor slice contours. This system worked, but the displays were poor, the interactive link was slow, the human interface in digitizing the CT scan cumbersome, and the disk capacity was inadequate for further development.

We then upgraded to a Data General Eclipse S140 minicomputer system and Ramtek Raster Image Display system. This system included a disk storage device of 192 Mbytes, which was initially adequate for stereotactic CT databases on several patients as well as the necessary programs for the procedure [3,4]. This was identical to the host computer and display system for a General Electric 8800 CT scanning unit (Independent Physicians Diagnostic Console (IPDC), General Electric Medical

Systems, New Berlin, WI). When General Electric upgraded their CT scanner to the 9800 series, a rewrite of the stereotactic software was necessary in order to take account of the different display formats and increased screen resolution inherent in this device. However, addition of stereotactic MRI, and stereotactic digital subtraction angiographic (DSA) databases to the CT database consumed 25–30 Mbytes bulk storage for each patient on the system. With a large volume of stereotactic procedures, there was barely room on computer disk storage to retain patient databases to accomplish the stereotactic operating room schedule for a single day. When surgery had been completed, patient's data had to be "dumped" from the disk in order to make room for other patients who were awaiting surgery that day. On a busy day, this process had to be repeated two or three times.

FURTHER UPGRADES

We upgraded to a Data General (DG) MV7800 super minicomputer system. This had 2 Mbytes of main memory and 700 Mbytes disk storage. In addition, the relatively slow input/output speed of the minicomputers in general for image processing, prompted us to acquire a Vicom VME image processing system (Vicom Systems Inc., Fremont, CA), which used the super minicomputer as its host computer. Unfortunately, programs for the minicomputer systems were written in FORTRAN 5, software for the DG MV7800 was in FORTRAN 77, and many display routines were in PASCAL. We had to upgrade our stereotactic software for this new system. Nevertheless, this was accomplished and the MV7800 system was on line in early 1987.

Shortly thereafter, Vicom Systems Inc. decided to change its image processing host computer from Data General systems to the Sun Microsystem 3/260 (Sun Microsystems Inc., Mountain View, CA). Continued support for the "obsolete" computer system then became a concern.

We changed computers again, and acquired a Sun 3/260, a UNIX-based system. The stereotactic software was modified yet again for the Sun 3/260 and the UNIX operating system. The software was rewritten into PASCAL and "C" programming languages. The Data General MV7800 was retained as a backup, primarily for bulk storage and patient database archiving.

Vicom Systems began supplying new imaging processing systems with a Sun 4/300 workstation host, and offered upgrades to its customers, which we acquired. Again software was modified for efficient operation on the Sun 4/300.

Therefore, at the present time, the computer system which supports volumetric stereotaxis consists of a Sun 4 workstation with a Vicom VME image processor.

STEREOTACTIC FRAME EVOLUTION

A new stereotactic system evolved from a Todd-Wells frame which had been modified for CT compatibility [16]. The present system and its predecessors in this evolutionary process were based on the arc-quadrant concept.

In an arc-quadrant stereotactic frame, the patient's head, fixed in a rigid headholder, is moved with three orthogonal degrees of freedom (x, y, and z) in order to position an intracranial target point into the focal point of a fixed sphere, which is defined by the arc-quadrant. A probe inserted perpendicular to the tangent of the arc-quadrant, and to a depth equal to its radius, will arrive at the focal point of the arc-quadrant. All approaches to the target point are therefore described by two angles: collar (angle from the horizontal plane), and arc (angle from the vertical plane). Thus, there are six simple mechanical adjustments: three axes (x, y, and z), two angles (collar and arc) and a probe depth. In addition, the patient's head in the headholder can be rotated to any position, which provides a comfortable working situation for the surgeon.

An "N"-shaped CT localization system was developed and eventually reported [5]. This was based on the inclined plane concept described by Goodenough *et al.* [17] and also used by Brown [18], Perry *et al.* [19], and Boethius *et al.* [20].

COMPASS™ STEREOTACTIC SYSTEM

The COMPASS™ stereotactic system (Stereotactic Medical Systems, New Hartford, NY) was specifically designed for volumetric tumor stereotaxis. The system consists of a fixed arc-quadrant, 3-D slide, and removable headholder. It can be fixed onto a semipermanent base unit or mounted onto the lateral support rails of a standard operating table (Fig. 22.1). The details of this system are presented in Chapter 6.

OTHER INSTRUMENTS FOR VOLUMETRIC STEREOTACTIC RESECTIONS

Stereotactic retractors

A stereotactic retractor system was developed for the COMPASS™ system. This consists of cylindrical retractors, dilators, and an arc-quadrant adapter [21]. The retractor is a thin-walled hollow cylinder, 140 mm in length and 2 cm in diameter. Indexing marks on the retractor shaft are provided for measurement of insertional depth with respect to the stereotactic arc-quadrant. The retractor cylinder is directed perpendicular to the tangent and toward the focal point of the stereotactic arc-quadrant. Dilators, which fit inside the retractor cylinder, are 1 cm longer than the retractor. The distal end of the dilator is wedge-shaped (like the bow of a ship), and spreads an incision to the diameter of the retractor, so that the retractor cylinder can be advanced.

The retractor maintains exposure and creates a shaft from the surface of the brain to the superficial aspect of deep-seated tumors. In addition, the retractor also has a known configuration (a cylinder). Since it is directed to a given depth by the stereotactic arc-quadrant, the distal end of the retractor also has a known location in stereotactic space. It therefore provides a fixed stereotactic reference structure in the stereotactic subglial field. Computer-generated slice reconstructions of the CT/MRI-defined tumor volume are related to the position of the distal end of the retractor [21].

Accessory instruments

A variety of custom-made extra-long instruments are necessary in the stereotactic resection of deep tumors. Bipolar forceps with a working shaft length of 150 mm are required to control bleeding in the surgical field when working

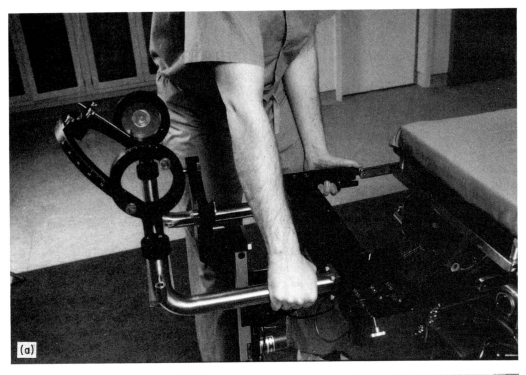

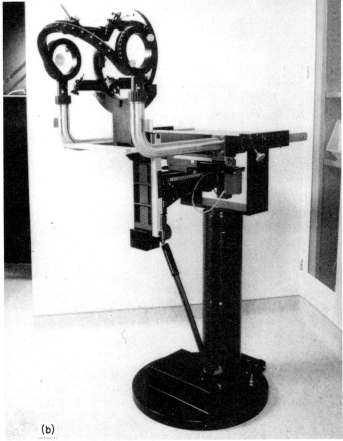

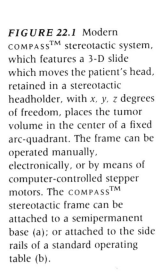

FIGURE 22.1 Modern COMPASS™ stereotactic system, which features a 3-D slide which moves the patient's head, retained in a stereotactic headholder, with x, y, z degrees of freedom, places the tumor volume in the center of a fixed arc-quadrant. The frame can be operated manually, electronically, or by means of computer-controlled stepper motors. The COMPASS™ stereotactic frame can be attached to a semipermanent base (a); or attached to the side rails of a standard operating table (b).

through the stereotactic retractors. In addition, 150–160 mm-long suction tips, dissectors, and alligator scissors are also used.

Heads-up display for the operating microscope

We developed a system by which the computer-generated slice images are transmitted to a small video monitor mounted on the operating microscope. This image, scaled to actual size, is optically superimposed on the surgical field viewed through the microscope. The computer-generated slice images displayed on the video monitor are scaled by a system of lenses to the desired size. Thus, through the microscope the surgeon sees the actual surgical field and the superimposed computer-generated CT- and MRI-based rendition of that field. In addition, when the image of the cylindrical retractor, reflected into the microscope by the heads-up display unit, is superimposed over the distal end of the retractor in the surgical field, the microscope is optically indexed to the stereotactic surgical field.

INTERACTIVE STEREOTACTIC RESECTION

With appropriate software for the transposition of volumetric information derived from axial stereotactic CT scans and MR images into 3-D space, the operating room computer system is used to monitor and display the position of stereotactically directed instruments in relation to computer-generated reconstructions of the tumor volume. The following will describe the instrumentation and methodology now employed for computer-assisted volumetric stereotactic extirpation of intra-axial lesions. The clinical results of these procedures will then be discussed.

Computer-assisted stereotactic laser microsurgical procedures are performed in three phases: database acquisition, treatment planning, and the interactive procedure. Because of the carbon fiber pin–osseous fixation system and micrometer measurement procedure which is described below, the stereotactic headholder is replaceable. Thus, following application of the headholder, the database acquisition, which consists of stereotactic CT, MRI, and DSA examinations, can be performed on one day. The

headholder can then be removed and later reapplied for the actual surgery, which is performed when convenient. This is a system which ensures efficient use of the operating room in a busy neurosurgical practice.

DATA ACQUISITION

Local anesthesia is employed for most stereotactic headholder application procedures. The headholder is secured to the patient's skull by the carbon fiber pin fixation system. After headholder placement, micrometer measurements are obtained which measure the exposed length of the carbon fiber pin extending beyond the fixed vertical support elements of the headholder. These measurements are recorded and used again when replacing the headholder for subsequent data acquisition or surgical procedures.

Following frame application, the patient undergoes stereotactic CT, MRI, and DSA examinations as follows.

A CT table adaptation plate receives the stereotactic headholder CT localization system, which consists of nine carbon fiber localization rods arranged in the shape of the letter "N," located on either side of the head and anteriorly, to create nine reference marks on each CT slice (Fig. 22.2). Stereotactic CT scanning is done on a General Electric 9800 CT scanning unit, gathering 5 mm slices through the lesion, utilizing a medium body format.

Stereotactic MRI examinations are performed on a General Electric 1.5 tesla Signa unit. The MRI localization system consists of capillary tubes filled with copper sulfate solution, which are arranged in basic "N"-shaped sets located bilaterally, anteriorly, posteriorly, and superiorly. These create reference marks on each transverse, coronal, or sagittal MR image, from which stereotactic coordinates may be calculated for any point on that image.

Stereotactic DSA is performed in each and every stereotactic tumor case, for two reasons. A DF adaptation plate fixes to the table of the General Electric DF 3000 and 5000 Digital Angiographic units and receives the stereotactic headholder. A DSA localization system consists of lucite plates, which contain nine radiopaque reference markers. This unit fixes to the base

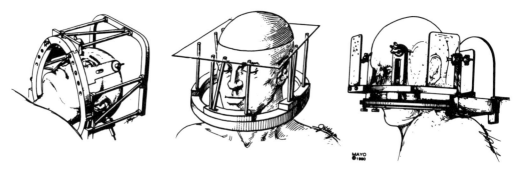

FIGURE 22.2 Stereotactic coordinates are determined by means of reference artifacts created on planar or projection images. The reference artifacts are produced by rods or radiopaque markers for planar (CT or MRI) or projection (DSA) modalities, which have known geometrical relationships.

ring of the stereotactic headholder and positions the lucite plates on each side of the patient's head and anteriorly and posteriorly. The radiopaque markers create 18 reference marks on each A/P and lateral DSA image (see Fig. 22.2). The mathematical relationships between the fiducial marks and their locations on the DSA images allow calculation of magnification in any depth plane, and allow establishment of a distortion correction grid, which corrects for non-uniformity of the images. The known distances between the reference marks on the lucite plates, the measured distances between those marks on the radiographs, the calculated magnification factors, and the distortion grid, permit calculation of the stereotactic coordinates for any point or points on intracranial blood vessels, but also allow display of the correct position of stereotactic target points and volumes which have been derived from CT and MRI on angiographic images.

DSA is performed utilizing the standard femoral catheterization and radiographic techniques used in diagnostic angiography. Orthogonal and 6° oblique arterial and venous phases are obtained in orthogonal and 6° rotated stereoscopic pairs. Indexing marks (6°) on the base ring of the stereotactic headholder base ring are aligned to ensure precise 6° rotation for the stereoscopic pair.

Surgical planning

Following data acquisition, the archived magnetic data tapes from the CT, MRI, and DSA examinations are transferred from the respect-

ive host computers and read into the operating room computer system. This computer system is located directly above the operating room equipped for stereotactic surgery. A treatment planning console is located above the operating rooms and in the induction room between the two stereotactic operating rooms (Fig. 22.3). The computer system can also be accessed from a keyboard or mouse/menu system in each operating room, or by means of a sterile joystick/menu system on the operating table.

The nine reference marks on each CT slice and MR image are detected automatically by an intensity detection algorithm. This suspends the position of each slice in a 3-D computer image storage matrix. The 18 reference marks on the arterial and venous DSA images are digitized by box cursor, which is manipulated by the mouse subsystem. This creates a series of matrices for each fiducial set (e.g. right and left on lateral views) on each image. Data is then added to each of these image matrices by manipulating the cursor and depressing the deposit key on the mouse. The computer reads the screen position of the cursor and transmits these screen coordinates, and deposits each point into the correct position within the appropriate image matrix.

The procedure used to create a tumor volume in stereotactic space has been described in more detail elsewhere [3,22,23]. Briefly, the surgeon first traces around the outline of the lesion defined by the various imaging modalities on all sequential slice images which show the lesion. Thus, a series of contours is established for the boundary defined by CT contrast enhancement,

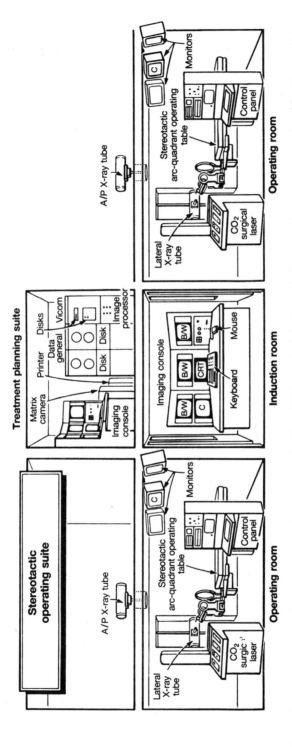

FIGURE 22.3 Arrangement of stereotactic operating rooms at the Mayo Clinic (author's institution). Two operating rooms are equipped for stereotactic surgery. Each is equipped with A/P and lateral fixed-tube laser collimated teleradiographic equipment, COMPASS™ stereotactic systems, and video display monitors suspended from the ceiling. A computer room, which houses the central processing unit and disk storage units with planning console, is located on the floor directly above the operating room. A second imaging console, located in an induction room between the operating rooms, is provided for intraoperative stereotactic calculations.

CT hypodensity T1- and T2-weighted signal abnormalities of the MRI and the Gadolinium-enhanced boundaries. Each of these digitized contours is suspended in computer image matrix. A computer program then interpolates intermediate slices at 1 mm intervals between the digitized contours. Volumes are created in defined stereotactic space by filling in each of the digitized and interpolated slices with 1 mm cubic voxels. Finally, a central target point is digitized on a CT or MRI slice. Stereotactic coordinates for this point are calculated. These coordinates (x, y, and z) are actually mechanical settings which position that point into the focal point of the stereotactic arc-quadrant frame. The interpolated tumor volume is constructed around that point, and all subsequent image displays and frame translations relate to that point.

Each volume is assigned an identifying gray level, so that slices through the matrix can display these individually or all together on a computer raster display monitor. However, before one can view these slice images, the angle of the slice and its position within the matrix must be specified. The former translates to the viewline and the latter is the slice depth. The viewline is the surgical approach to a central point within the tumor volume (which is positioned in the focal point of the stereotactic arc-quadrant), defined mathematically and expressed in angles from the horizontal and vertical planes, which are, in fact, collar and arc angle settings on the stereotactic frame respectively.

The slice depth refers to a plane perpendicular to and along that viewline, expressed in millimeters above or below the central target point. The next step is to define the viewline by selecting the surgical approach.

The stereotactic surgical approach to the lesion is planned, taking its 3-D shape and important overlying cortical regions, subcortical white matter pathways and vascular structures into account. Ideally, tumors should be approached through non-essential brain tissue and in a direction parallel to major white matter fiber tracts. In addition, deep sulci, localized stereotactically from stereotactic MRI or stereoscopic DSA, provide a route for the approach to, and exposure of, deep-seated lesions. In this

case an entry point in the superficial aspect of the sulcus is selected, and the trajectory or viewline is determined from target and entry points.

In summary, the actual surgical approach (or viewline) is expressed in stereotactic frame adjustments (collar = angle from the horizontal plane; arc = angle from the vertical plane), which access a selected point within the interpolated tumor volumes from an entry point on the surface of the brain. The CT- and MRI-defined tumor volumes, residing within the image storage matrix, are sliced perpendicular to the intended surgical approach angles.

There is one more option which frequently proves useful — patient rotation. The base ring of the COMPASS™ stereotactic headholder is circular, and the patient's head can be rotated to any position which will provide a comfortable working position for the surgeon. Indexing marks at 5° intervals on the base ring align with a reference mark on the yoke of the 3-D slide system. Thus a patient with a right central laterally lying tumor is operated on in the left-side-down lateral decubitus body position, with the head and base ring of the headholder rotated to 270°. This rotation parameter is entered into the computer, which adjusts the x, y, and z stereotactic frame settings, and updates arc and collar angles to account for this rotation. Therefore, the final viewline will depend on patient rotation, arc, and collar angles.

Surgical procedures

The technical aspects of the surgical procedure will depend on whether the lesion is located superficially or deeply. In both procedures, the patient is positioned and the base ring fixed in the receiving yoke of the 3-D slide system at the proper rotation position after the x, y, and z adjustments for the target have been inputted. The computer-generated slice images will serve as a *guide* to help a surgeon identify the plane between tumor and surrounding brain tissue.

In the approach to superficial lesions, the stereotactic instrument is used to center a circular trephine of known diameter over the tumor. The relationships between the computer display of the circular trephine, superimposed by the "heads-up" display onto the actual trephine in the surgical field, and slices from the CT- and/ or MRI-defined tumor volumes, will orient the surgeon during dissection around and removal of the neoplasm with the CO_2 laser. Deep tumors are removed through a cylindrically shaped retractor, utilizing a stereotactically directed and computer-monitored CO_2 laser.

Superficial lesions

Procedural aspects The patient is placed under general endotracheal anesthesia. The stereotactic headframe is replaced using the same pin holes in the skull, pin placements, and frame micrometer settings utilized during the data acquisition phase. The patient is then positioned in the stereotactic frame. The frame rotation angle is set and entered into the computer program, and the computer calculates frame adjustments which place the center of the tumor into the focal point of the stereotactic arc-quadrant accounting for this rotation. After prepping and draping the head, the stereotactic arc-quadrant is positioned. The selected arc and collar approach angles are set on the instrument. Through a stab wound in the scalp a pilot hole is drilled in the outer table of the skull by a stereotactically directed $\frac{1}{8}$ inch drill. The scalp is then opened by a linear incision. A craniotomy is performed using a power trephine centered on the pilot hole. The size of the trephine selected is equal to or slightly larger than the largest cross-sectional area of the tumor viewed from the selected surgical approach angles, which have been determined during the planning phase.

The computer displays, into the "heads-up" display unit of the operating microscope, the configuration of the trephine in relationship to the reformatted tumor outlines (Fig. 22.4). The surgeon then superimposes the graphics image of the trephine over the actual trephine in the surgical field, using the most superficial computer-generated tumor slice as a template. A section of cortex having the same size and configuration as the computer-generated image is removed with bipolar forceps and scissors. We have found that cortex is non-viable when

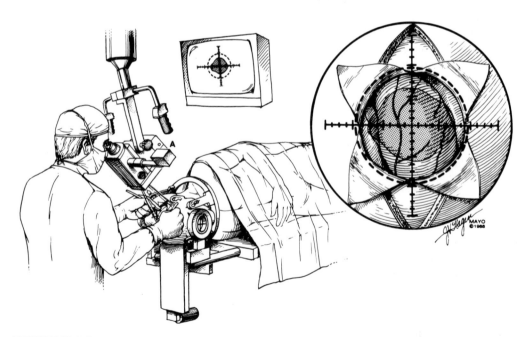

FIGURE 22.4 Stereotactic craniotomy for superficial tumor. A computer-generated image corresponds to the outline of a stereotactically placed trephine as well as the imaging-defined limits of the lesion. These are scaled and superimposed upon the surgical field by the heads-up display unit to aid the surgeon in identifying and developing a plane around a superficial lesion. From Kelly [8].

tumors extend to within 1 cm of the surface. A plane is then developed around the tumor utilizing a CO_2 laser or bipolar forceps.

During tumor resection, the computer displays successive slice configurations of the lesion at successively deeper levels. It is best to first isolate the lesion from surrounding brain tissue and keep the specimen intact. The surgeon interacts with the computer by means of a sterile joystick, a controller system mounted on the operating table, and the menu system which is displayed in the microscope by means of the heads-up display unit. The interior of the lesion should not be entered until late in the procedure, because the walls of the lesion may collapse in on themselves and render subsequent computer-generated slice images no longer accurate. We have found that intermediate and high-grade gliomas can be removed as intact specimens with negligible bleeding. In addition, infiltrated areas of brain parenchyma in low-grade gliomas located in non-essential brain tissue can also be resected in a similar manner.

Deep tumors

The open stereotactic approach to periventricular basal ganglia or thalamic tumors requires stereotactic retractors, extra long bipolar forceps, and dissecting instruments.

The stereotactic retractors are mounted on an internal stereotactic arc-quadrant. The position of these retractors is also indicated on the computer display terminal in the operating room, and in the "heads-up" display unit of the operating microscope (Fig. 22.5). The position of the cylindrical retractor is shown as a circle in the computer display in relationship to the tumor slice. During surgery, the computer-generated image of the retractor is superimposed on the actual view of the retractor in the operating microscope.

A variety of surgical approaches have been developed for various deep tumor locations. These include transcortical, trans-sulcal, trans-sylvian, and interhemispheric exposure. The actual approach selected depends on the proximity of the tumor to deep sulci, which can be

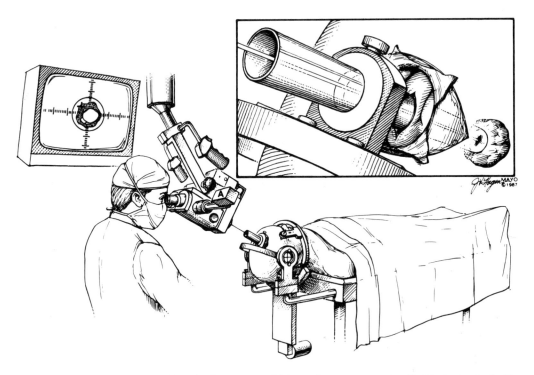

FIGURE 22.5 Stereotactic resection of a deep tumor which employs a stereotactic cylindrical retractor held on the arc-quadrant. The computer monitor demonstrates the position of the distal end of the retractor with respect to slices through the tumor volume, cut perpendicular to the surgical viewline. From Kelly [8].

split microsurgically and spread wide enough to provide adequate exposure. The approach to thalamic tumors depends on whether they are located anteriorly (and thus approached anterosuperiorly), posterodorsally (and exposed through the lateral ventricle by way of the superior parietal lobule), or posteroventrally (and approached posterolaterally). The issue here is the preservation of normal thalamic tissue. Multiplanar MRI is invaluable in defining the anatomic relationships between tumor and normal structures, in order to select the best surgical approach trajectory for stereotactic craniotomy.

The stereotactic resection of deep tumors is performed under general anesthesia, and the patient is replaced in the stereotactic head holder and positioned in the stereotactic frame. The selected target point within the tumor volume is positioned into the focal point of the stereotactic arc-quadrant. In cystic tumors, intraventricular tumors, or those near the ventricular system, the following step may be necessary in order to monitor possible movements of the tumor during the procedure. A series of 0.5 mm stainless steel reference balls are deposited at 5 mm intervals along the surgical viewline in the tumor by a stereotactically directed biopsy cannula inserted through a $\frac{1}{8}$-inch drill hole in the skull. A/P and lateral

radiographs are obtained (Fig. 22.6). The position of these steel balls on subsequent radiographs, following exposure of the lesion, may indicate shifts in the position of the tumor, which can be adjusted in the computer software for updated accurate tumor slice images.

The scalp is opened with a linear incision. A 1½ inch trephine craniotomy is performed and a cruciate opening of the dura accomplished. A linear incision is made in the cortex and then the subcortical white matter incision is progressively deepened with the stereotactically directed CO_2 laser. Alternatively, a convenient sulcus can be split microsurgically and the cortical incision made in the depths of this sulcus.

The direction of the subcortical incision should be through non-essential brain tissue and in a direction parallel to major white matter fibers. As the incision is deepened, the stereotactic retractor is advanced to maintain the developing exposure.

The computer has calculated the range of the tumor along the surgical viewline. At the outer border of the tumor, the laser beam is deflected laterally, a dilator placed through the retractor, and the retractor is advanced. This creates a shaft from the surface to the outer border of the tumor. Using the computer display as a guide, the surgeon creates a plane of dissection around the lesion with the laser, advances the retractor,

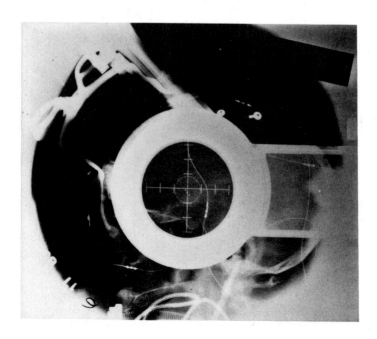

FIGURE 22.6 In cystic tumors, or those located near the ventricular system, a series of stainless steel balls are occasionally placed by means of a stereotactically directed cannula. A/P and lateral teleradiographs are obtained to document their position. Shifts in their position, detected by subsequent radiographs, indicate movement of the tumor volume in intracranial space. Appropriate adjustments of the tumor volume can be made within the 3-D imaging-derived computer matrix, so that updated slice images depict the actual position of the tumor.

and deepens the incision circumscribing the tumor. Tumor tissue within the retractor is then removed with 65–85 W of defocused laser power. The tumor is removed slice by slice, extending from the most superficial slices to the deepest. Hemostasis is secured, utilizing the extra long bipolar forceps. A/P and lateral teleradiographs are obtained to document the progress of the procedure and record possible movements of the reference balls (which are removed as they are encountered during the procedure).

Tumors larger than the retractor opening can be removed as follows. First, one side of the tumor is positioned under the retractor and, with the laser, the surgeon creates a plane between this side of the tumor and brain tissue. The display image is then translated on the computer display terminal to position the other side of the lesion under the retractor. The computer calculates new stereotactic frame adjustments, which are duplicated on the stepper motor-driven slide mechanism of the frame by means of a remote control panel. This side of the tumor is then separated from brain tissue with the laser. After isolating the lesion from surrounding brain tissue, it may then be vaporized by laser as described above.

Ultimately, a cavity is produced in the brain by removal of the lesion. This may be monitored by A/P and lateral teleradiographs, and these may be compared to coronal and sagittal examinations of CT data through the tumor. The cavity produced should resemble the configuration of the tumor in location, shape, and size.

Results

Between August 1984 and August 1989, 374 patients underwent computer-assisted stereotactic craniotomies. Lesion locations are illustrated in Fig. 22.7 and histology, mortality, and morbidity are listed in Table 22.1. Patients ranged in age from 2 to 78 years, with an average age of 46.8 years.

Preoperative neurologic examinations were normal in 181 patients. This included 63 patients who presented with seizures. The remaining 193 patients had a preoperative neurologic deficit. Neurologic examinations performed at discharge from the hospital, or 2 weeks following surgery, revealed that 116 of the 193 patients with preoperative deficits had improved from their preoperative levels. In addition, all of the 63 patients presenting with seizures were seizure-free on medications at the 3-month follow-up examination. Admittedly, longer follow-up will be necessary in this group before any definitive statements regarding long-term seizure control can be made.

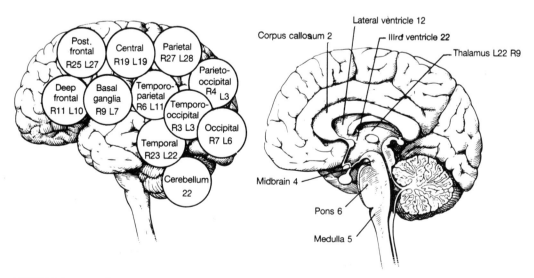

FIGURE 22.7 Localization of 374 lesions resected by computer-assisted stereotactic technique, August 1984–August 1989.

TABLE 22.1 Histologic findings in 374 stereotactic craniotomies

	No.	Total no.	Mortality (%)	Morbidity (%)
Glial neoplasms		205		
Astrocytomas:				
Grade 4	71		1.4	8
Grade 3	15		—	13
Grade 2	15		—	33
Grade 1	5		—	—
Pilocytic astrocytomas	45		2.0	8
Oligodendrogliomas	32			
Oligoastrocytoma	13		—	3
Subependymoma	2		—	—
Ependymoma	4		—	—
Medulloblastoma	1		—	—
Neurocytoma	2		—	—
Non-glial tumors		113		
Metastatic	65		—	6
Meningioma	15		13.0	6
Lymphoma	7		—	—
Choroid plexus papilloma	1		—	—
Ganglioglioma	4		—	—
Colloid cyst	18		—	—
Hemangioblastoma	2		—	—
Teratoma	1		—	—
Non-neoplastic mass lesions		56		
Vascular lesions	36		—	12
Abscess	3		—	—
Cysticercosis	1		—	—
Hematoma	2		—	—
Tuberous sclerosis	4		—	—
Glial scar (epilepsy)	5		—	—
Radiation necrosis	5		—	—
Total		374		

One-hundred and sixty-seven patients were neurologically unchanged postoperatively. Of these 167 patients, 110 had been normal preoperatively, and remained normal postoperatively, and 57 patients had preoperative neurologic deficits which did not improve postoperatively.

Morbidity and mortality

Twenty-eight patients were neurologically worse postoperatively: nine patients were neurologically normal preoperatively and had deficits postoperatively; 16 additional patients experienced worsening of a deficit noted at the preoperative neurologic examination. Postoperative deficits were due to the surgical approach or local perilesional trauma. In 12 of these 28 patients, postoperative neurologic deficits were consistent with neuronal injury along the surgical approach. For instance, eight patients with medial temporal or posterior ventral thalamic lesions sustained a permanent contralateral superior quadrantopsia, and two others had a homonymous hemianopsia following the temporo-occipital approach necessary to resect their lesions. A trans-Sylvian exposure of a left subinsular metastatic tumor produced a contralateral arm dyspraxia in another patient. Finally, a transvermian exposure of a midline cerebellar thrombosed arteriovenous malformation resulted in increased gait apraxia.

The remaining 16 patients who were worse following surgery had deficits consistent with local trauma inflicted in resecting the neoplasm, or disruption of the parenchymal blood supply. Most often, this occurred in high-grade glial neoplasms with peritumoral tumor cell infiltration.

In this series of 374 patients, three deaths occurred within 1 month following surgery: one from massive brainstem edema following removal of a ventral thalamic astrocytoma with brainstem infiltration apparent on MRI; and two from massive pulmonary embolization; one 2 weeks after resection of a large left lateral ventricle meningioma; and the other 6 days after resection of a thalamic glioblastoma.

Postoperative imaging

Figure 22.8 presents representative pre- and postoperative imaging studies in some of the patients in this series. It is clear that a significant

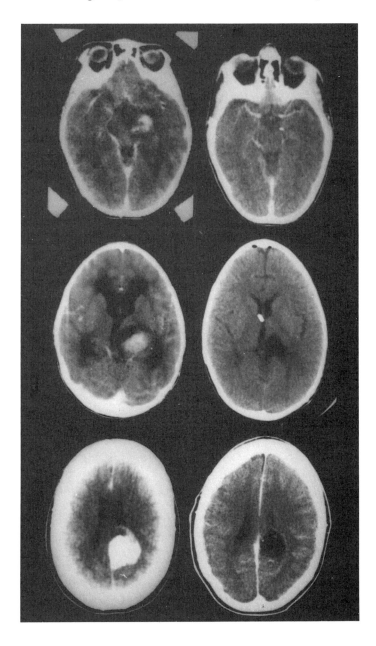

FIGURE 22.8 Pre- (left) and postoperative (right) CT scans in patients with pilocytic astrocytomas, resected from (top) left anterior ventral thalamus; (middle) posterior lateral thalamus; and (bottom) left deep parietal area. All of these patients were neurologically intact following surgery.

amount, if not all, of the tumor detected by the preoperative stereotactic imaging studies can be removed by this method. The long-term followup on the various histologic subgroups of patients has been dealt with in many other publications [5−9,23], and will not be repeated here.

Discussion

One can do stereotactic tumor resections without a computer. We did it. A computer is not essential for stereotactic tumor surgery. Unfortunately, many of the calculations necessary for volumetric stereotaxis and graphic methods for image reconstruction can take hours to perform. In addition, once formulated, intraoperative modifications of the surgical plan, such as changing the viewline, are not really practical using manual methods because of this time factor.

We have found minicomputers or workstations desirable in tumor stereotaxis because they can save surgeons a great deal of time. Target points are calculated instantaneously and imaging-defined tumor volumes are interpolated in seconds to minutes. Cross-registration of points and volumes between CT, MRI, and DSA can be done in real-time [7, 23−27]. The computer makes interactive image displays possible during the actual surgical procedure. In fact, the computer, more than any other factor, makes volumetric stereotactic procedures practical and time-efficient.

There are many computer systems on the market, ranging from microprocessor-based personal computers, through minicomputer and workstations, to super computers. Slow computers in terms of input−output speed and random access memory (RAM) are relatively inexpensive. Computers with high capacity buses with fast input−output speeds and capacious memories are much more expensive.

In theory, most point-in-space and volumetric stereotaxis could be done on contemporary personal computers. The large RAM capacity in many 80386 ('386) machines allows problems to be solved entirely within RAM, where communications are infinitely faster than disk access. Nonetheless, these '386 machines are still much slower, and their capacities are much more limited, than in more expensive minicomputers and workstations. In the selection of a computer system there will always be a trade-off between efficiency time (e.g. during imaging processing and interactive operations) and expense of the hardware.

The computer-interactive surgical technique described in this chapter helps the surgeon maintain 3-D surgical orientation during subcortical procedures. It enables finding the lesion, but also helps the surgeon stay oriented within the lesion. The method can be thought of as an adjunct to standard non-stereotactic neurosurgery: the surgeon not only visualizes and derives information from the surgical field as usual, but also has the added stereotactic information provided by the computer-generated image displays, which demonstrate where the plane between lesion and surrounding brain tissue should be. Furthermore, the surgical approach is simulated on the computer beforehand, and the safest approach possible is selected after appreciating the various anatomic relationships displayed by the imaging system. Therefore, tumors in important subcortical areas may thus be approached in a preplanned way through non-essential brain tissue, and the resection of the lesion is precise. Finally, the actual surgery usually requires less operating time because everything has been planned out beforehand.

With computer-assisted volumetric stereotactic microsurgery, it is possible to resect any preselected volume digitized from CT or MRI. The complex nature of the usual intermediate and high-grade glial neoplasms limits the outright benefit which can be derived from this procedure in these cases. The tumor tissue component of high-grade glial lesions corresponds to the volume defined by contrast enhancement on CT scanning [26−29]. This can be resected. However, some form of adjuvant therapy must be directed at neoplastic cells remaining in the surrounding intact parenchyma, which on CT corresponds to the hypodense zone surrounding the area of contrast enhancement. Nevertheless, in selected cases, a significant reduction of tumor cell burden in high-grade glial neoplasms may favorably influence survival and response to external radiation and chemotherapy [30].

Lesions comprised primarily of infiltrated parenchyma are stereotactically resectable only when they are located within expendable brain tissue. Tumor tissue components do exist in some non-pilocytic low-grade glial lesions. However, tumor tissue in these cases is hypodense on CT scanning and indistinguishable from parenchyma infiltrated by tumor cells [27]. The only method by which the limits of tumor tissue can be determined in these low-grade lesions is by serial stereotactic biopsy, which is done as a separate procedure prior to computer-assisted stereotactic laser craniotomy.

The resection of circumscribed lesions from superficial and deep seated intra-axial locations is very straightforward. For example, pilocytic astrocytomas and metastatic tumors can be completely removed with minimal morbidity from any subcortical location, including the thalamus, by this method. In addition, other circumscribed low-grade glial tumors, thrombosed vascular malformations, and cavernous hemangiomas can be excised totally and these patients can derive significant benefit, frequently in the control of seizures.

In conclusion, computer-assisted volumetric stereotactic craniotomy provides several advantages over conventional freehand neurosurgical techniques in the management of intra-axial mass lesions. First, the stereotactic method maintains surgical orientation as the procedure extends below the cortical surface, the approach being preplanned to disrupt as little important brain tissue as possible. Beyond the gross appearance of a tumor and its apparent margins on visual inspection at surgery, the computer display images provide additional information to the surgeon of where tumor boundaries lie in relationship to surrounding brain tissue. The computer-assisted volumetric stereotactic method allows us to resect as much of a lesion as we choose to remove, and to simulate the surgical approach beforehand. Limitations on resections of glial neoplasms lie in the constraints established by the disease process itself: there may be unresectable intact parenchyma which is infiltrated by isolated tumor cells. Patients with histologically circumscribed glial and non-glial tumors, and non-neoplastic lesions, are the best candidates for computer-assisted stereotactic volumetric resection.

References

1 Kelly, P.J., Alker, G.J. Jr & Goerss, S.J. Computer-assisted stereotactic laser microsurgery for the treatment of intracranial neoplasms. *Neurosurgery* **10**: 324−31 (1982).

2 Kelly, P.J., Alker, G.J. Jr & Zoll, J.G. A micro-stereotactic approach to deep seated arteriovenous malformation: case report and technical note. *Surg. Neurol.* **17**: 260−2 (1982).

3 Kelly, P.J., Alker, G.J. Jr, Kall, B. & Goerss, S. Precision resection of intra-axial CNS lesions by CT-based stereotactic craniotomy and computer monitored CO_2 laser. *Acta Neurochir.* **68**: 1−9 (1983).

4 Kelly, P.J., Kall, B., Goerss, S. & Earnest, F. Computer-assisted stereotaxic resection of intra-axial brain neoplasms. *J. Neurosurg.* **64**: 427−39 (1986).

5 McGirr, S.J., Kelly, P.J. & Scheithauer, B.W. Stereotactic resection of juvenile pilocytic astrocytomas of the thalamus and basal ganglia. *Neurosurgery* **20**: 447−52 (1987).

6 Kelly, P.J., Kall, B.A. & Goerss, S.J. The results of CT-based computer assisted stereotactic resection of metastatic intracranial tumors. *Neurosurgery* **22**: 7−17 (1988).

7 Kelly, P.J. Stereotactic technology in tumor surgery. In: Black, P. (ed.) *Clinical Neurosurgery*, Vol. 35, pp. 215−53. Baltimore: Williams & Wilkins (1987).

8 Kelly, P.J. Volumetric stereotactic surgical resection of intra-axial brain mass lesions. *Mayo Clin. Proc.* **63**: 1186−98 (1988).

9 Kelly, P.J. Stereotactic imaging, surgical planning and computer assisted volumetric resection of intracranial lesions: methods and results. In: Symon, L. (ed.) *Advances and Technical Standards in Neurosurgery*, Vol. 17, pp. 77−118. New York: Springer-Verlag (1990).

10 Moore, M.R., Black, P.McL., Ellenbogen, R., Gall, C.M. & Eldredge, E. Stereotactic craniotomy: methods and results using the Brown−Roberts−Wells stereotactic frame. *Neurosurgery* **25**: 572−8 (1989).

11 Kelly, P.J. & Alker, G.J. Jr. A method for stereotactic laser microsurgery in the treatment of deep seated CNS neoplasms. *Appl. Neurophysiol.* **43**: 210−15 (1980).

12 Kelly, P.J. & Alker, G.J. Jr. A stereotactic approach to deep-seated CNS neoplasms using the carbon dioxide laser. *Surg. Neurol.* **15**: 331−4 (1981).

13 Kelly, P.J., Olson, M.H. & Wright, A.E. Stereotactic implantation of ^{192}Iridium into CNS neoplasms. *Surg. Neurol.* **10**: 349−54 (1978).

14 Kelly, P.J., Olson, M.H., Wright, A.E. & Giorgi, C. CT localization and stereotactic implantation of ^{192}Ir into CNS neoplasms. In: Szikla, G. (ed.) *Stereotactic Cerebral Irradiation*, pp. 123−8. Amsterdam: Elsevier/North-Holland Biomedical Press (1979).

15 Goerss, S., Kelly, P.J., Kall, B. & Alker, G.J. Jr. A computed tomographic stereotactic adaptation system. *Neurosurgery* **10**: 375−9 (1982).

16 Kelly, P.J., Goerss, S.J. & Kall, B.A. Evolution of contemporary instrumentation for computer-assisted stereotactic surgery. *Surg. Neurol.* **30**: 204−15 (1988).

17 Goodenough, D.J., Weaver, K.E. & Davis, D.O. Potential artifacts associated with the scanning pattern of the EMI scanner. *Radiology* **117**: 615−20 (1975).

18 Brown, R.A. A computerized tomography−computer graphics approach to stereotaxic localization. *J. Neurosurg.* **50**: 715−20 (1979).

19 Perry, J.H., Rosenbaum, A.E., Lunsford, L.D., Swink, C.A. & Zorub, D.S. Computed tomography guided stereotactic surgery: conception and development of a new stereotactic methodology. *Neurosurgery* **7**: 376−81 (1980).

20 Boethius, J., Bergstrom, M., Greitz, T. & Ribbe, T. CT localization in stereotactic surgery. *Appl. Neurophysiol.* **43**: 164−9 (1980).

21 Kelly, P.J., Goerss, S.J. & Kall, B.A. The stereotactic retractor in computer-assisted stereotactic microsurgery: a technical note. *J. Neurosurg.* **69**: 301−6 (1988).

22 Kelly, P.J., Kall, B.A. & Goerss, S.J. Transposition of volumetric information derived from computed tomography scanning into stereotactic space. *Surg. Neurol.* **21**: 465−71 (1984).

23 Kelly, P.J. Stereotactic biopsy and resection in thalamic astrocytomas. *Neurosurgery* **25**: 185−95 (1989).

24 Kall, B.A., Kelly, P.J., Goerss, S.J. & Earnest, F. Cross-registration of points and lesion volumes from MR and CT. *Proceedings of the 7th Annual Conference Institute of Electrical and Electronic Engineers Engineering in Medicine and Biology Society, Chicago, IL,* pp. 939−42. (1985).

25 Kelly, P.J., Kall, B., Goerss, S. & Alker, G.J. A method of CT-based stereotactic biopsy with arteriographic control. *Neurosurgery* **14**: 172−7 (1984).

26 Kelly, P.J., Daumas-Duport, C., Kispert, D.B., Kall, B.A., Scheithauer, B.W. & Illig, J.W. Imaging-based stereotactic serial biopsies in untreated intracranial glial neoplasms. *J. Neurosurg.* **66**: 865−74 (1987).

27 Kelly, P.J., Daumas-Duport, C., Scheithauer, B.W., Kall, B.A. & Kispert, D.B. Stereotactic histologic correlations of computed tomography- and magnetic resonance imaging-defined abnormalities in patients with glial neoplasms. *Mayo Clin. Proc.* **62**: 450−59 (1987).

28 Burger, P.C., Dubois, P.J., Schold, S.C. Jr *et al.* Computerized tomographic and pathologic studies of the untreated, quiescent, and recurrent glioblastoma multiforme. *J. Neurosurg.* **59**: 159−68 (1983).

29 Daumas-Duport, C., Scheithauer, B.W. & Kelly, P.J. A histologic and cytologic method for the spatial definition of gliomas. *Mayo Clin. Proc.* **62**: 435−49 (1987).

30 Hoshino, T., Barker, M., Wilson, C.B., Boldrey, E.B. & Fewer, D. Cell kinetics of human gliomas. *J. Neurosurg.* **37**: 15−26 (1972).

chapter 23

Computer Image Display during Frameless Stereotactic Surgery

David W. Roberts, John D. Pavlidis, Eric M. Friets, Erin Fagan, and John W. Strohbehn

Introduction

Neurosurgical stereotactic systems conventionally employ a frame which is affixed to the patient's head, and which serves the dual, integrated purposes of defining a spatial coordinate system and of mechanically guiding a surgical instrument, such as a radiofrequency electrode or biopsy needle, to a predetermined point within the brain. As the role of navigational assistance expands beyond special applications and begins to be appreciated in open neurosurgical procedures, the means by which that assistance is made available to the surgeon is evolving beyond mechanically directed probes oriented towards target points [1,2]. Video displays, either adjacent to the surgical field or superimposed upon the field through an operating microscope, obviate the need during craniotomy for frame-held instrumentation. If a non-mechanical means is adopted to effect spatial registration between imaging studies, the operative field, and the video display, then the need for the frame (whose other purpose — definition of a spatial coordinate system — is thus achieved) can be eliminated altogether.

A project to develop such a system was begun at Dartmouth in 1981, and in 1984 a working prototype was first employed clinically [3–7]. The component systems of this prototype — from imaging data storage and processing to spatial calculation and graphic display — are all entirely dependent upon (and, indeed, made possible by) computers. For purposes of economy, the first configuration of the system employed five already available computers, including an IBM PC wheeled into the operating room for a given case. Today, the system runs on a single Vicom VME image processing workstation (Vicom Systems Inc., Fremont, CA), consisting of a Sun 3/160 microcomputer with an enhanced backplane of image processing hardware, which communicates with the computer via a high speed data bus.

The concept of frameless spatial registration

Central to any stereotactic procedure is the concept of spatial registration, the process by which the locations of the imaging information, the surgical field, and the guided instrumentation can be defined with respect to one another. Most frame-based systems accomplish this by having localizable portions of the frame identifiable on the same computed tomography (CT) or magnetic resonance imaging (MRI) image that contains the target point. By measuring on that image the relationship between the frame and the target, the system enables delivery of an instrument to that target. In a frameless system, the spatial relationship between imaging information and instrumentation in the operating room can be defined by a common set of reference points on the patient that are visible during both the imaging and the start of the operative procedure. These points, or fiducials, enable one to readily move between the coordinate system of the imaging study and that of the operating room. A non-imaging ultrasonic rangefinder (Science Accessories Corporation, Model GP-8-3D, Southport, CT) is used to measure distances in the operating room without mechanical linkages, and the set of ultrasonic microphones fixed above the surgical field defines the operating room (OR) coordinate space, within which the location of ultrasound generators (called spark gaps) can be accurately determined. Used first on fiducial points and then on the operating microscope, these spark gaps effect the necessary spatial registration.

Data acquisition, transfer, and processing

CT, MRI, and angiographic studies may alone or in combination be the source of imaging data used by the system. Prior to imaging, a minimum of three and as many as five fiducial points on the patient's scalp are arbitrarily selected. Their locations are constrained only by the requirement that they be in line of sight of the rangefinder microphone array at surgery; in practice, this usually means that points are selected over the hemisphere ipsilateral to the surgical approach. At each point the scalp is shaved and a small mark placed, much as tattoos are employed in radiation therapy. If a distinctive natural landmark is evident on the skin, that may be employed. For CT scanning, 5 mm glass beads are taped over the fiducial points. Capsules containing copper sulfate are used for MRI, and small steel spheres are employed for angiography. For CT and MRI scanning, the study must cover the region of surgical interest as well as all of the fiducials. Any slice thickness may be used but, as the greatest error in the system lies in this parameter, thin slice thickness is desirable. For angiography, a plexiglass box is attached to the patient table (though not to the patient), such that fine steel wires embedded in its sides will be visible on the study. These wires enable the geometric relationships between central beam, fiducials, and angiographic objects of interest to be determined.

Following CT, MRI, or angiography, the radiodetectable markers overlying the fiducial points are removed. With indelible fiducial marking, subsequent surgery may be scheduled for any time after the study. Transfer of the imaging data to the Vicom is accomplished by a separate tape drive for CT, by Ethernet for MRI, and by a digitizing tablet for angiography.

At some point prior to surgery, processing of the image data on the Vicom is performed. Using a straightforward interactive video graphics subprogram, the fiducials and object(s) of anticipated surgical interest — such as the outline of a tumor, the desired extent of a planned lobar resection, or an aneurysm — are specified by the surgeon. In the typical case of an outlined tumor, a triangulated volume dataset is then created from the set of stacked contours; this is important in the subsequent task of reformatting the image information into planes perpendicular to the surgeon's line of sight.

The operative procedure

At the time of surgery, the patient is placed on the standard operating room table in three-point pin fixation, identically to the way he would be prepared for any craniotomy at our institution. Attention is given, as noted above, to assuring visibility of the fiducial points to the overhead microphone array. The array itself comprises three ultrasonic microphones (sensitive to 55–60 kHz), approximately 100 cm apart, attached to an arm movable on the overhead light track. When the patient has been positioned, the optimal position of the array over the patient's head is checked and the arm locked in place. Registration of the fiducial points is now performed, requiring on average several minutes. The hand-held spark gap of the ultrasonic rangefinder is sequentially positioned and fired at each of the scalp fiducial points. For each point, multiple slant ranges are determined, and the system is programmed to accept only data with a certain standard error. The transformation matrix necessary to relate the coordinates system of the imaging study to that of the microphone array is immediately generated, and a measure of the accuracy of the system and the registration step can be quickly obtained by holding the spark gap over the fourth or fifth fiducial point. The scalp is then prepared and draped in the conventional manner.

When the Zeiss OPMI 1H operating microscope is prepared prior to the operation, two special pieces of equipment are attached. The first is an adapted beam splitter (originally intended as an artist's drawing tube) to which is attached a JVC miniature cathode ray tube (CRT), weighing approximately 500 g; this will provide the graphic display of navigational assistance superimposed on the surgical field. A simple alignment test, in which a video pattern is superimposed on the cross-hairs of the microscope ocular, may be performed at this time. Also attached to the microscope prior to its draping is a bracket receptacle at the level of the objective lens (Fig. 23.1).

After draping of the microscope, a sterile Y-shaped bracket, holding three spark gaps in a triangular array of side 30 cm, is attached to the receptacle through the drape-bag. In the system's original configuration, the spatial relationship between the microscope's spark gaps and the focal point and oriented plane had been determined in a separate step during each case. The newly machined bracket and receptacle are precision fitted with reproducible alignment, and the previous step has been eliminated. When the operating microscope is now brought over the surgical field, and at each subsequent repositioning, the microscope spark gaps are fired and its position determined.

Graphic display

Navigational guidance may be provided for the operating surgeon in one of three different ways. The simplest and original method of stereotactic data presentation is the superimposed display of any outline information which spatially should lie in the microscope's focal plane. To accomplish this, the system first calculates that focal plane, reformats the processed imaging data into a corresponding

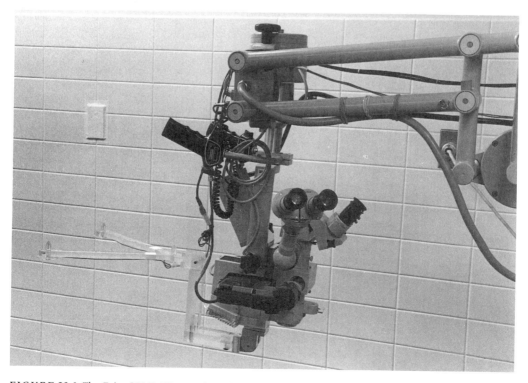

FIGURE 23.1 The Zeiss OPMI-1H operating microscope has been adapted by the addition of a Y-shaped bracket (holding three spark gaps) and a miniature CRT attached to a modified beam-splitter. From Roberts *et al.* [4].

plane, and then displays the boundaries of any objects of interest in that plane on the CRT, such that they are superimposed in correct location, scale, and orientation (Fig. 23.2). Should the surgeon's interest lie deep to the focal plane, any other reformatted plane parallel to the microscope's focal plane may be called. This function is obviously most useful in locating pathology not visible on the cortical surface and during tumor resection.

A second very practical function enables quick location of a small object of interest, whose depth or even general position may not be immediately apparent to the surgeon. When called, this function draws a line connecting the focal point (in the center of the field of view) with a point representing the projection of the center of the object of interest onto the microscope's focal plane. This has been particularly convenient when a tumor lies outside the microscope's field of view. While the length of the line is given, segmentation of the line into

quarters allows quick, visual extrapolation of its endpoint. The distance of the projection up onto the focal plane is also given, providing the surgeon with an easy appreciation for its depth.

The third method of displaying information utilizes a monitor on a shelf in the operating room, rather than the microscope's optical display system. At any time during the microscope's employment, the location of the operating microscope's focal point can be displayed as a cursor on the appropriate CT or MRI unreformatted image. Similar to the locating function of recently developed robotic arms [8], this display enables orientation with respect to the full grayscale original image, as well as viewing by operating room personnel away from the microscope.

Error analysis and phantom testing

Accuracy of the system has been studied through both error analysis and simulation of

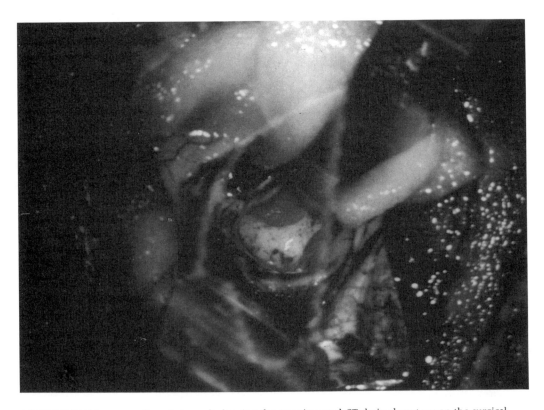

FIGURE 23.2 Intraoperative photograph showing the superimposed CT-derived contour on the surgical field during tumor resection. From Roberts *et al.* [5].

operative use with two phantoms [7]. In the former, sources of error can be considered as either "experimental" (e.g. errors in distances determined by the ultrasonic rangefinder) or "algorithm-induced."

The calculation of distance by the ultrasonic rangefinder requires a temperature-dependent velocity factor, estimated by the commercially available rangefinder by a temperature sensor at one microphone. As wide gradients of temperature characterize the vertical space above the operative field, an early modification of the system was to use a pilot pole for determination of velocity. A spark gap and microphone have been mounted on this vertically aligned pole at a precisely measured, fixed distance. Each time a slant-range is measured (either from a spark gap held at a fiducial or from a spark gap on the microscope), the pilot pole spark gap is also fired. The velocity calculated from the pilot pole is then used for calculating the slant-range.

Measurements of typical spark-gap-to-microphone distances using calipers have been within ± 0.2 mm of the means of most sets of rangefinder determinations. The standard deviation of 100 rangefinder determinations (an often used number of determinations in practice) has been < 0.1–0.2 mm. This level of accuracy, in combination with other measurements, such as that of the distances between the microphones over the surgical field, enters into algorithms that ultimately locate points in the three-dimensional (3-D) coordinate space of the operating room. Computer simulations, in which variables of measurement accuracy and geometric configurations may be studied, have shown an average position error of 0.6 mm. An important modification of the algorithms arising from this analysis was the change from an operating room coordinate system based on the microscope's spark gaps to one based on the overhead microphones (whose separation is approximately three times that of the spark gaps). This step alone decreased average error by 34%.

Determination of the transformation matrix between image space and OR space is also dependent upon the accuracy of the rangefinder in measuring the locations of the fiducials during the spatial registration step.

For a 0.2-mm slant-range error, an error of 0.8 ± 0.3 mm can be expected in the system's ability to locate a point, such as an additional check fiducial.

The greatest source of error has been found to lie in the resolution of the imaging data. Comparing the above errors with those deriving from a CT scan, whose resolution within a slice may be between 0.5 and 1.0 mm, and along the scanner's z axis between 1.5 and 2.5 mm, one may readily appreciate the limitations imposed by the imaging information. The accuracy of any stereotactic system can never exceed that of the imaging information with which it works.

Phantom studies, using a $18 \times 10 \times 10$-cm plexiglass block with fiducial points and test triangles inscribed with a milling machine accurate to 0.025 mm, have assessed system accuracy independent of errors introduced at imaging. An average error of 1.2 ± 0.4 mm has been found in locating a test point, and of 3.0 ± 0.6 mm in projecting a contour. A second phantom, consisting of a staircase within a lucite shell, has been CT scanned with 1.5-mm slice thickness, enabling simulation of an entire operative procedure. Error in locating a test point has averaged 2.0 ± 0.5 mm; that in superimposing a contour has averaged 1.7 ± 1.0 mm.

Clinical experience

Use of the system during operative procedures since 1984 has been oriented towards assessment of its performance, in terms of accuracy, its ease of use in the clinical operating room environment, and its general utility in a variety of applications. Cases have been limited to those in which stereotactic guidance might have been useful, but not in which safe completion of the procedure would have been dependent upon performance of the system.

Accuracy during clinical applications has generally been slightly less than during phantom testing in a more controllable environment. In our early surgical experience, errors in excess of 20 mm were sometimes recorded. Numerous improvements, including thinner CT and MRI slice thicknesses, decreased temperature gradients and air turbulence through control of the ventilation system, the above-described modification of the OR coordinate system and the introduction of the pilot pole have led to an average error of approximately 5 mm. While less than the accuracy of frame-based systems, and insufficient for many of the functional applications of conventional stereotaxy, this performance has been satisfactory for navigational guidance to small subcortical lesions or to boundaries of resection for larger tumors.

With respect to feasibility, the system and its components have performed favorably in the operating room. The spark gap bracket has not been obtrusive over the adjacent surgical field and drapes; line-of-sight difficulties with the spark gaps and microphones have been infrequent. The quality of the video image through the beam splitter has been satisfactory, and the superimposed contours have been readily appreciated. Graphics more complicated than lines and contours have been suboptimal when superimposed upon a heterogeneous surgical field.

Of equal concern to the physical encumbrances imposed by such a system has been the issue of adding to the time of a surgical procedure. Monitoring of the microscope's position, reformatting of image data, and display of information within the microscope currently require less than 1 minute. As this process is independent of the surgeon, who generally may continue to work under the microscope as he would conventionally, this imposes no particular delay. The lengthiest step in the system's application, but one that precedes the start of surgery, is that of registering the fiducials. Through both practice and some software changes, this step can now be accomplished in a few minutes; a test of system accuracy at this stage using an additional fiducial takes an additional minute. The biggest improvement with regard to facility of use has been in the attachment of the spark gap bracket to the microscope. As already described, the original system had required a potentially inaccurate 5 minute step, to determine the spatial relationship between the bracket's spark gaps and the focal point and plane of the microscope, immediately following fixation of the bracket. The precision-milled attachment assembly eliminates that step altogether.

Independent of the inaccuracies and encumbrances of the described prototype, the frameless stereotactic operating microscope was developed to illustrate a conceptual idea. Perhaps the most important aspect of its assessment in this regard is in the clinical utility a variety of surgical experiences has suggested. As anticipated, guidance to small lesions — most typically, but not limited to, solitary metastases to be resected — has been extremely helpful. Guidance in determining the extent of resection in larger tumors, usually malignant gliomas, has also been of practical benefit. Assistance during craniotomy for aneurysm clipping was potentially useful in one of two instances, but experience in vascular cases remains insufficient. An unexpected but helpful application has been in corpus callosotomy procedures for intractable seizure disorders, where accurate determination of the extent of ongoing section may be more precise than other methods.

Conclusions

A frameless computer-based stereotactic system has been developed that can provide navigational guidance to the surgeon in the form of CT, MRI, and angiographic information, superimposed on the surgical field in the correct location, scale, and orientation. The operating microscope remains freely movable, its position determining the reformatting of imaging data (the reverse of conventional stereotactic systems). Mean accuracy with phantom testing has been 2−3 mm, and that during clinical procedures approximately 5 mm. Utility appears to be greatest in (but not limited to) guidance to small subcortical or deep lesions.

References

1 Kelly, P.J., Alker, G.J. Jr. & Goerss, S. Computer-assisted stereotactic laser microsurgery for the treatment of intracranial neoplasms. *Neurosurgery* **10**: 324−31 (1982).

2 Kelly, P.J. Volumetric stereotactic surgical resection of intra-axial brain mass lesions. *Mayo Clin. Proc.* **63**: 1186−98 (1988).

3 Hatch, J.F., Roberts, D.W. & Strohbehn, J.W. Reference-display system for the integration of CT scanning and the operating microscope. In: Kuklinski, W.S. & Ohley, W.J. (eds) *Proceedings of the Eleventh Annual Northeast Bioengineering Conference.* New York: Institute of Electrical and Elec-

tronic Engineers (1985), pp. 252−4.

4 Roberts, D.W., Strohbehn, J.W., Hatch, J.F., Murray, W. & Kettenberger, H. A frameless stereotaxic integration of computed tomographic imaging and the operating microscope. *J. Neurosurg.* **65**: 545−9 (1986).

5 Roberts, D.W., Strohbehn, J.W., Friets, E.M., Kettenberger, J. & Hartov, A. The stereotactic operating microscope: accuracy refinement and clinical experience. *Acta Neurochir.* (suppl.) **46**: 112−4 (1989).

6 Friets, E.M., Strohbehn, J.W. & Roberts, D.W. Improved accuracy for the frameless stereotaxic operating microscope. In: LaCourse, J.R. (ed.),

Proceedings of the Fourteenth Annual Northeast Bioengineering Conference, pp. 47−9. New York: Institute of Electrical and Electronic Engineers (1988).

7 Friets, E.M., Strohbehn, J.W., Hatch, J.F. & Roberts, D.W. A frameless stereotaxic operating microscope for neurosurgery. *Institute of Electrical and Electronic Engineers Trans. Biomed. Eng.* **36**: 608−17 (1989).

8 Watanabe, E., Watanabe, T., Manaka, S., Mayanagi, Y. & Takakura. Three-dimensional digitizer (neuronavigator): new equipment for computed tomography-guided stereotactic surgery. *Surg. Neurol.* **27**: 543−7 (1987).

24

Robotic-aided Surgery

Ronald F. Young and Yik S. Kwoh

Introduction

Since 1980, robotic technology has been applied to many industrial situations in which consistency, accuracy, and cost-effectiveness are the primary considerations. The most common uses of robots include automotive and electronic assembly. Robots are also useful in situations where the environment is hazardous to human beings, or in an environment so clean or sterile that it is difficult to achieve in the presence of human beings. Only recently have robots been considered as potentially useful in neurosurgery.

Major advantages of robots include their great accuracy and flexibility. Researchers from different parts of the world, such as USA, Germany, Canada, France, Japan [1–3], and others, have independently used robotic surgical assistance for stereotactic surgery.

Stereotactic surgery is a technique for guiding a probe or other instrument to a predetermined point in the nervous system, without directly viewing the surgical site. Referencing is provided by landmarks in images from X-ray, computed tomography (CT), magnetic resonance imaging (MRI), etc., correlated against some physical landmarks. This chapter presents an example of CT-guided robotic stereotactic surgery, using N-shape locators mounted on a headframe as reference landmarks. Reference marks along two axes are used to locate and

position surgical instruments. To visualize the brain landmarks a CT scan is used, providing two-dimensional (2-D), high-resolution, axial pictures that show detailed soft-tissue anatomy inside the cranial vault and the spinal cord.

Use of the standard stereotactic headframe presents the surgeon with certain problems: the manual adjustments required by the frame are time-consuming, making frequent trajectory modifications difficult. The difficulties of reading the CT scan data, and setting appropriate parameters on the frame between surgeon and patient may result in an awkward arrangement. This chapter describes the development of a surgical procedure using a programmed robot arm to replace the stereotactic frame. Driven by a computer, the arm offers substantial flexibility, speed, and accuracy, which allows the surgeon to manipulate the probe trajectory conveniently in a variety of directions. The surgeon has flexibility in choosing the trajectory, and in addition he can instantly see and monitor the needle tip on CT images. The result is expected to be increasingly sophisticated stereotactic procedures.

Stereotactic surgery is a technique that has been developed and used for almost 80 years. Horsley and Clarke first invented the three-dimensional (3-D) stereotactic machine [4,5]. Since this pioneering effort, many pieces of stereotactic equipment have been devised [6–8]. In the early stereotactic surgeries, the road map to the target was provided by conventional X-ray pictures that were often enhanced by contrast material.

In the late 1970s, the integration of stereotaxis with CT scanning provided a much more powerful tool for surgeons. The new technique used high-resolution axial 2-D pictures to guide the probe to the target with unsurpassed accuracy. Several groups have developed CT-aided stereotactic headframes for intracranial operations [9–11]. The brain is ideally suited for such procedures because of the availability of rigid skull fixation and the absence of physiologic motion.

Until now, all previous stereotactic procedures have involved some stereotactic "frame." However, the use of a frame poses several problems. The manual reading and setting of the frame parameters is a slow process. It is tedious and error-prone when frequent maneuvers are required. A motorized frame could help solve this problem, but such a system tends to be heavy unless one needs to achieve accuracy in micrometers. A frame is usually designed only for the head or body. Although a frame intended for application to both the head and body has been designed, its performance to date has not been satisfactory. A robotic system, however, can be applied to the body as well as the head.

The fixed radius arc of a frame also lacks the flexibility that surgeons prefer. For example, the surgeon often wishes to place the probe holder as close as possible to the patient, which requires a small arc. But if one builds a frame with the required small arc, it cannot be used with an oversized patient. Further, each frame, depending on its structure and design, has its unreachable corners. Occasionally, the desired trajectory is within one of these forbidden zones of the frame. Finally, the frame structure hampers the surgeon's view of the patient and makes some surgical procedures difficult.

In the course of many stereotactic procedures conducted at Memorial Medical Center of Long Beach from 1980 to 1984, it became evident that reading the scales on the frame, and adjusting the frame according to the computer output, was a tedious and time-consuming procedure, especially in the case of tumors which required an approach from several different directions.

Adjustments after the first trajectory setting were difficult because the frame had already been draped under sterile conditions. The multiple time-consuming and manual adjustments of the frame motivated the search for a new procedure, one that was potentially faster, more automated, more flexible, more reliable, and more accurate, a procedure that could be used for both the body and the head. The solution appeared to be the radical replacement of the stereotactic frame — a device more than 80 years of age — by a high-precision, versatile, computer-controlled, latest generation robot, fully interfaced with the CT scanner and with the probe guide at its end effector.

The new stereotactic technique eliminates the above shortcomings by using a robot to replace a frame. Driven by a computer with sophisticated stereotactic software, such a system demonstrates advantages in accuracy, flexibility, time consumption, and convenience.

The robot system

In order to choose a robot suitable for stereotactic purposes, several issues must be considered. The robot arm must have substantial maneuvering capability. Ideally, stereotactic surgery requires the surgeon to have complete freedom to position the arm and its probe. In addition, the arm must have an appropriate reach in order to provide an unobstructed support of the probe over the entire area. It must be sturdy enough to provide very stable probe trajectory control, and should have sufficient fail-safe features to prevent it from causing harm and damage should it malfunction.

The robot system and its backup must be highly reliable to avoid breakdowns during surgery. The size and the weight of the robot arm should be as small as possible. The robot is a surgical tool that the surgeon should be able to move about quickly during an emergency.

The first phase of this project was a careful evaluation of the industrial robots available on the market, in order to determine whether a robot with enough dexterity, accuracy, and reliability to operate in the surgical environment was available. After a long screening procedure, although the ideal robot was not available on the market, we have felt that the robot best suited to our purpose was the PUMA 260. These considerations led to the choice of the PUMA 260 robot system by Unimation Inc., a company which was later sold to Westinghouse and subsequently sold to Stäubli AG (Stäubli International, Switzerland). This robot system consists of a mechanical arm and an electronic controller. The mechanical arm has six joints. Each joint is driven by a permanent magnet DC servomotor through a gear train. The major hardware parameters for the PUMA 260 robot are summarized in Fig. 24.1 and Table 24.1.

The decision to use the PUMA 260 robot involved, among other things, the following considerations. The PUMA 260 is a programmable, computer-controlled, versatile robot. It has been especially designed for accurate, delicate work, yet it is sturdy enough to provide a very stable trajectory. The PUMA 260 motions are similar to those of the human body and can be described in human terms: waist, shoulder, elbow, wrist, flange rotation, and wrist bend. This robotic arm has the smallest footprint or support base of those commercially available, and yet it provides a sufficient work coverage. The PUMA 260 is designed to work with human beings and at human tempos, so that it will mesh with existing surgical procedures. It has a relative accuracy of 0.05 mm, and has been devised to be very versatile; its computer is compatible

with a variety of imaging computers currently used in the biomedical field. The robot is safe: the waist, shoulder, and elbow joints are equipped with spring-applied, solenoid-released brakes, which are automatically clamped should any mechanical or electrical defect occur. Recently, a request was made to Stäubli AG to add three more brakes to the last three joints. The ideal robot should have a fault-tolerant design. Should any of the electronic components fail, a backup exists which will automatically assume function. In addition, the brakes are designed such that, whether arm power is on or off, the braking action will not cause joint movement. This safety feature ensures that the arm will not move during stereotactic surgery because the arm power is off. All servomotors incorporate optical incremental encoders that provide position and velocity feedback to the robot's servo system. Recently, a clean room version (Class 10) of the same arm has become available. The clean room PUMA 260 is more suitable for surgical applications.

As shown in Fig. 24.2, a custom-made probe holder is attached to the end effector of the robot arm so that the surgeon can guide the probe. The sleeve of the probe holder makes fine tuning of the probe possible. This feature was designed to offer additional flexibility to the surgeon. However, because of fine con-

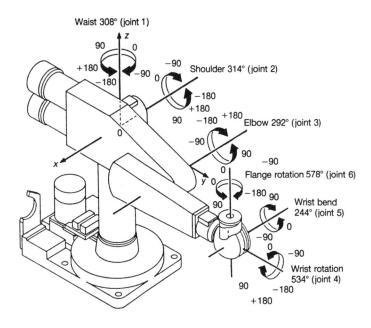

FIGURE 24.1 The Unimation PUMA Mark II Robot 260 series provides the precise, repeatable positioning required for stereotactic neurosurgery. Reprinted with permission Robotics Age, © 1985.

TABLE 24.1 Major parameters of PUMA 260

	Parameters
Robot Arm	
Axes	Six revolute axes
Clearance required	Spherical volume with shoulder at center. 0.47 m (18.5 inch) radius to hand mount flange
Drive	Electric DC servomotor
Maximum inertia load (including gripper)	Wrist rotation (J4) not exceeding 1.0 inches ounce^{-1} s^{-1} Wrist bend (J5) not exceeding 1.8 inches ounce^{-1} s^{-1} Flange rotation (J6) not exceeding 0.5 inches ounce^{-1} s^{-1}
Position repeatability	± 0.05 mm (± 0.002 inch) within primary work envelope
Tool velocity	1.0 ms^{-1} (3.3 feet s^{-1}) maximum load within primary work envelope
Software movement limits	
Waist — joint 1	$-184-124$ (308°)
Shoulder — joint 2	$-247-67$ (314°)
Elbow — joint 3	$-56-236$ (292°)
Wrist — joint 4	$-223-355$ (578°)
Wrist — joint 5	$-122-122$ (244°)
Wrist — joint 6	$-222-312$ (534°)

trollability of the robot arm, one can achieve the fine tuning by software control of the robot if desired, rather than by hand. In functional neurosurgery, where fine control is necessary, a microadjustment end effector can be designed to fit the PUMA 260. A quick release mechanism allows the probe to be separated from the robot arm. This feature is useful for multiple targets, and is also necessary for body stereotactic procedures where movement continues after the probe is inserted.

The electronic robot controller contains the built-in electronics for the robot system. The "brain" of the controller is a DEC LSI-11 minicomputer. The robot's operating system software (named VAL) supports both serial and parallel input/output peripheral devices, such as a CRT terminal, a floppy disk, and a manual

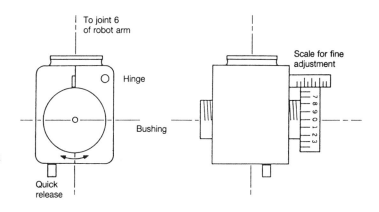

FIGURE 24.2 In stereotactic neurosurgery, the end effector is a custom-made holder for surgical probes. Fine adjustment of the probe is provided by a threaded bushing with vernier scale. Reprinted with permission Robotics Age, © 1985.

control unit. The controller also contains digital and analog circuits to manipulate the robot in several modes through buttons and a speed-control switch on the unit. When the panic button is depressed, all processes are stopped and every joint of the robot arm is frozen. The VAL operating system also constantly monitors the robot. For example, if the robot is diverted from its programmed task for a short time, VAL will sense the discrepancy and turn off the arm power automatically for safety reasons.

Since the LSI-11 microcomputer is designed for robot control only, it lacks the software needed for stereotactic computational programs. Even the latest version of VAL, the UNIVAL, does not accommodate the stereotactic programs. In addition, the robot system has to communicate with a CT scanner. Hence a host computer is used to store the scanned images and to run the stereotactic software. The host Data General Eclipse or DEC 11/34 mini-computer communicates with the LSI-11 via a standard RS-232 link. The surgeon interacts with the host computer, using the stereotactic procedure software developed for this purpose. Recent progress has implemented the stereotactic program on the IBM PC for higher performance and added reliability, while lowering the cost of maintenance compared with the method of using the minicomputers. The linking or interface between the CT scan, host computer, IBM PC, and the robot is shown in Fig. 24.3.

Improving the absolute positioning accuracy of the robot

While the commercially available PUMA 260 robot proved accurate, enough for operations on large tumors (say 0.5 cm) located in non-critical areas of the brain, it soon became evident that operating on smaller-sized lesions located deep in the brain would require some improvement in the accuracy [12].

Unimation Inc. specifies that the PUMA 260 robot has a relative accuracy of 0.05 mm. Relative accuracy is also referred to as "repeatability", which is a measurement of the deviation between a position previously held by the end effector and the position to which it returns on repetitive motion.

In such an application as CT-guided surgery, in which the robot is guided by some external sensory device, the notion of accuracy should refer to an external reference frame. The accuracy (or absolute accuracy) of a robot arm is defined as the mismatch between, on the one hand, the actual position of the end effector and, on the other hand, the end effector position as it has been specified by its coordinates in some external reference frame.

The repeatability tolerance is less than the accuracy. The difference between accuracy and repeatability stems from the fact that all robot arms within the same family are not identical. Because of finite precision manufacturing, the link parameters of a particular robot within a family do not have exactly the nominal values of the robot family. Repeatability is a characteristic of a robot arm family; accuracy is a characteristic of a particular robot within the family. For this reason manufacturers specify repeatability, rather than accuracy. However, the accuracy tolerance can be brought to about the same level as the repeatability tolerance, provided the imperfections in the robot can be compensated for. This process is referred to as "calibration of the robot," or improvement of its absolute position accuracy. Without compensation for the inherent geometric errors of the

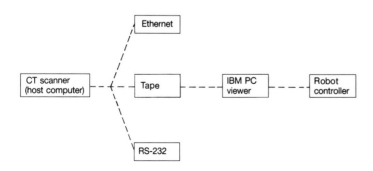

FIGURE 24.3 The linking between CT scan and the robot. The link can be made by one of the three methods shown.

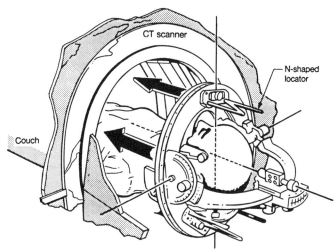

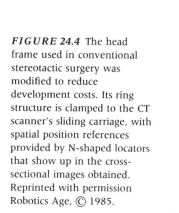

FIGURE 24.4 The head frame used in conventional stereotactic surgery was modified to reduce development costs. Its ring structure is clamped to the CT scanner's sliding carriage, with spatial position references provided by N-shaped locators that show up in the cross-sectional images obtained. Reprinted with permission Robotics Age, © 1985.

particular robot being used, the probe tip could be as much as a few millimeters from the specific targets. However, for some delicate neurosurgical applications, the consensus among neurosurgeons is that submillimeter accuracy is required, particularly for functional neurosurgery. The purpose of our calibration is to compensate for the robot error in order to reach submillimeter accuracy.

The essential factor limiting the absolute accuracy of a particular robot within a family is the imprecise knowledge of the robot's geometry. In a certain sense, the offset between nominal and actual kinematics must be compensated for. The basic assumption of the calibration is that manufacturing errors can be compensated for by adjustment of the four link parameters: the joint angle, link length, link

shift, and link twist. Essentially, one applies software compensation to adjust the joints, so that one achieves correct and accurate position at the end effector.

In order to reduce the development costs, a previously built stereotactic headframe was used as part of this development. With the arc removed, the ring structure supports the patient's head with a head rest and four stainless steel-tipped pin screws. Three N-shaped locators, mounted on the ring, determine the location of the scanned images. The ring in turn is attached to the scanner couch's sliding surface. This set-up is shown in Fig. 24.4.

The PUMA 260 robot is bolted to a pedestal. After CT images are taken, the patient is translated or slid out of the scanner to the robot's work area. Then the N-shaped locators are

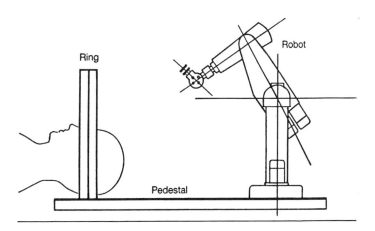

FIGURE 24.5 The robot pedestal is attached to the metal ring. Reprinted with permission Robotics Age, © 1985.

removed and the robot pedestal is attached to the metal ring, as shown in Fig. 24.5.

Next, the surgeon indicates a target point on one of the CT images. Using the trace of the N-shaped locators on the image and the known position of the ring, the x, y coordinates of the target are transformed into the robot's 3-D coordinate system. Next, the surgeon maneuvers the robot arm to designate an appropriate entrance point on the skull. He also determines the approximate entry trajectory by directing the probe holder, as illustrated by Fig. 24.6. Such maneuvers may be accomplished either by pushing buttons on the manual control unit or by setting the robot in the "Free" mode and manually manipulating the robot arm.

Stereotactic software is then used to direct the robot arm to align the probe holder with the trajectory determined by the entrance point and the target. Initially, the robot is driven in such a manner as to be a safe distance from the head. By pushing two buttons, the surgeon may control the robot so that the probe holder moves in or out along the trajectory (Fig. 24.7), as close to the head as desired. The surgeon may use the buttons on the manual control unit to alter the trajectory. Computer software maintains the probe holder trajectory line, constantly pointing at the target, as seen in Fig. 24.8. Once the trajectory is determined, the probe holder is removed so that the surgeon can use the robot arm as a stable guide to create a burr hole or other opening through the skull.

After the burr hole is drilled, the robot can be programmed to retract to its standby position. As soon as the surgeon completes the burr hole, the robot can be summoned back to the trajectory that it left. The probe holder and the probe are remounted on the robot arm and the surgeon is prepared for probe insertion. At this moment the surgeon can still modify the probe trajectory for slight adjustments. For example, a main artery might be avoided by a quarter-inch shift. The surgeon can fine-tune the final trajectory by pushing buttons on the manual control unit, in a manner similar to the use of a joystick. The stereotactic program maintains the probe direction, aiming at the target constantly.

Once the final trajectory is determined to the surgeon's satisfaction, he locks the robot arm by turning off the arm power electric switch. Turning off the arm power will automatically activate all internal brakes. In the final configuration, the surgeon inserts the probe manually. A threaded sleeve, mounted on the probe holder with a scale, allows the surgeon to further increase or decrease the computed probe length.

In such cases as hypothermia therapy or interstitial brachytherapy, the surgeon may need to access many targets through different paths. The above procedure can be repeated as many times as necessary. Stereotactic software can direct the robot arm to access targets in parallel trajectories or along any trajectory desired. After insertion, a quick release mechanism on the probe holder permits the probe or catheter to separate from the robot arm, so that the arm can move to another trajectory for reinsertion.

Comparison of the robotic stereotaxis system and the system using a manually adjustable frame

The robotic system has several important advantages over the frame-oriented system. The robotic system is capable of fast, easy trajectory adjustments, and is extremely flexible in its ability to allow for trajectory modifications. Such capability offers the surgeon a versatile tool. Sophisticated stereotactic operations can be performed by the surgical team with less effort and time.

The robot eliminates human error. The reading and setting of parameters on the stereotactic frame constitutes the major source of errors in a frame-oriented stereotaxis system. The robotic stereotaxis system does not require human intervention, and hence eliminates the possibility for gross error originating from this source.

Robotic stereotaxis can be applied to both head and body. No existing stereotactic frame can be applied to both the head and the body. Robotic stereotaxis has no fixed radius arc constraints. The arc structure in a stereotactic frame has two drawbacks: (1) the surgeon cannot position the probe holder at an arbitrary distance from the patient; and (2) in the case of the body frame system, the arc is sensitive to an oversized patient. The robot arm system has none of the above constraints. When the surgeon needs a guide for probe insertion, the robot arm assists: it is a capable assisting tool, at the same time

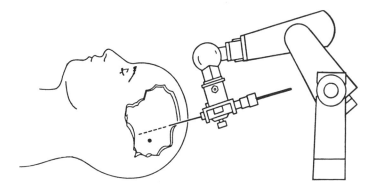

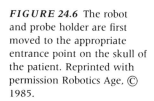

FIGURE 24.6 The robot and probe holder are first moved to the appropriate entrance point on the skull of the patient. Reprinted with permission Robotics Age, © 1985.

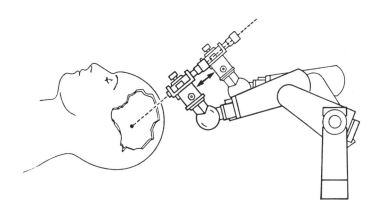

FIGURE 24.7 Using CT scan information, the surgeon selects a target point. Trajectories for the arm are then computed which will keep the probe centerline coincident with a desired centerline intersecting the target point. Reprinted with permission Robotics Age, © 1985.

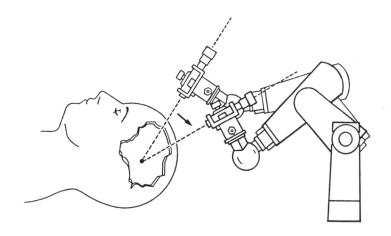

FIGURE 24.8 During alignment and set-up, the software in the main computer keeps the probe holder's centerline pointed at the target. Reprinted with permission Robotics Age, © 1985.

occupying a minimum amount of space. When not in use, the robot arm can be removed from the area between the surgeon and the patient, and the surgeon can access a large open surgical field.

The robot allows for a wide variety of access angles. The robot discussed in this chapter has six degrees of freedom. Hence, it offers an arbi-

trary trajectory at an arbitrary location within its working area. It has a wider choice of accessing angles than can be incorporated in a frame. The robotic system is capable of superior accuracy. Although the precision provided by a stereotactic frame has proved satisfactory, with an angular precision of ± 2 arc-seconds in a typical headframe set-up, the robot arm can provide an even higher degree of accuracy. The robot arm is capable of placing probes within a Cartesian coordinates precision of ± 0.05 mm.

Since the robot has precise position feedback at all times, under the appropriate software guidance, the surgeon can monitor exactly the position of the tip and track of a probe in reference to the CT scan images. As soon as the surgeon moves the arm, the effect can be seen on the CT scan images. The surgeon can use the robot to measure, monitor, and plan. It is difficult to implement all these features with a stereotactic frame.

The robot can also be programmed to provide a "zero gravity" environment, which will be used in conjunction with the planning process just before probe insertion. "Zero gravity" means that the robot controller provides just the sufficient amount of servo currents to balance the arm in free space. Therefore, the surgeon can push the arm into any position effortlessly. As soon as the surgeon removes his hands, the robot will stay where it was without falling under the effect of gravity. The surgeon can check the trajectory with the robot suspended in space, so that he can physically observe the geometry of the situation. In addition he can also see the planned needle trajectory with respect to the CT scan images in real time. Such a dynamic and interactive feedback verification on CT images is not easily achievable with a stereotactic frame arrangement.

Finally, however, the robot does have new problems to be considered. For instance, it may reach a point or trajectory in many different ways. One must choose the preferred path required by safety and/or convenience requirements into the computer; at present, it is considered time-consuming. Such a problem can be handled reasonably well by three precautionary measures: (1) the robot is allowed to move at a speed sufficiently slow that a human can react in time; (2) the computer program is allowed to move the robot arm only at a distance sufficiently far from the patient to avoid injury; and (3) the manual control unit is kept within easy access. In an emergency, the panic button can bring the robot system to a complete stop.

Conclusions

The robotic stereotactic procedure provides the surgeon with a more convenient tool to position probes than does the stereotactic frame. The software developed for these procedures is not overly complex. We believe robotic stereotaxis may eventually become the core of an integrated computerized system for delicate surgery.

The PUMA 260 robot may not be the ideal robot for use in stereotactic operations. However, it is currently the best among candidates that can be acquired with reasonable resources. The original intent of the present research effort was to demonstrate the effectiveness of using a robot as a replacement for a stereotactic frame. However, we have progressed beyond that stage. The robotic stereotactic system should continue to improve, in both hardware and software, to become a better assistant for the surgeon performing stereotactic surgeries. Recently, the possibility of implementing two robot arms has been investigated. The range of possible applications of robotics to surgery is only limited by our imagination.

References

1 Kelly, P.J., Kall, B.A. & Goerss, S.J. Special stereotactic techniques: stereotactic laser resection of deep-seated tumors. In: Heilbrun, M. Peter (ed.) *Stereotactic Neurosurgery, Vol. 2: Concepts in Neurosurgery*, pp. 233−9. Baltimore: Williams & Wilkins (1988).
2 Doll, J., Schlegel, W., Pastyr, O., Sturm, V. & Maier-Borst, W. The use of an industrial robot as a stereotactic guidance system. *Computer Assisted Radiology, Proceedings of the International Symposium on Computer Assisted Radiology*, pp. 374−8 (1987).
3 Benabid, A.L. Research work done at Laboratoire de Neurobiophysique-Inserm U 318, Grenoble Cedex, France. (Personal communication.)
4 Horsley, V.A. & Clarke, R.H. On the intrinsic fibres of the cerebellum, its nuclei and its effect tracts. *Brain* **28**: 12−29 (1905).
5 Horsley, V.A. & Clarke, R.H. The structure and functions of the cerebellum examined by a new method. *Brain* **31**: 45−124 (1908).
6 Ingram, W.R., Ranson, S.W., Hannett, F.I. *et al.* Results of stimulation of the tegmentum with the Horsley-Clark stereotaxis apparatus. *Arch. Neurol. Psychiatr* **28**: 512−41 (1932).
7 Leksell, K. The stereotactic method and radiosurgery of the brain. *Acta Chir. Scand.* **102**: 315−9 (1951).

8 Barcia-Salorio, J.L., Barbera, J., Broseta, J. & Soler, F. Tomography in stereotaxis: a new stereo-encephalotome designed for this purpose. *Acta Neurochir.* (suppl.) **23**: 77−83 (1977).

9 Brown, R.A. A computed tomography−computer graphics approach to stereotactic localization. *J. Neurosurg.* **50**: 715−20 (1979).

10 Brown, R.A., Roberts, T.S., Osborn, A.C. *et al.* Stereotactic frame and computer software for CT-directed neurosurgical localization. *Invest. Radiol.*

15: 308−312 (1980).

11 Spiegel, E.A. Development of stereoencephalotomy for extrapyramidal diseases. *J. Neurosurg.* **24**: 433−9 (1966).

12 Kwoh, Y.S., Hou, J., Jonckheere, E.A. & Hayati, S. A robot with improved absolute positioning accuracy for CT-guided stereotactic brain surgery. *Institute of Electrical and Electronics Engineers Trans. Biomed. Eng.* **35**(2): 153−60 (1988).

25

Computer-driven Robot for Stereotactic Neurosurgery

Alim L. Benabid, Stéphane Lavallée, Dominique Hoffmann, Philippe Cinquin, Jacques Demongeot, and François Danel

Introduction

Computerization and robotization of stereotaxy are inherent in the basic principles of stereotaxy. These principles encompass a natural evolution towards precision, repetition, automation of parts or even of entire procedures, automatic adaptation of procedures to specific, anatomic, parameters of the patient, reports of procedure parameters to control databases such as anatomic atlases, and interactivity and feedback processes between the databases and the current procedure. A six-axis robot has been specially designed for stereotactic procedures, according to a previously reported program [1,2]. The history of stereotaxy [3] is already rich in examples of such attempts at motorization, automatization, and computerization. Indeed, the present burst of computer and information technology has boosted this original tendency [4] and made possible the realization of what was, some years ago, a science fiction concept. At the Edinburgh meeting of the Society for Stereotaxy and Functional Neurosurgery in 1972, computerizations of atlases were already reported; later, computerization of stereotactic calculations was attempted or achieved through computed tomography (CT)-adapted stereotaxy [5–12], and in 1982 Kelly [13] described the first routine application of computer-assisted neurosurgery, foreseeing the potential of such an approach. In the 1990s this concept will

undoubtedly come to maturity and extend widely to the general field of computer-assisted medicosurgical procedures. Current problems concerning ethics and safety, already brought to public attention [14], have to be kept in mind and resolved.

Structure of the robot system

RATIONALE

The structure of the Grenoble robot system is a logical consequence of the needs, difficulties, and frustrations which are experienced during the daily practice of stereotaxy applied to a wide variety of diseases, such as brain tumors, dyskinesias, pain, and epilepsy. This led to a list of prerequisites, used to outline the project. The system had to be:

1 Precise and reliable.

2 Capable of performing every kind of routine stereotactic procedure using the same frame and equipment.

3 Driven from various types of neuroradiologic images, such as X-rays, CT, magnetic resonance imaging (MRI), from which the target would be defined with submillimeter accuracy.

4 Safe, and permanently subject to human control, for safety reasons as well as for iterative corrections of the programmed trajectory.

5 Capable of including subroutine softwares which could be applied to sophisticated but

stereotyped procedures, such as thalamic approaches for thalamotomies or electrode implantations, based on simple radiologic landmarks.

6 Subsequently integrated into a larger system, including, if needed, other kinds of neuro-imaging as well as databases such as computer-resident atlases.

7 A possible first step towards other therapeutic applications, such as multibeam convergent irradiation and computer-guided "open neurosurgery." In addition, the project needed to consider the development of user-friendly human/computer interfaces, versatility towards future applications, and the maintenance of reasonable costs compatible with conventional hospital practice.

The system which is described here, as it is presently used in daily routine practice at the Grenoble University Hospital, comprises a robot, physically linked to a stereotactic frame, and driven by a computer according to target coordinates provided by a digitizing table. This basic system can be connected to a digitized angiography system, to the main computer of an MR imager through an Ethernet network, and to a central computer where these images are processed, three-dimensional (3-D) pictures are generated, and stereotactic atlas data are stored.

THE STEREOTACTIC FRAME

Until now, the frame used in Grenoble has been the Talairach frame, consisting of a base plate holding four pillars bearing the verniers of the pins. Any other kind of frame can be used, provided that exact placement of the patient is possible and that the calibration and definition of inaccessible areas, due to the external features of the frame, have been established for that particular frame. The frame is mounted on a rotating ring, which allows complete examination of the ventricular system by taking X-rays in the supine, lateral, and recumbent positions. The rotating system is itself mounted on a solid base firmly attached on the floor and to the base of the robot. The center of the frame is situated at the crossing point of the beams of two X-ray tubes, permanently positioned at 3.5 m from the frame, one on the ceiling of the

operating room for anterior–posterior (A/P) pictures, and the other one on a wall of the room for lateral views.

THE ROBOT

Description

The robot used at the present time is a six-axis robot (Fig. 25.1) which, on the basis of an industrial model, has been specially redesigned to meet the specific requirements of stereotaxy. The position encoders on each axis have been set to 200 000 encoding pulses per turn, to achieve a resolution of $360°/200\,000 = 1.8 \times 10^{-3°}$. High reduction gears have been incorporated in order to reduce the maximal speed (about 0.02 turns s^{-1} on each axis) and, most of all, to eliminate the risk of back-driving when the servocontrol and the power of the motors are cut off. The dimensions of the various parts of the robot are human-like and allow a comparable spatial field of action, in half a sphere around the head of a patient in the recumbent position. The robot is fixed on a solid base screwed on the floor. The trunk of the robot, 30 cm high, can turn 270° around its vertical axis. The shoulder, which is at 100 cm above the floor (at the same height as the patient's head), holds the arm, which is 35 cm long and has 180° freedom of movement. The forearm, 45 cm long, is connected to the arm by the elbow which is able to turn through 270°, and is terminated by a wrist, made of three combined axes, having respectively a freedom of 270°, 180°, and 270° for the first, second, and third axes. The end plate of the wrist is adaptable to specific tools or "hands," which can be designed for special tasks. At the present time, a universal holder can be mounted on this end-plate and features a tungsten shaft, in the axis of which can be inserted a drill or guide tubes, the diameters of which are adapted to several tools such as electrodes, biopsy samplers, needles, and cannulas. On this holder, a micromanipulator can be mounted to drive microelectrodes during functional surgery recording sessions. A calibration cage made of two pairs of parallel plexiglass plates, each containing nine lead beads, can also be mounted on the end-plate at the time of calibration, which is the initial step in all procedures.

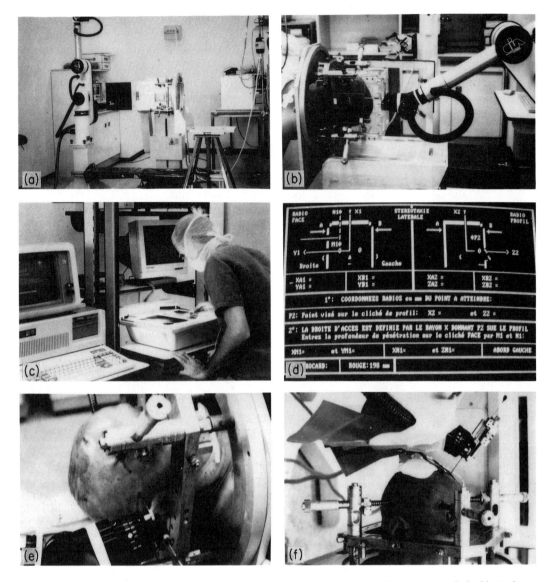

FIGURE 25.1 Overview of the system. General set-up: the robot, in the stand-by position, is linked by its base to the five-legged stereotactic frame; (b) the calibration cage is held around the patient's head by the robot's arm; (c) command consoles: an IBM PC-AT (left) is equipped with softwares for coordinate transformation and trajectory computation. A digitizing table (right) is used to sample the coordinates of the target and of the fiducial markers; (d) display of a menu during data acquisition of the target; (e) biopsy under lateral approach; (f) double oblique approach for thalamic implantation.

Command module

The command module is basically an IBM PC-AT computer, in which a designated robot programming card has been inserted. The PC is loaded with a program file containing a calibration file, a function translating the Cartesian coordinates given by the operator, through either the digitizing table or the mouse of the digitized angiography system, into the six angle coordinates of the robot, a file of the spatial data describing the inaccessible areas (the robot's trajectory to the final target must avoid certain areas containing obstacles, such as frame super-

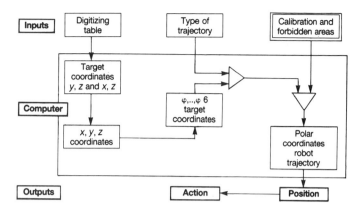

FIGURE 25.2 Flow chart of the program and computer files. φ = robot's six angles.

structures), and subroutine files to achieve specific purposes (such as calculation of the thalamic approach for thalamotomies or electrode implantations using ventricular landmarks: anterior and posterior commissures, top of the thalamus, midline, laterality) (Fig. 25.2).

Data acquisition

At the present time, all data are fed into the command computer via the digitizing table, from X-rays taken during the procedure. These data are of two kinds:

1 Calibration data: the X-ray pictures taken with the calibration cage positioned by the robot around the head of the patient show the images of the lead beads (Fig. 25.3), which are digitized and their coordinates introduced into the data file.

2 Target data: the positions of the target, or targets, which are plotted on the same pictures, are also digitized.

This system is currently being replaced by a digitized subtraction angiography (DSA) system (Digital Design, Saphyr system), which is used to collect all neuroradiologic images and display them on monitors, and to store in the central DSA memory the coordinates of every point on the pictures. Using a mouse, it is possible to move a cursor onto the target point and to sample and store the coordinates of this point. The step of using the digitizing table is therefore avoided, which has the advantages of time saving, higher precision, and the future possibility of automated detection of given features, such as the lead beads, for example.

Current performances of the system and achievements

GENERAL PROCEDURE

At the present time, the complete procedure consists of the following steps. Under local or general anesthesia, depending upon the type of planned stereotaxy, the patient is placed on the frame. The four pins of the frame are inserted into burr holes through the skull and the numbers on the pin-holding verniers are recorded. The calibration cage is mounted on the endplate of the robot's hand, and the initial step of the program orders the robot to place the cage around the patient's head. X-ray pictures are taken which show the lead beads and the fiducial markers of the frame on the same images. The calibration method was inspired by the two-plane method used for camera calibration [15], which was applied to robot model calibration [16] using a modified Denavit–Hartenberg model [17], the parameters of which were estimated with a non-linear least-squares algorithm. Angiograms and ventriculograms are then performed and the target point is determined. In the case of a tumor, data from the MRI are transferred onto the stereotactic ventriculogram (see Chapter 17), and a biopsy track is chosen which is compatible with the vessels, as shown on the angiograms. In the case of thalamic implantation, the target is drawn according to Taren *et al.*'s scheme [18]. In all cases, the landmarks used to define the target are digitized.

The program is run and computes the parameters of the trajectory, which are displayed

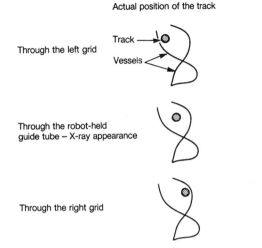

Actual position of the track

Through the left grid

Track

Vessels

Through the robot-held
guide tube – X-ray appearance

Through the right grid

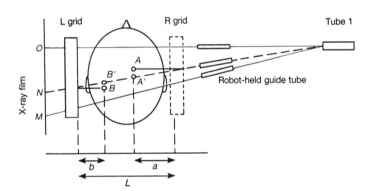

FIGURE 25.3 Alignment of
the guide tube along with the
X-ray beams. Due to the
parallax effect, a projected track
chosen in a vascular-free
window will be actually more
anterior when the probe is
introduced into a hole of the
right grid, and more posterior in
the left grid, as the grids are not
perpendicular to X-ray beams
except to the central beam itself.
As the guide tube of the robot is
positioned and aligned along
the beam passing through the
target, the projection of the
vessels is not distorted by
parallax, and the track will
actually be situated with respect
to the vessels exactly as shown
on the X-ray picture.

for control and eventually for validation. Careful attention is paid to avoid any error: the difference between the recalculated and real positions of the lead beads is displayed and must be accepted by the operator before proceeding to the next step.

When the proposed trajectory has been accepted, the program is able to drive the robot in the vicinity of its final position and hold it on stand-by. During this time, the robot arm and hand are dressed with a sterile plastic bag. A new validation from the surgeon starts the final approach at lower speed, during which the robot can be stopped instantly, at any time, if needed. X-rays are taken in order to control the actual position of the guide tube, as compared to the planned position. If this position is different from what was decided, the error can be measured and corrected, using a subroutine

which allows iterative and calibrated displacements. (Work is in progress to automatically adjust the robot to the final position, via automatic detection of the image of the probe holder on digitized radiograms and comparison with the theoretical target.) When the position is considered correct, the power of the command module is shut down, preventing any unexpected move of the robot during the last phase of the procedure, the robot holding its planned position without any possibility of changing it.

During the last phase, the skin is opened in front of the guide tube. A 2.3 mm hole is drilled into the skull through the guide tube, and the appropriate tool (biopsy sampler, electrode, cannula, etc.) is inserted down to the previously calculated depth, while X-rays are taken to check the accuracy of the track. For obvious security reasons during this experimental period of the robot's development, all penetrating procedures, although they could be performed by the robot itself, are manually performed, the robot at this stage being used only as a guide tube holder, to prevent any accidents while a probe is inside the brain.

At the end of the procedure, the inserted tool is hand-withdrawn and the robot is reactivated. A final subroutine drives it back to its initial resting position.

INTRINSIC PERFORMANCES

Precision

In the absence of any resistance or stress, the precision of the robot essentially depends on the zone involved by the trajectory. In most of these operation zones, the precision (defined as the precision of execution after giving spatial coordinates of the target as well as the mean deviation during repetition tests) is about 0.1 mm. In some special zones, such as the left anterior temporal or at the level of the vertex, the precision is much lower, and iterative displacements of about 2 or 3 mm can be needed. This is due to the positions of the joints the robot has to take in order to achieve the required trajectory. A new program card, as well as additional calibration procedures and the above-mentioned automatic feedback control, will suppress these inaccuracies.

Limits and drawbacks

No definitive statement can be made concerning limitations and drawbacks, since the robot is under permanent experimental investigation and improvement. At the present time, the procedure is still rather slow due to the extensive control steps which are followed for obvious ethical and safety reasons. Introduction of digitized radiography will significantly shorten the duration of these steps. Dangerous steps, such as drilling the skull, or the introduction and progression of a tool into the brain, could theoretically be performed by the combined six axis movements of the robot. This would essentially need strain gauges to detect the changes in resistance between successive structures (e.g. bone and brain), or against an obstacle (vessel,

bone, or calcified lesion). However, it is safer to use a seventh axis, driven by a linear motor.

CURRENT APPLICATIONS

From March 1st 1989 to March 1st 1990, 113 robotized stereotactic procedures were performed in various situations. For the last 50 of these, the surgical team was sufficiently trained to pilot the robot without the in-room assistance of roboticians and technicians, which demonstrates the convivial level of software development, already user-friendly, compatible with routine clinical use without an overly-apparent experimental impact in the operating room. The patients were informed that a robot was to be used, that security procedures were set up which avoided any risk, and they were told the extent and limits of its action. In all cases, they were confident and considered the robot as a new and sophisticated tool designed to improve surgery. Actually, the outcome of each patient was not influenced by the use of the robot, which did not introduce any additional risk during the procedure. It is possible to say that, on the contrary, the increased precision of execution of the decided trajectories, as well as easier decision-making due to a larger freedom of choices, often made the procedure safer.

Tumor biopsies (77 cases)

For several years [19,20], pretherapeutic stereotactic investigation of brain tumors has become increasingly popular and is currently aimed at diagnostic purposes, using serial biopsies as well as spatial localization, before conventional neurosurgery, for debulking the tumor mass, or before stereotactic implantation of isotope seeds or wires for interstitial brachytherapy. In these cases, the procedure essentially consists of the choice of a target central to the tumor core, and of a trajectory which is the safest depending on the brain structures and blood vessels surrounding the tumor. In our practice, we most often use a lateral approach and choose the trajectory according to the vessels as shown in stereotactic angiography. The point representing the lateral projection of the biopsy trajectory is digitized, and its coordinates

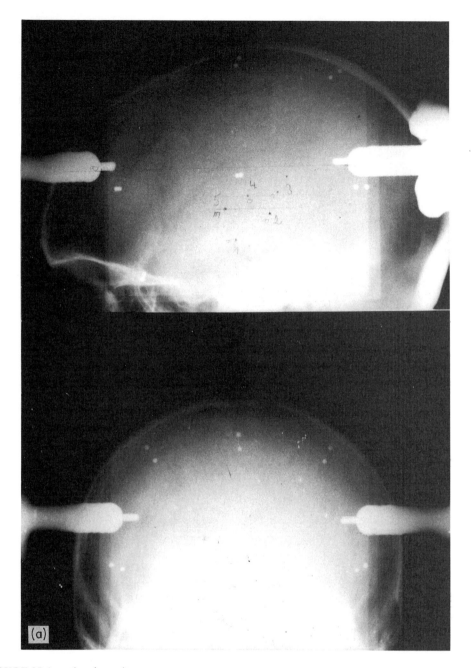

FIGURE 25.4 *continued opposite.*

are therefore available to the robot central unit in the command module, which computes and proposes a trajectory which, if validated by the neurosurgeon, is executed. The guide tube is set in a position which is checked by X-rays. The subroutine *lateral approach* has calculated, from the X-ray image of the calibration cage beads, the position of the central X-ray beam, which is perpendicular to the faces of the cage and along which no parallax is induced. Therefore, the program may calculate the parallax error for any point not situated on this central X-ray beam, and provides the robot with the data necessary to align the guide tube along the

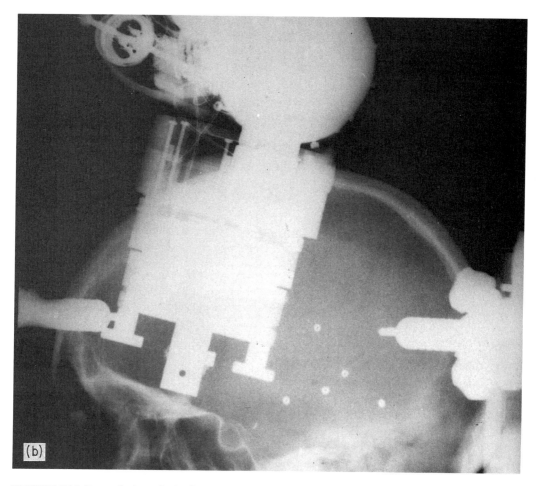

FIGURE 25.4 X-rays during robotized procedures. (a) Calibration cage: image magnification is different for beads of the left and right sides. (b) SEEG electrodes: when the robot has reached its final position, a control X-ray is taken, and the accuracy of the guide tube placement is checked. If necessary, a correction is made by iterative displacements, prior to drilling the final trajectory.

X-ray beam passing through the target point. This has the advantage of creating a trajectory which is co-linear to this X-ray beam, and which will have with the surrounding structures, such as blood vessels, the same relationships as shown on the X-ray picture (Fig. 25.3). If needed, iterative displacements of the guide tube can be achieved via the keyboard of the driving computer, which allows one to choose on a menu the amplitude (0−100 mm, with a 0.1 mm precision) of the displacements, the x, y and z coordinates on which they are desired, and their speed (from 5% to 100% of the maximal speed).

In 62 patients, this lateral approach was used to take 180 samples. In 15 patients, a double oblique trajectory (as described below) was used, mainly to reach tumors of the midline, such as in the pineal region or in the IIIrd ventricle.

Stereo-electroencephalographic (SEEG) investigations of epileptic patients (five cases) (Fig. 25.4)

Stereo-electroencephalography consists of introducing into the brain of an epileptic patient several depth electrodes with 5−15 contacts in a row, at precise locations depending on the clinical features of the epileptic seizures, and aimed at determining the extent of the epileptic focus and its propagating paths, with a view to surgical excision. These sites are chosen according to these clinical considerations, as well as to the permitted areas based on the angiograms. They are digitized in the same way as for lateral biopsies and the guide tube is positioned by the robot as previously described. The robot has a special subroutine which provides the possibility of feeding the program with all the desired sites of SEEG electrode implantation (usually 5–10, with sometimes one contralateral electrode) at the same time, and of subsequently positioning the guide tube. As for biopsies, drilling the holes, insertion of holding screws through the guide, and insertion of the electrodes into the central hole of the screws is still performed manually. Five patients underwent this procedure and had 35 electrodes inserted in this way.

Brachytherapy (five cases)

Introduction of permanent ^{125}I seeds or ^{192}Ir wires is, in terms of stereotactic procedure, very similar to biopsy sampling, and has been performed five times in this series of robot-operated patients. [125]I brachytherapy (three patients) in our protocol is made by permanent implantation of a unique seed of 12.5 mCi of ^{125}I, to deliver 60 Gy over a 35-mm diameter spherical surface in small low-grade gliomas. Brachytherapy with ^{192}Ir is very similar to SEEG investigations, as it requires the insertion of removable adjustable catheters [21,22], and has been performed in two patients of this series (one by lateral approach and one by oblique approach). The possibility of positioning the robot guide tube at any desired distance from the scalp makes this procedure, as well as SEEG electrode insertion, much easier than using the conventional grids of the Talairach frame, which requires the design of specific devices [23,24].

Midline stereotactic neurosurgery

Oblique approaches are needed mainly when the target is in the midline area, either for biopsies of midline tumors (pineal gland, IIIrd ventricle area), or for functional surgery of the basal ganglia (Parkinson's disease, chronic pain).

We used this approach to treat two patients with deafferentation pain by chronic somatosensory thalamic stimulation, and 20 patients suffering from dyskinesias (15 Parkinson's disease, five dyskinesias of other origins) by permanent thalamic VIM (ventral nucleus intermedius) stimulation. As the disease is often bilateral, 29 thalamic sides were implanted in this series of patients. The interest in using a robot is particularly well demonstrated in this type of procedure: the target, mainly the VIM nucleus in our dyskinesia patients [25,26], is principally defined on the basis of anatomic landmarks (the anterior and posterior commissures of the IIIrd ventricle, the top of the thalamus, and the midline), using a geometrical paradigm [18] and given lateralities [27]. A subroutine has been written which computes the VIM spatial coordinates from these landmarks as digitized on the ventriculograms, and then positions the robot. Control X-rays are taken with a mock probe inserted into the guide tube against the skin, and corrective displacements can be performed if needed. This saves a considerable amount of time, especially when bilateral electrodes are inserted. During this procedure, the exact target is precisely located using a first trajectory, based on the same landmarks, which crosses the VIM nucleus while recognizing its boundaries by semi-microelectrode recording. A further step in robotization of this procedure is in progress; this will drive the electrode micromanipulator from the robot computer and will report the calculated position of the electrode tip on the ventriculogram, as well as on stereotactic atlas maps.

OPERATIVE COMPLICATIONS

Only complications relevant to the use of the robot in the above-described procedures are taken into account in this chapter, and obviously, surgical complications due to biopsy sampling, electrode introduction, isotope implantation or deep brain stimulation, when they happen, as well as the therapeutic results of these procedures, cannot be attributed to use of the robot. In this series of 113 patients, we did not observe any complication which would have been eventually induced by the use of a robot.

Positioning was always possible as intended with the expected precision, within the limits of visual detectability on X-ray controls by the surgeon's eye. There was no displacement of the guide tube during penetrating procedures (or any unwanted displacement during previous steps when the robot was not deactivated). In addition, there was no limitation of execution of the intended program due to robot use itself.

It is important to note that during this clinical experience the robot was considered as safe as conventional stereotactic procedures. Moreover, the flexibility of its positioning made the choice of trajectories easier and thus, the overall procedure was safer.

Perspectives

This chapter describes the state of the art of robotics in neurosurgery in our department, as currently performed in the daily routine. Future perspectives which have recently been presented in the literature on robotics in medicine are applicable, and for some of them adaptation to our system is in progress.

STATE-OF-THE-ART

Due to progress in informatics, image processing, and robot technologies, medical and surgical applications of robots will rapidly become more diversified in the coming decade. The pioneering work of Kelly [4,8,9,13,28−35] and of Young [36] and Kwoh et al. [37−39] has opened up the field and is extensively described in this book. Work has been reported by other authors in neurosurgical stereotaxy [40] and in diverse medical applications [41], but is still at the laboratory experimental level. To our knowledge, with the exception of Kelly's and our own work, no other experience in routine robotized neurosurgery has thus far been reported.

SHORT-TERM PERSPECTIVES

Seventh axis

Penetration of the probe could be driven by the robot, even in the present state of development. However, the robot's linear advance has not been refined to within millimetric precision, because the method used to generate linear advance involves iterative computation of a succession of points on a line. New software will provide a more linear generation of trajectory, which could be used to drive a probe into the brain. However, another solution is more easily available. On the "wrist" of the robot, the sterilizable tool, which is at the present time a guide tube, can be replaced by a motorized tool, such as a drill or a micromanipulator used for the insertion of a biopsy sampler, an electrode, or a cannula. The final positioning of the probe can therefore be driven by the computer and integrated into the general software of the robot. A particularly interesting feature will be the provision of a feedback input of the spatial localization data of the tip of the probe and its display on X-rays, operating diagrams, or on stereotactic brain atlas maps.

Digitization and automated adjustment

Digitized X-ray images have already been used in stereotaxy [42]. At the present time, the data are taken from X-rays (angiograms, ventriculograms) by manual digitization of landmarks on a digitizing table. A Digital Design image processor (Saphyr) has been set up in the operating room and processes the images taken by a fluoroscope (28 cm in diameter) and a Hamamatsu TV camera. The data provided on X-ray films and manually digitized are now directly available from the digital data bank of the image processor, and can be sampled on the video display using a mouse-driven cursor. An automated procedure is being set up to recognize the images of the lead beads of the calibration cage, and to perform the calibration step automatically. A similar approach is possible to detect the image of the hole of the guide tube, to compare it with the designated position, and to compute the necessary iterative displacements for adjusting the final position of the guide tube exactly as desired.

Computer-resident atlas

This was among the first applications of computers to neurosurgery [43]. The basal ganglia area of the Schaltenbrand and Wahren atlas

[44] has been digitized, and the various anatomic structures have been named. An algorithm involving 3-D-spline functions has been designed [45] and provides 3-D reconstruction of these structures. The planned or actual trajectories can be displayed on these maps as intersections of the track with every plate or as a recalculated plane including the whole track.

MIDDLE TERM PERSPECTIVES

Use of 3-D images

3-D reconstruction algorithms [45] have been successfully applied to MRI and CT scan images. Connection of the image processor of the operating room with the VAX computer of our Department of Informatics will make possible the availability in the operating room of these 3-D images and their matching with the stereotactic X-ray images. Direct choice of the target from the MRI and CT-scan pictures of the pathologic target will therefore be possible.

Vascular collision

A further step is planned to recognize the blood vessels and detect the theoretical hit points between them and the intended trajectory. This will provide an aid to decision-making. Current approaches to solve this important problem are detailed in this book (Chapter 17) and elsewhere [46–50].

Open surgery

The final goal of computer-assisted surgery is to achieve intraoperative control of surgical tool position with respect to the pathologic lesion, such as a tumor. As a result of stereotactic investigations, the tumor is precisely located with respect to the fiducial markers of the frame. It is therefore possible to place the patient in an operating frame and take advantage of a surgical robot for the tasks of spatial localization and guiding the surgeon's tools during "open field" surgery. This is in the same perspective as Kelly *et al.*'s approach [11], which has already demonstrated the advantages of such a procedure [31–35]. Intermediate solutions have been also reported to guide surgical trephination [51,52]

or during the intracerebral procedure, using ultrasound localization [53–56].

Conclusions

The stereotactic robot has to be considered as a first step in the more general approach of computer assisted medico-surgical procedures. The development of such a system opens the way to an integrated system linking image databases, theoretical reference databases (such as computer-resident stereotactic atlases), and surgical procedures, during either stereotactic or "open" surgery. The long-term goal is to build an interactive system, allowing surgical procedures during which the surgeon knows at every moment where he is, what he is doing, and what structures his actions involve, via a feedback mechanism in which the data banks are continually fed with new information gathered during the procedure.

References

1 Benabid, A.L., Cinquin, P., Lavallée, S., Le Bas, J.F., Demongeot, J. & de Rougemont, J. Computer-driven robot for stereotactic surgery connected to CT scan and magnetic resonance imaging. *Appl. Neurophysiol.* **50**: 153–4, (1987).

2 Lavallée, S. Gestes médico-chirurgicaux assistés par ordinateur. Thèse Sciences Mathématiques, Université Joseph Fourier, Grenoble (1989).

3 Gildenberg, P.L. Whatever happened to stereotactic surgery? *Neurosurgery* **20**(6): 983–7 (1987).

4 Kelly, P.J., Kall, B.A., Goerss, S. & Earnest, F. Present and future developments of stereotactic technology. *Appl. Neurophysiol.* **48**: 1–6 (1985).

5 Brown, R.A. A computerized tomography-computer graphics approach to stereotactic localization. *J. Neurosurg.* **50**: 715–20 (1979).

6 Colombo, F., Angrilli, F., Zanardo, A., Pinna, V., Alexandre, A. & Benedetti, A. A universal method to employ CT scanner spatial information in stereotactic surgery. *Appl. Neurophysiol.* **45**: 352–4 (1982).

7 Gildenberg, P.L., Kaufmann, H.H. & Krishna Murthy, K.S. Calculation of stereotactic coordinates from the computed tomographic scan. *Appl. Neurophysiol.* **45**: 443–8 (1982).

8 Goerss, S.J., Kelly, P.J., Kall, B.A. & Alker, G.J. A computed tomographic stereotactic adaptation system. *Neurosurgery* **10**(3): 375–9 (1982).

9 Kall, B.A., Kelly, P.J., Goerss, S.J. & Earnest, F. IV. Cross-registration of points and lesion volumes from MR and CT. *Proceedings of the 7th Annual Meeting of Frontiers of Engineering and Computing in Health Care*, pp. 935–42 (1985).

10 Kelly, P.J., Kall, B.A. & Goerss, S.J. Transposition of volumetric information derived from computed tomography scanning into stereotactic space. *Surg. Neurol.* **21**: 465−71 (1984).

11 Mundinger, F., Birg, W. & Klar, M. Computer-assisted stereotactic brain operations by means including computerized axial tomography. *Appl. Neurophysiol.* **41**: 169−82 (1978).

12 Perry, J.H., Rosenbaum, A.E., Junsford, L.D., Swink, C.A. & Zorub, D.S. Computed tomography-guided stereotactic surgery: conception and development of a new stereotactic methodology. *Neurosurgery* **7**: 376−81 (1980).

13 Kelly, P.J., Alker, G.J. & Goerss, S. Computer-assisted stereotactic laser microsurgery for the treatment of intracranial neoplasms. *Neurosurgery* **10**: 324−31 (1982).

14 Asimov, I. *I, Robot.* New York: Doubleday (1950).

15 Gremban, K.D., Thorpe C.E. & Kanade T. Geometric camera calibration using systems of linear equations. *Proceedings of the Institute of Electrical and Electronic Engineers International Conference on Robotics and Automation*, pp. 947−51. Philadelphia: Institute of Electrical and Electronics Engineers (1988).

16 Roth, Z.S., Mooring, B.W. & Ravani, B. An overview of robot calibration. *Institute of Electrical and Electronics Engineers' J. Robotics Automation* **3**(5): 377−85 (1987).

17 Denavit, J., Hartenberg, R.S. & Evanston, I.L.L. A kinematic notation for lower-pair mechanisms based on matrices. *J. Appl. Mechanics* **55**: 215−21 (1955).

18 Taren, J., Guiot, G. Derome, P. & Trigo, J.C. Hazards of stereotaxic thalamotomy. Added safety factors in corroborating X-ray target localization with neurophysiological methods. *J. Neurosurg* **29**: 173−82 (1968).

19 Ostertag, C.B., Mennel, H.D. & Kiessling, M. Stereotactic biopsy of brain tumors. *Surg. Neurol.* **14**: 275−83 (1980).

20 Daumas-Duport, C., Monsaingeon, V., Szenthe, L. & Szikla, G. Serial stereotactic biopsies: a double histological code of gliomas according to malignancy and 3-D configuration, as an aid to therapeutic decision and assessment of results. *Appl. Neurophysiol.* **45**: 431−7 (1982).

21 Gutin, P.H., Phillips, T.L., Wara, W.M., *et al.* Brachytherapy of recurrent malignant brain tumors with removable high activity [125]iodine sources. *J. Neurosurg.* **60**: 61−8 (1984).

22 Benabid, A.L., Chirossel, J.P., Mercier, C., *et al*, Removable, adjustable, and reusable implants for stereotactic interstitial radiosurgery of brain tumors. *Appl. Neurophysiol.* **50**: 278−80 (1987).

23 Olivier, A. Double-headed stereotaxic carrier apparatus for insertion of depth electrodes. *J. Neurosurg.* **65**: 258−9 (1986).

24 Bouvier, G., Saint Hilaire, J.M., Giard, N., Lesage, J., Cloutier, L. & Beique, R. Depth electrodes implantation at Hospital Notre-Dame, Montreal.

In: Engel, J. Jr (ed.) *Surgical Treatment of the Epilepsies*, pp. 589−94. New York: Raven Press (1987).

25 Benabid, A.L., Pollak, P., Louveau, A., Henry, S. & de Rougemont, J. Combined (thalamotomy and stimulation) stereotactic surgery of the VIM thalamus nucleus for bilateral Parkinson's disease. *Appl. Neurophysiol.* **50**: 344−6 (1987).

26 Benabid, A.L., Pollak, P., Hommel, M., Gaio, J.M., de Rougemont, J. & Perret, J. Traitement du tremblement parkinsonien par stimulation chronique du noyau ventral intermédiaire du Thalamus. *Rev. Neurol. (Paris)* **145**(4): 320−3 (1989).

27 Tasker, R.R., Organ, L.W. & Hawrylyshyn, P. Investigation on the surgical target for alleviation of involuntary movement disorders. *Appl. Neurophysiol.* **45**: 261−74 (1982).

28 Kelly, P.J. & Alker, G.J. A method for stereotactic laser microsurgery in the treatment of deep-seated CNS neoplasms. *Appl. Neurophysiol.* **43**: 210−5 (1980).

29 Kelly, P.J. & Alker, G.J. A stereotactic approach to deep-seated central nervous system neoplasms using the carbon dioxide laser. *Surg. Neurol.* **15**: 331−5 (1981).

30 Kelly, P.J., Alker, G.J., Kall, B. & Goerss, S. Method of computed tomography-based stereotactic biopsy with arteriographic control. *Neurosurgery* **14**: 172−7 (1984).

31 Kelly, P.J. Technical approaches to identification and stereotactic reduction of tumor burden. In: Walker, M.D. & Thomas, D.G.T. (eds) *Biology of Brain Tumor*, pp. 237−343. Boston: Martinus Nijhoff (1986).

32 Kelly, P.J., Earnest, F., Kall B.A., *et al.* Surgical options for patients with deep-seated brain tumors: computer-assisted stereotactic biopsy. *Mayo Clin. Proc.* **6**: 223−9 (1986).

33 Kelly, P.J., Kall, B., Goerss, S. & Alker, G.J. Precision resection of intraaxial CNS lesions by CT-based stereotactic craniotomy and computer monitored CO_2 laser. *Acta Neurochir.* **68**: 1−9 (1983).

34 Kall, B.A., Kelly, P.J. & Goerss, S.J. Interactive stereotactic surgery system for the removal of intracranial tumors utilizing the CO_2 laser and the CT-derived database. *Institute of Electrical and Electronics Engineers Trans. Biomed. Eng.* **32**: 112−6 (1985).

35 Kall, B.A., Kelly, P.J. & Goerss, S. Comprehensive computer-assisted data collection treatment planning and interactive surgery. *Proceedings of the Society of Photo-optical Instrumentation Engineers, Medical Imaging* **767**: 509−14 (1987).

36 Young, R.J. Application of robotics to stereotactic neurosurgery. *Neurol. Res.* **9**: 123−8 (1987).

37 Kwoh, Y.S., Reed, I.S., Chen, J.Y., Shao, H.M., Truong, T.K. & Jonckheere, E.A. New computerized tomographic-aided robotic stereotaxis system. *Robotics Age* **7**: 17−22 (1985).

38 Kwoh, Y.S., Hou, J., Jonckheere, E.A. & Hayati, S.

A robot with improved absolute positioning accuracy for CT-guided stereotactic brain surgery. *Institute of Electrical and Electronics Engineers Trans. Biomed. Eng.* **35**(2): 153−60 (1988).

39 Kwoh, Y.S. & Young, R. Robotic-aided surgery. In: Kelly, P.J. & Kall, B.A. (eds), *Computers in Stereotactic Neurosurgery*. Oxford: Blackwell Scientific Publications (1992). (Chapter 24, this volume.)

40 Doll, J., Schlegel, W., Pastyr, O., Sturm, V. & Maier-Borst, W. The use of an industrial robot as a stereotactic guidance system. *Comput. Assist. Radiol.* **79**: 374−8 (1987).

41 Vidal, P., Hache, J.C., Hayat, S., Guerrouad, A., Ben Gayed, M. & Lepers, B. Un microtélémanipulateur chirurgical applicable en neurologie et en ophthalmologie. Congrès Institut d'Informatique et de Rercherche au Intelligence Artificielle de Marseille, Marseille. Productique Hospitalière (1988).

42 Peters, T.M., Clark, J.A., Olivier, A., *et al.* Integrated stereotaxic imaging with CT, MR imaging, and digital subtraction angiography. *Radiology* **161**: 821−6 (1986).

43 Kall, B.A., Kelly, P.J., Goerss, S.J. & Frieder, G. Methodology and clinical experience with computed tomography and a computer-resident stereotactic atlas. *Neurosurgery* **17**: 400−7 (1985).

44 Schaltenbrand, G. & Wahren, W. *Atlas for Stereotaxy of the Human Brain*, 2nd edn. Stuttgart: Thieme (1977).

45 Cinquin, P. Application des fonctions splines au traitement d'images numériques. Thèse d'état de Sciences Mathématiques, Université Joseph Fourier, Grenoble (1987).

46 Suetens, P., Jansen, P., Haegemans, A., Oosterlink, A. & Gybels, J. 3D reconstruction of the blood vessels of the brain from a stereoscopic pair of subtraction angiograms. *Image Vision Comput.* **1**(1): 43−51 (1983).

47 Cloutier, L., Nguyen, D.N., Ghosh, S., *et al.* Simulator allowing spatial viewing of cerebral probes by using a floating line concept. *Symposium on Optical and Electro-Optical Applied Science and Engineering*, Cannes, France (1985).

48 Camillerapp, J., Leplumey, J. & Walter, A. Acquisition of a 3D model of the cranial vascular system from two stereoscopic pictures. AFCET, Antibes 16−20 Nov, 1987.

49 Smets, C., Vandermeulen, D., Suetens, P. & Oosterlinck, A. A knowledge-based system for the 3D reconstruction and representation of the cerebral blood vessels from a pair of stereoscopic angiograms. *Proceedings of the Society of Photo-optical Instrumentation Engineers Medical Imaging III* **1092**: 130−8 (1989).

50 Venaille, C., Mischler, D., Coatrieux, J.L. & Catros, J.Y. Reconstruction 3D de reseaux vasculaires en angiographie. *Proceedings of the 7th Congress AFCET-RFIA*, pp. 1533−47. Paris (1989).

51 Kosugi, Y., Watanabe, E., Goto, J., *et al.* An articulated neurosurgical navigation system using MRI and CT images. *Institute of Electrical and Electronics Engineers Trans. Biomed. Eng.* **35**(2): 147−52 (1988).

52 Roberts, D.W., Strohbehn, J.W., Hatch, J.H., Murray, W. & Kettenberger, H. A frameless stereotaxic integration of computerized tomographic imaging and the operating microscope. *J. Neurosurg* **65**: 545−9 (1986).

53 Berger, M.S. Ultrasound-guided stereotaxic biopsy using a new apparatus. *J. Neurosurg.* **65**: 550−4 (1986).

54 Iseki, H. & Amano, K. CT-guided stereotactic surgery in combination with intra-operative monitoring by sector type ultrasonography. *Asian Med. J.* **28**(3): 157−67 (1985).

55 Masuzawa, H., Kamitani, H., Sator, J. *et al.* Intra-operative application of sector scanning electronic ultrasound in neurosurgery. *Neurol. Med. Chir. (Tokyo)* **21**: 277−85 (1981).

56 Tsutsumi, Y., Andoh, Y. & Inoue, N. Ultrasound-guided echo biopsy for deep-seated brain tumors. *J. Neurosurg.* **57**: 164−7 (1982).

part   *VI*

Future Possibilities

chapter 26

Future Possibilities

Patrick J. Kelly

Introduction

Competition within the computer industry produces ever more powerful and capacious computer systems for less cost. No industry in the history of mankind has undergone the advancement exhibited by the computer industry in the past 40 years. For example, if aircraft development had kept pace with computer evolution, a commercial airliner could circle the globe in $2\frac{1}{2}$ hours and the cost of the airline ticket would be $1.35. In addition, information systems tend to feed on themselves and develop in an exponential fashion. Each development is basically the product of all that has preceded it. Because of the explosion in information systems and technology, we are truly living in a renaissance more significant in impact and scope than any other in history. We will be catapulted into the distant future faster than any generation ever. Medicine will also benefit.

Progress is inevitable in robotics, electronics, lasers, optic ultrasonic imaging, and superconducting magnetic technologies, to name a few. In particular, further progress is inevitable in computer technology. Computers will provide the direct and indirect substrate for incorporation of many technologies into medicine and neurosurgery in general, and stereotactic neurosurgery in particular.

Because of computers, all of neurosurgery, indeed all branches of surgery, may ultimately become stereotactically based: three-dimensionally (3-D) controlled interventions on 3-D defined target volumes. Advances in computer technology and software will make stereotaxis practical, time- and cost-efficient, and thereby irresistible to most neurosurgeons.

Imminent computer developments

Graphics

Basically, stereotactic applications center on the manipulation of images. Graphic manipulations require large computer memories. Currently there is a trend toward connecting microcomputers and minicomputers into networks for picture archiving and communication systems. As computers are becoming faster, larger, and more competitively priced, larger memories and faster input/output speeds are becoming available to the medical community. A major advantage of larger capacity and faster input/output speeds is that higher-level language functions can be supported and truly user-friendly software interfaces are practical. High-level languages are essential for convenient and time-efficient software development.

One major problem in imaging-based computer-assisted stereotaxis rests with the wide variety of computer hardware devices, display and reconstructive software on the various computed tomography (CT), magnetic resonance imaging (MRI), and digital angiographic devices. In order to work with these systems, one must obtain the proprietary code from the manufacturer of the imaging system, and spend resources rewriting display software in order to be able to use the images within a surgical computer system. However, the American College of Radiology (ACR) and the National Electrical Manufacturers Association (NEMA) have been negotiating with the manufacturers of the various medical imaging systems. They have developed a standärd for transferring images and associated information between devices from different companies. If this so-called ACR and NEMA standard is adopted by all manufacturers, a direct communication data link between imaging host computers and surgical host computers would be possible without specific software development.

Several research laboratories are developing distributor processors where multiple central processing units (CPUs) operate in parallel on a defined problem. Parallel processing enhances the ability of the computer to process data quickly. The host processor transmits commands to coprocessors. The coprocessors perform the operations and notify the host processors when the operations have been completed. As an example, the voxel processor is a device which employs several processors; each processor is responsible for processing reconstruction of part of a medical image. Each part is then returned to the host processor for display of the final image. This technology currently has limited image resolution. However, it is likely that thousands of CPUs will be combined in the future for high resolution 3-D imaging. With such systems it is conceivable that one CPU could be responsible for each pixel on the screen. This system could operate tens of thousands of times faster than current imaging systems, and true real-time applications and interactive real-time two-dimensional (2-D) and 3-D image displays would be possible.

Stereotactic image displays

A major problem in surgical planning is imposed by the fact that computers can only display 3-D information on a 2-D screen. Therefore, 3-D objects, such as interpolated tumor volume or surrounding anatomic structures, can be visualized by only three methods, none of which is totally satisfactory. First, a series of sequential slices through the data matrix can be displayed on the 2-D display screen. Thus, a complex 3-D volume is displayed in a series of 2-D images, sliced perpendicular to some arbitrary viewing line.

Second, a shaded surface display of an object, e.g. a tumor or the skull, can be constructed by means of a shading algorithm, which provides a qualitative illusion of a 3-D image. In fact, a movie can be created of these images as the object is rotated about a defined axis within a computer storage matrix and each of these images is displayed rapidly and in sequence. Such displays provide a 3-D concept of the lesion and its anatomic environment. These images cannot yet be used quantitatively in stereotaxis, but do make impressive pictures and may be used in surgical simulations.

Finally, a stereoscopic pair of these shaded surface displays can be generated and presented to the viewer. The observer views the paired image with crossed eyes, prisms, or a stereoscopic merge unit which blends the stereoscopic pair into a 3-D picture. Furthermore, a 3-D cursor can be used to determine stereotactic coordinates within these images.

Holographic displays

A projection holographic display of combined imaging data could provide a true and accurate 3-D picture of the lesion and its relationship to surrounding anatomic structures. These images can be life-sized and are free of distortion. The surgeon could actually place a ruler within a hologram and measure the distance between two structures, for example, and expect that the measurements taken from these images would be accurate.

The problem with holography is that it now takes days to produce a quality projection hologram. It is a tedious photographic process, and holograms usually require a high-power laser light source and a stable surface which is free of vibration. Nevertheless, there are several companies working on turn-key systems that will generate projection holograms in a matter of minutes. These proposed systems usually require a computer which generates sequential slice data, and displays these slices on a high-resolution liquid crystal display unit, which is shifted for each image a precise distance by a stepper motor-controlled slide system. Holograms could then be built up from serial slice images generated by a computer, or the actual raw CT and MRI image data. Blood vessels could be first suspended within a 3-D image matrix, derived from stereoscopic stereotactic angiograms or MRI angiography. The matrix could then be sliced and subsequent sequential image displays used to create a hologram of the blood vessels in space also.

With holography it is practical to superimpose databases from several sources. For example, stereotactic CT, MRI, and angiography could be combined into a single holographic image. It would therefore be possible to have a single white light hologram of the entire combined stereotactic imaging database. This holographic "plate" would project a true life-sized transparent image of the patient's brain.

Display of this image would be very straightforward — a diffraction grating light box which could be mounted alongside the X-ray view-boxes in the operating room. Thus, during an operation, the stereotactic surgeon could refer to the patient's CT, MRI, and angiogram, as well as a projection holographic image of all of the databases combined in a display which represents precise 3-D stereotactic space. Furthermore, there is a possibility that we will be able to interact in real-time with computer-generated holographic displays.

Some computer laboratories are now in the process of developing holographic display terminals. These would have resolution far beyond those 3-D computer displays of the vibrating mirror variety which have been around for about 10 years. We are discussing computer-generated real-time 3-D holographic displays. The application of the vibrating mirror type displays has been limited in stereotaxis because of the poor resolution provided by them.

Computer-generated holograms have been possible for over 10 years. Computers can generate, on a plotter, an image which would have programmed into every pixel a diffraction coefficient that would deflect light of a given

wavelength, and produce the interference pattern necessary to produce the holographic effect. The compositions for each pixel of such an image are substantial. Therefore, the resolution of these images has been crude because of limited computer memory available in systems used to generate them. Since computers are becoming faster and more capacious, and multiple parallel processors are now practical, resolution of these computer-generated holographic images has improved substantially. In theory they may ultimately have resolutions similar to high quality 2-D raster display images. In addition, a special liquid crystal-based diffraction display terminal is presently under development so that these images can be displayed on a computer screen.

The major advantage of such hardware, beyond image quality, would be the ability to interact with the holographic display in real-time. Thus, a surgeon could plan a 3-D operation within a true 3-D image. In addition, during an operation, the operating room computer system could display the position of stereotactically positioned surgical instruments within that 3-D holographic display.

Software developments

Computers do not understand English (or French, or German, etc.). They understand a binary code of 0s and 1s. The order of the 0s and 1s which enable a computer to do something is controlled by a binary assembler which is, in turn, directed by low-level language, such as machine or assembly language. These languages are not anything like English either. However, an excellent computer programmer, who understands these low-level languages, can produce relatively simple programs in assembly language which will run fast and efficiently, and consume minimal space within the CPU to do so. Nevertheless, few neurosurgeons will ever understand machine or assembly language, and not many computer scientists want to write programs in these low-level languages, either. Therefore higher-level language programs have been developed over the years, which are translated into lower-level languages by the appropriate compiler or interpreter. The following is a brief list and description of the common languages used in medical imaging.

High-level languages

C This is a general purpose high-level language, originally developed for UNIX-based operating systems. It is a structured language which produces high speed executable code. It is well suited for graphics applications. C is now very popular in the personal computer (PC) market-place and is used in graphics processing.

PASCAL Language developed in the late 1960s for programming teaching machines. It is a block-structured language and it reads more like "English" than other languages. Many graphics routines in modern imaging systems are in PASCAL and C.

FORTRAN Formula Translation (FORTRAN) is a mathematic application language. It is used in rapid computations and employed within the scientific community. In general, FORTRAN generates rapid codes for a variety of scientific applications. Many versions of FORTRAN have been developed, e.g. FORTRAN 4, FORTRAN 5, FORTRAN 77.

BASIC This is a simple language which was used in early microcomputers. It was constructed so that a line of code could be translated into a set of machine language instructions a line at a time. BASIC code executes slowly because every instruction must be decoded each time it is executed. It has limited scientific and graphic applications. It could be used to store office records, clinical data, etc.

Other programming languages, such as SNOBOL and COBOL, are used in the business community for report generation and business applications. They are not applicable to medical image processing or stereotaxis.

Low-level languages

Assembly or machine level language This mnemonic language is one step above the binary code (or 0s and 1s) that the computer CPU uses for manipulating memory registers directly. Programs written in Assembly language run faster than programs written in high-level languages. This is because instructions need not be interpreted first by the high-level language compiler. However, assembly language programs are cumbersome and difficult to write. In addition, assembly or machine level programs are not portable from one machine to another unless their processor's instruction sets are upward compatible.

Some of the above languages sound more like English than others, but are still a long way from providing a neurosurgeon not familiar with programming with a means of getting a computer to do what he or she wants. A computer scientist who knows the format and structure of the language is still necessary in order to write code and make the program work. That, therefore, is the problem: computer scientists. Until this human interface between neurosurgeon and computer can be eliminated, there will always be a general reluctance for stereotactic and general neurosurgeons to accept the computer as a useful operating room instrument.

Computer scientists

What is wrong with computer scientists? Nothing personally. However, their time is expensive, and writing and debugging computer code is labor-intensive and exacting. Good computer scientists do this efficiently, bad ones do it slowly or not at all. Good computer scientists who can efficiently produce executable code are a rare breed in medical circles. Good ones are usually hired away by industry at twice or three times the salary offered by a hospital or university medical departments. Indeed, even university computer science departments have problems attracting and keeping qualified faculty, which further limits the supply of qualified colleagues in computer science.

Second, computer scientists speak a different language than neurosurgeons. They may not be able to understand the tasks the stereotactic neurosurgeon proposes to them until the task is presented in terms familiar to them. For example, one cannot say to a computer scientist "I want to determine stereotactic coordinates for a blood vessel detected on a stereoscopic pair of an angiogram." The neurosurgeon will have to explain what a stereotactic coordinate system is, what an angiogram is, derive methods for measuring the blood vessel, derive a reference system for radiographs from which to derive coordinates, select the appropriate equations to determine magnification and image distortion, and equations to determine 3-D distance. Finally, the neurosurgeon will have to list the actual procedure in a logical step-by-step method which also defines how data will be inputted and outputted. This the computer scientist will understand.

Computer scientists experienced in working with neurosurgeons will gradually learn a great deal about the problems, background methods, and calculations in stereotactic neurosurgery. Neurosurgeons experienced in working with computer scientists will eventually learn how to present a problem to them so that they can derive the algorithms and flow charts from which to develop code. However, the "learning curves" for neurosurgeon and computer scientist take time to come to fruition. The point is that a neurosurgeon cannot just choose a computer scientist "off the street" and expect him or her to write useful and executable code from the very first day.

Therefore, the problem is not necessarily the computer scientist *per se*, but rather the language barrier between neurosurgeons and computer scientists. However, younger neurosurgeons are becoming more computer-literate. Some are capable of doing rudimentary programming. Nonetheless, this only reduces the time necessary for the "learning curve" which enables neurosurgeons and computer scientists to talk to each other. It does not get to the basic root of the problem: the necessity for the middleman (i.e. the computer scientist) between neurosurgeon and computer.

USER-FRIENDLY SOFTWARE

Certainly neurosurgeons can use computers in the operating room on a day-to-day basis by means of "user-friendly" software and convenient input/output devices. Once this "user-friendly" software has been developed and thoroughly debugged, the surgeon can indeed work directly with the computer. The computer scientist should no longer be necessary. In fact, more and more stereotactic neurosurgeons are currently using on a regular basis these "packaged" programs for point-in-space and volumetric stereotaxis.

STEREOTACTIC FACULTY POSITIONS FOR COMPUTER SCIENTISTS

Computer-assisted stereotaxis is, and always will remain, "a work in progress." New ideas will be generated by continued use and experience with the methods. New software will always be required. Use of the computer for repetitive calculations and image displays only is to ignore the tremendous potential of the computer as a tool: the potential for continued and progressive development of our field. Thus at present a competent computer scientist remains a necessity in any stereotactic development program.

In addition, computer manufacturers continue to supply us with faster, more capacious and, in terms of cost : performance ratio, more inexpensive hardware, for which existing software must be modified. Who will modify this software? Upgrading software can be a tedious and difficult endeavor for someone not familiar with the original software and source codes. Obviously, the computer scientist who developed the original program can upgrade software for a new machine faster and far easier than someone else. Therefore, for the time being, we are better off keeping "middlemen" within our departments, whether we like it or not.

Stereotactic neurosurgeons may consider creating a faculty position in sections of stereotactic neurosurgery for a full-time computer scientist. However, we must constantly come up with ways to keep these people interested. In addition, can we generate the money necessary to pay them the salaries they deserve and which are competitive with what they would earn elsewhere? Perhaps, but there are alternate solutions to maintaining full-time computer scientists within our section of stereotactic neurosurgery.

THE NEUROSURGEON AS PROGRAMMER

Neurosurgeons could learn to write their own computer programs. However, this is a ridiculous solution. Writing programs in FORTRAN, C or PASCAL is complex, time-consuming, and requires tremendous attention to detail. It is not something we can do between cases in the operating room, for example. Furthermore, it takes time to become a good computer programmer and time to learn the "tricks" which make a good computer scientist efficient. A young neurosurgeon's time is better spent learning to be a good clinician and surgical technician. Learning high-level computer languages, and plodding through the development of massive programs for complex image displays, is an inefficient use of a neurosurgeon's time. Nonetheless, there may be a couple of ways that a neurosurgeon could do some of his or her own programming, without having to learn PASCAL, C or FORTRAN. Our colleagues in computer science must help us get started on both of the following avenues.

Block task programming

First, let us consider how a good computer program is structured. Basically, a program is a logical series of tasks which are executed in order and which produce the final result: the calculation of stereotactic coordinates, display of an image, or whatever. Each task in the program is performed by a small subprogram: subroutines which are called by the main program when required.

Stereotactic neurosurgeons will wish to modify the main program as the development of his or her stereotactic system proceeds. Therefore, we will require a user-friendly means of modifying the main program. This can be done by simply adding or deleting subroutines, or changing their order within the main computer program. This could be executed in many ways.

For example, a displayed menu could list the various options and the subroutines which have been written previously and are available. Each subroutine would perform a defined task: for example, to read and to display an MR image, or to digitize fiducials, etc. These subroutines could be added into an existing skeletal program to provide further operational options.

After using the "main" program for several months for simple calculations of a point in space, a surgeon now wishes to incorporate the ability to utilize stereotactic angiographic data. Subroutines for the display of digital angiograms

or calculation of stereotactic coordinates from them could be purchased, loaded onto the stereotactic computer system, and included in the menu. The surgeon could display the "blocks" or steps in the main program, and then insert these new subroutines in the appropriate place. Other subroutines could be rearranged if desired.

After the various blocks of the new "program" were assembled, the surgeon could finally select a "compile" box in the main menu. This would first ask for a new name for this custom program, and then compile it. This new program could be recalled and used, or modified further, at any time.

Thus, the software proposed above would be a program which would allow a surgeon to change it or to create and compile a new program, utilizing only a menu, mouse, and cursor.

In order to construct such a thing, a computer scientist would have to understand and write programs for all of the possible tasks a surgeon might want to have a computer perform. However, in reality there is a finite and predictable number of tasks in medical imaging and stereotactic neurosurgery.

Super-high-level languages

As stated above, computers understand binaries: 0s and 1s. Programming languages are ultimately translated to binary code by means of compilers. Compilers are basically translation tables which convert statements or commands in high-level languages to symbols in machine language; the symbols in machine languages are translated into 0s and 1s by the assembler. The compiler is a program in itself. It requires a significant chunk of random access memory (RAM) to do its job. However, with the increasing RAM capacities which are now available, super-high-level compilers, which would translate everyday English into a high-level computer programming language, are a very real possibility in the future.

The development of these compilers would require an extensive programming effort which would employ, among other things, artificial intelligence algorithms. The reason for the latter is that there are many ways in which to say the same thing. However, computers have no imagination. They must receive their instructions in a precise and defined format. Therefore, an extensive library of possible synonymous input options would have to be created. These would be translated by the computer into specific instructions, in the correct format that the computer will understand and act upon. In addition, elaborate internal lists of steps would have to be associated with even the simplest commands, such as "Display the radiograph." Inherent in a command as seemingly simple as this, for example, would include in a "list maker" the commands: (1) "Check to see that a digital version of the radiograph exists on the storage disk"; (2) "Transfer the file of the radiograph to the central processing unit"; (3) "Transfer it from the CPU to the image display matrix"; (4) "Read pixel 1,1"; (5) "Display pixel 1,1 in position 1,1 on the display screen at intensity I"; (6) "Read pixel 1,2"; etc. This may seem complicated to some. But the beauty of a computer is that once the program has been written and debugged, it will run all of this over and over again. Therefore a command such as "display the radiograph" will be instantaneously translated into all of the above steps.

What would happen if the neurosurgeon said "Let me see the X-ray?" Obviously this would come under the function of the translator, which would have a glossary of all possible input options, and would interpret this to mean "Display the radiograph," and then invoke the "list maker," which would provide the various logical steps listed above and "Display the radiograph."

Input devices

Computer scientists enter code or instructions into a computer by means of a keyboard. Few neurosurgeons will accept that. If neurosurgeons really have to type in computer code or commands, as computer programmers do now, we cannot expect much development to come from them, even if there is a simplified high-level language compiler. Typing on a keyboard is one option for data or instruction input, albeit a tedious one. A mouse, cursor, and menu system would be easier to use, faster, and would find greater acceptance. But menus by necessity must have a limited number of options, or they become unwieldy. Obviously they cannot cover

all possible command options. Could we simply just talk to the computer? The answer to that is yes.

Voice recognition programs are already available, even in inexpensive microprocessor based systems. Some of these have a vocabulary of several thousand words. In addition, voice recognition programs will provide the security required (for example, a neurosurgeon may not appreciate having the cleaning lady talking to the computer and manipulating its database). Furthermore, even with today's technology, the computer could even respond to the surgeon in English (or French, or German, or Vietnamese, if required). Anyone who has obtained a telephone number from the directory assistance in a large city has had a computer answer them with relatively high quality speech.

Interactive communication

Surgeons must not only communicate with the computer to write programs, they must also interact with them on-line during stereotactic surgical procedures, during surgical planning, and during data input. How is this done? Obviously commands can be inputted by means of the keyboard, by means of a mouse cursor, and menus and icons. The latter is used quite effectively in modern workstations.

All of these are satisfactory for data input and during surgical planning. However, keyboards and mouse−cursor systems are cumbersome to use during the course of an operation. The surgeon must either break scrub to use the computer or relay his or her commands to an assistant who, in turn, inputs these to the computer by keyboard or mouse, cursor and menu system. As an alternative, a sterilely draped mouse or joystick can be prepared on the operating table so that the surgeon doesn't have to break scrub to activate the cursor and the menu system. Admittedly, all of these interactive options are cumbersome.

As stated above, we have available technology which will permit verbal interaction with the computer system. This possibility may sound similar to the plot of science fiction movies. Nonetheless, with voice recognition and computer-generated speech, verbal interchange between surgeon and operating room computer system is possible even now. One must simply acquire the interface hardware ("off-the-shelf") and write the software.

Consider the following interchange. The surgeon enters the operating room equipped with a microphone, connected to a multiplex board, which transmits his or her digitized speech patterns and content to the computer. Basically the dialog would be very similar to the interactive interchanges which are currently displayed in the menu system of the COMPASS computer system illustrated in Chapter 16. The only difference here is that the questions posed in the menu displayed on the screen in Chapter 16 are passed through a voice synthesizer, and outputted by means of a loudspeaker in the operating room. The surgeon's responses are received through the microphone, and the words compared through a microphone to a speaker with a digitizer, which translates the sound waves to analog voltages. Thus voltages are passed through an analog-to-digital converter, and into a buffer which compares phonemes and matches them with an existing digital template of the surgeon's voice pattern, in order to reconstruct each word. Finally, these words are compared to a resident glossary within the computer. The words used are either present in that glossary, and thus indicate one of several appropriate responses, or they are not present, in which case the computer responds with "I don't understand..." and requests clarification. This or a similar system would be very convenient to use during the course of an operation, especially during volumetric resections.

With this system the surgeon could verbally request not only displays of approach trajectory on sequential CT or MRI slice images, but reformatted images, especially next or prior slice image volume at resections, and could request image translations, and so on. Furthermore, the surgeon could voice-activate movements of the stereotactic frame, which positions the patient's head within the fixed arc-quadrant, in order to position a different portion of the tumor under the stereotactically directed retractor.

Stereotactic robotics

Robots are machines which are programmed to perform repetitive tasks and are now used extensively in industry. In fact, some industrial robots have a precision of ± 25 μm; certainly more precise than most available stereotactic instruments. There are four general robotic device types:

1 Cartesian, or x, y, z type. In this device the tool moves on a 3-D slide system which defines each of the axes x, y, and z. In fact, the COMPASS stereotactic system is a Cartesian robot (see Chapter 21).

2 Cylindrical arm type. In this device an arm is raised or lowered on a cylindrical shaft and rotates about that shaft. The arm extends or retracts from a housing on the cylindrical shaft. For example, this type of device is used on an assembly line for moving objects from one point to another.

3 Spherical robot. The extendable arm can pivot or rotate about a fixed base unit.

4 Articulated arm or revolute type. This device is the one that most consider a candidate for a surgical robot, probably because it resembles human anatomy more than the other types listed above. There are multiple flexion/extension joints which provide six or seven degrees of freedom; combinations involve rotation at the base (or waist), flexion/extension of the shoulder and elbow, and rotation about the wrist joint.

In all of the robotic types, each joint or movement is electronically controlled by stepper motors or servomotors. In addition, feedback of joint position is supplied to the host computer by means of an optical encoder on each joint.

Certainly some robots could be adapted for surgical applications. For example, an operating microscope could be suspended from a surgical robot. The robotic device would position the microscope in precise 3-D space. The position of the microscope, and thereby its field of view, would thus be known and transmitted to the surgical computer system. The computer could then display, with respect to the position of the actual surgical field, a preoperatively derived image of what the surgical field should look like, gathered from CT/MRI/DSA data.

Magnetic sensors similar to those found on helicopter gunships could be attached to the surgeon's cap just as they are fixed to the gunner's flight helmet. These could transmit the position of the surgeon's head in 3-D space to the operating room computer system, so that the robotically controlled microscope could be directed whichever way the surgeon's head is pointing. In addition, sensors in the ocular lenses of the microscope could be used to continuously achieve the proper focal length between microscope and field of view. This also is similar to technology already used in the defense industry. For example, on jet fighter aircraft, sensors in the pilot's eyeshield measure the interpupillary distance of the pilot's eyes to rapidly aim the guns of the airship.

If the robotically positioned microscope has a known and constantly updated position in space, and this is indexed to a precise point and oriented to a defined plane on the patient, a stereotactically derived database can always be related to the surgical field viewed through that microscope. The axis of the microscope defines the viewline, as discussed in Chapter 21.

Imaging-based renditions of the surgical field, scaled for the particular magnification being used, can be displayed to the surgeon in several ways. One efficient method for this is by means of the "heads-up" display device, described in Chapter 22 (p. 300). Thus the surgeon would overlay the scaled image of the surgical field upon the actual surgical field in order to identify tumor boundaries, anticipate important blood vessels which may be near or beneath the plane of surgery, etc. Voice-activated computer commands would prompt projection into the microscope, a 3-D reconstructed angiogram reformatted to the viewline and level of the surgical field, for example, or a menu, etc.

Stereotactic digitization of surgical instruments

In the past, stereotactic calculations were simple, and based on the fact that effective instruments are directed intracranially by means of a stereotactic frame. For example, one may easily determine the 3-D position of the working end of a lesioning probe, or a cylindrical retractor mounted on an arc-quadrant or positioning bow of a stereotactic instrument. This information can be easily transferred to stereotactic radiographs, or CT or MRI scans. As an intermediate step, one can also transmit this information to the computer, and have the computer display the position of the instrument on an appropriate image, as a cursor or some other defined indicator. However, this procedure is somewhat cumbersome, since a

human interface is required: someone must enter manually certain parameters from which the computer can calculate the position of the stereotactic instrument. In an arc-quadrant system, one must enter the arc and collar angles and the probe depth, in order to have the computer calculate the 3-D position of its tip and indicate its position on the appropriate image display.

Automatic sensors, such as optical encoders, could be used to provide the input data to the computer: this would be faster and more convenient. But this solution is appropriate for instruments which are *attached* to the stereotactic frame itself. That is not really convenient either.

Neurosurgeons truly need systems which will give the stereotactic coordinates of *hand-held* instruments within the operative field. Before they are universally accepted, these systems must be convenient, produce instantaneous results, and be totally free of any human interface: the surgeon moves the instrument and the computer display shows that movement immediately and accurately. In fact it may be this facility alone that makes stereotaxis irresistible to general neurosurgeons. If a surgeon had immediate feedback on the position of the tip of a sucker or bipolar forceps with respect to the CT- or MRI-defined tumor boundaries, few neurosurgeons could pass this up. But how could we calculate and transmit to the operating room computer system the position of hand-held surgical instruments which are not attached to the stereotactic frame?

A fiberoptic calibration system developed by NASA and Ames Research Laboratory quantitatively measures deflection of fiberoptic bundles. These fiberoptic bundles are small and can be attached to any flexible structure. Basically, the system detects where the fiberoptic shaft is being bent, how far it is being deflected, and in what direction. It is thus possible to obtain 3-D coordinates for the tip of the fiberoptic shaft. At present this device is being used in a digitizing glove worn by an astronaut, in order to control, by movements of the astronaut's hand and fingers, a remote robotic device in space machinery. In fact, a toy manufacturer uses a crude version of the same technology in an interactive action glove supplied with a videogame.

This technology may be adapted to provide the 3-D position of any instrument which is connected by a flexible cord such as a bipolar forceps or suction tip. Several of these bundles could be incorporated into the electrical cord of a bipolar cautery, or onto a suction tubing, in order to provide the deflection information in three or more planes. Supplied with these data and given the length of the forceps and suction tip, computers could calculate coordinates in 3-D space. The computer could output in numbers, or on a real-time display, the final stereotactic coordinates for the distal (or working) end of the forceps or sucker. The position of these instruments could be indicated in relationship by means of a cursor or some other indicator on the display screen. Furthermore, such a system could be zeroed by simply touching a reference point having known stereotactic coordinates on the stereotactic frame. How could we determine coordinates for instruments which are not connected to a long cord?

The stereotactic position of dissectors, scissors, or forceps in the surgical field could be determined in several ways; here is just one. The shaft of each instrument could be fitted with two microbattery-powered light-emitting diodes (LEDs) having a specific emission frequency. The distance between the LEDs would be known, as would the length and configuration of the instrument. Biplane video cameras with appropriate magnification would transmit to the operating room computer system the images of the surgical field, viewed from precise anterior–posterior (A/P) and lateral projections, and in each image the two LEDs would be evident. The images would be placed in 2-D image matrices by frame grabbers. An intensity detection scan would register the position of each LED in A/P and lateral matrix. The computer could calculate the inclination between the two LEDs and measure their position in the surgical environment. Since the length and configuration of the instrument are known, the computer could determine the position of the tip of the instrument within the surgical field.

On-line stereotactic radiation therapy

Some companies and institutions are developing variable aperture collimators for linear acceler-

ators. Such a device could vary the beam configuration of the accelerator during an arc rotation sequence, to allow further tailoring of the radiation dosimetry to conform to the shape of the lesion being treated. A host computer system, similar to that described elsewhere in this volume, could present a "beam's-eye view" of the tumor, and this could be used to activate the variable collimator, such that the beam's configuration would conform to the precise cross-sectional shape of the tumor, viewed from that particular direction. Through an appropriate interface, this would be accompanied through electronic or hydraulic connections. In the latter, stepper motors could activate the master hydraulic cylinders, which would in turn transmit the position to a slave cylinder, utilized to set the position of a collimator tooth in a multiple tooth collimator array on the linear accelerator.

Frameless stereotaxy

The concept of a stereotactic frame is sacred to stereotacticians and oppressive to non-stereotactic neurosurgeons. Stereotactic frames are cumbersome and stereotactic calculations time-consuming. In addition, stereotactic frames require a database acquisition procedure. This frequently necessitates repeating CT, MRI, and angiographic examinations, which may already have been performed in making the initial diagnosis. Could the stereotactic frame be eliminated? Could diagnostic imaging be used as the stereotactic database?

Let us consider what a stereotactic frame does. A stereotactic frame establishes a coordinates system. This allows transformation of the 3-D coordinate system of the imaging studies into stereotactic space. Computers provide a mechanism for performing rapid transformation functions; transforming the coordinates system of the imaging studies to the coordinates system of the patient, and back again.

All we have to do is define the coordinates system in both patient and database. This can be done with reference markers, applied to the patient's head or scalp, which would be visible on the imaging studies and indexed into the operating room computer system by means of a 3-D digitizer. However, this method requires that the imaging studies be done with the markers in place. Therefore, in most cases these imaging studies must be repeated prior to surgery. More capacious computer systems will render this unnecessary.

CT, MRI, and angiography are precise 3-D databases which fill a volume in space. The patient's brain, cranial vault, and envelope of skin and muscle also fill a volume in 3-D space. Theoretically the real volume (the patient) should superimpose precisely on the imaging-defined volume. We can represent the imaging-defined volume by inputting the diagnostic studies into the operating room computer system. This will establish a 3-D voxel-based matrix, and derive a coordinates system based on its center of gravity. How do we establish the 3-D matrix and coordinates system for the patient's head held, say, in a Mayfield head-holder and not in a stereotactic frame?

First, A/P and lateral radiographs could be obtained and digitized which would define the bony cranial vault in two projections. The imaging-based database could be transformed (rotated, translated, and scaled) so that the cranial vault, defined by CT, superimposes on the cranial vault defined by the biplane radiographs.

Alternatively, intensity detection algorithms on the MR database can define the surface of the patient's scalp. In the operating room, bi-plane automatic laser scanners could establish, with a series of spline functions and tiling algorithms, the real configuration of the surface of the patient's scalp. This would define a surface within a computer-defined image matrix. Finally, the computer could perform a transformation function which would translate, rotate, and ultimately superimpose the MRI-defined surface with that defined by the laser scanners in the patient.

A surgeon could then use a 3-D digitizer in order to input the position of set landmarks, e.g. the external auditory canals, the nasion, and indicate these positions on an image display of the patient. This would then permit transformation of digitizer coordinates to the CT- and MRI-derived database. Thus, at any time during a surgical procedure, the surgeon could touch the digitizer to the surgical field, and the computer could indicate, by cursor, the position of the digitizer tip on CT or MRI slices. It could

also project a cursor into a 3-D graphics display, projected stereoscopically into both ocular viewing ports of an operating microscope by means of a "heads-up" display device. However, there are many other options for "frameless stereotaxy" provided by capacious, high-speed computers.

The operating room itself could be the stereotactic frame, with a real world coordinates system. All objects within it, including the patient's head, would have object coordinates systems which could easily undergo transformation to the real world coordinates system of the operating room. Laser scanners could provide to the operating room computer system precise 3-D information on the location and configuration of the patient's head, then skin incisions, craniotomy defects, etc. Multiple video monitors with appropriate filters could detect the positions of surgical instruments (including the microscope) equipped with instrument-specific LED patterns, and transmit these positions to the computer system. The computer would note the instrument positions on a shaded graphics display reconstructed from the preoperative database.

In addition, these instruments could be identified by an LED pattern similar to a bar code. These instruments could be passed to the surgeon not by a scrub nurse, but by a voice-activated robotics device which would efficiently select the appropriate instrument from a precise location on the sterile overhead table and pass it to the surgeon. It would pass it to the surgeon in the same way every time, and return it to its former position on the scrub table. This robot nurse would be immune to boredom, anxiety, and verbal abuse.

Conclusions

The above represents only a short list of the many possible applications of computers in future stereotactic neurosurgery. However, these developments are predictable extensions of what is already possible, and indeed in operation, in various non-medical industries. We cannot predict the impact on stereotaxis of revolutionary developments in other disciplines which may be easily adaptable for stereotactic surgery. For example, few could have anticipated the profound impact on stereotactic surgery of the development of CT scanning.

New computer systems, optical storage devices, and efficient means of electronic data transfer are being developed at a rapid rate.

Stereotactic neurosurgeons must keep abreast of high technological developments and keep an open mind on how useful they could be in the stereotactic operating room.

Index

Page numbers in *italics* refer to figures. Those in bold refer to tables.